Rhinitis

Guest Editor

MICHAEL A. KALINER, MD

IMMUNOLOGY AND ALLERGY CLINICS OF NORTH AMERICA

www.immunology.theclinics.com

Consulting Editor
RAFEUL ALAM, MD, PhD

August 2011 • Volume 31 • Number 3

SAUNDERS an imprint of ELSEVIER, Inc.

W.B. SAUNDERS COMPANY

A Division of Elsevier Inc.

1600 John F. Kennedy Blvd., ● Suite 1800 ● Philadelphia, PA 19103-2899.

http://www.theclinics.com

IMMUNOLOGY AND ALLERGY CLINICS OF NORTH AMERICA Volume 31, Number 3

August 2011 ISSN 0889-8561, ISBN-13: 978-1-4557-1105-5

Editor: Rachel Glover
Developmental Editor: Donald Mumford

Immunology and Allergy Clinics of North America (ISSN 0889-8561) is published quarterly by Elsevier Inc., 360 Park Avenue South, New York, NY 10010-1710. Months of issue are February, May, August, and November. Periodicals postage paid at New York, NY and additional mailing offices. Subscription prices are $272.00 per year for US individuals, $392.00 per year for US institutions, $129.00 per year for US students and residents, $334.00 per year for Canadian individuals, $187.00 per year for Canadian students, $486.00 per year for Canadian institutions, $379.00 per year for international individuals, $486.00 per year for international institutions, $187.00 per year for international students. To receive student/resident rate, orders must be accompanied by name of affiliated institution, date of term, and the *signature* of program/residency coordinator on institution letterhead. Orders will be billed at individual rate until proof of status is received. Foreign air speed delivery is included in all *Clinics* subscription prices. All prices are subject to change without notice. **POSTMASTER:** Send address changes to *Immunology and Allergy Clinics of North America*, Elsevier Health Sciences Division, Subscription Customer Service, 3251 Riverport Lane, Maryland Heights, MO 63043. **Customer Service: 1-800-654-2452 (U.S. and Canada); 314-447-8871 (outside U.S. and Canada). Fax: 314-447-8029. E-mail: journalscustomerservice-usa@elsevier.com(for print support); journalsonlinesupport-usa@elsevier.com (for online support).**

Reprints. For copies of 100 or more, of articles in this publication, please contact the Commercial Reprints Department, Elsevier Inc., 360 Park Avenue South, New York, New York 10010-1710. Tel. (212) 633-3812, Fax: (212) 462-1935, e-mail: reprints@elsevier.com.

Immunology and Allergy Clinics of North America is covered in MEDLINE/PubMed (Index Medicus), Current Contents/Life Sciences, Science Citation Index, ISI/BIOMED, Chemical Abstracts, and EMBASE/Excerpta Medica.

Printed in the United States of America.

Contributors

CONSULTING EDITOR

RAFEUL ALAM, MD, PhD
Veda and Chauncey Ritter Chair in Immunology, Professor, and Director, Division of Immunology and Allergy, National Jewish Health; and University of Colorado Health Sciences Center, Denver, Colorado

GUEST EDITOR

MICHAEL A. KALINER, MD
Medical Director, Institute for Asthma and Allergy, Chevy Chase; Medical Director, Institute for Asthma and Allergy, Wheaton, Maryland; Clinical Professor of Medicine, George Washington University School of Medicine, Washington, DC

AUTHORS

ROBERT K. BUSH, MD
Professor (Emeritus) of Medicine, Department of Medicine, University of Wisconsin-Madison, Madison, Wisconsin

JONATHAN CORREN, MD
Associate Clinical Professor of Medicine, University of California, Los Angeles; Allergy Medical Clinic, Los Angeles, California

LINDA COX, MD
Associate Clinical Professional of Medicine, Nova Southeastern University School of Osteopathic Medicine, Davie, Florida

MARK S. DYKEWICZ, MD
Director, Allergy and Immunology; Professor of Internal Medicine, Section of Pulmonary, Critical Care Allergy and Immunologic Diseases, Department of Internal Medicine; Director, Fellowship Program in Allergy and Immunology, Center for Human Genomics and Personalized Medicine Research, Wake Forest University School of Medicine, Winston-Salem, North Carolina

GARY N. GROSS, MD
Clinical Professor of Internal Medicine, Division of Allergy and Immunology, University of Texas Southwestern Medical School; Staff Physician, Dallas Allergy and Asthma Center, Dallas, Texas

FLAVIA C.L. HOYTE, MD
Clinical Instructor, Division of Immunology and Allergy, National Jewish Health, Denver, Colorado

MICHAEL A. KALINER, MD
Medical Director, Institute for Asthma and Allergy, Chevy Chase; Medical Director, Institute for Asthma and Allergy, Wheaton, Maryland; Clinical Professor of Medicine, George Washington University School of Medicine, Washington, DC

ROHIT K. KATIAL, MD, FAAAAI, FACP
Professor of Medicine; Director, Allergy/Immunology Program, Division of Immunology and Allergy, National Jewish Health, Denver, Colorado

NATALIYA M. KUSHNIR, MD
Clinical Director, Allergy and Immunology Clinic of East Bay, Berkeley; Director, Breathmobile of Northern California, Oakland, California

ELI O. MELTZER, MD
Co-Director, Allergy and Asthma Medical Group and Research Center; Clinical Professor of Pediatrics, University of California, San Diego, San Diego, California

LANNY J. ROSENWASSER, MD
Dee Lyons/Missouri Endowed Chair in Pediatric Immunology Research; Professor of Pediatrics, Allergy-Immunology Division, Children's Mercy Hospital; Professor of Pediatrics, Medicine, and Basic Science, University of Missouri-Kansas City School of Medicine, Kansas City, Missouri

RUSSELL A. SETTIPANE, MD
Clinical Associate Professor of Medicine, Brown University, Alpert Medical School, Providence, Rhode Island

RICARDO A. TAN, MD
California Allergy and Asthma Medical Group, Los Angeles, California

DANA WALLACE, MD
Associate Clinical Professor of Medicine, Nova Southeastern University School of Osteopathic Medicine, Davie, Florida

Contents

The immune response to an allergen depends on an initial sensitization process, with future exposures triggering a 2-part allergic response including an early and late phase. The process by which an allergen is recognized has become clearer. Similarly, the roles of the preformed mediators responsible for many of the signs and symptoms of the early-phase response have been elucidated. Recent work also has shed some light on the cells and mediators involved in the late-phase reactions. This article discusses some of this recent work and reviews the basics behind of all of the stages of the allergic response.

This review focuses on the poorly understood condition of nonallergic rhinopathy (NAR) at a clinical level, with an eye on current optimal treatment. NAR is the new designation for the conditions formerly referred to as vasomotor rhinitis or nonallergic idiopathic rhinitis. The clinical characteristics and differential diagnosis are provided in detail in this review, and the disease should now be characterized sufficiently for clinical studies.

It is important to consider a comprehensive differential of possible rhinitis types when considering the diagnosis of chronic rhinitis, including at least 9 subtypes of nonallergic rhinitis: drug-induced rhinitis, gustatory rhinitis, hormonal-induced rhinitis, infectious rhinitis, nonallergic rhinitis with eosinophilia syndrome, occupational rhinitis, senile rhinitis, atrophic rhinitis, and nonallergic rhinopathy. This article focuses on some of the most common types of chronic rhinitis, including mixed rhinitis (allergic and nonallergic overlap), rhinitis medicamentosa, hormonal rhinitis, rhinitis of the elderly, and gustatory rhinitis.

The nose has a limited repertoire of responses regardless of the triggers. These responses primarily serve as a protective mechanism for the lower respiratory tract. Although the nasal reactions to pollens, particles, and pollution may have a beneficial effect for the lower airway, they create symptoms in some individuals that lead to significant morbidity. The symptoms of allergic rhinitis extend far beyond the nose, and the morbidity associated with rhinitis is significant. The nasal symptoms of rhinitis and their causes are the focus of this review.

Epidemiologic, genetic, immunologic, and clinical studies show a close relationship between allergic rhinitis and asthma, food allergy, and atopic dermatitis. Rhinitis and sinusitis often coexist and are commonly referred to with the term rhinosinusitis. These conditions are also linked in the so-called atopic march, which is the sequential appearance of atopic manifestations starting with atopic dermatitis and later followed by food allergy, allergic rhinitis, and asthma. Allergic rhinitis and asthma are now increasingly being approached diagnostically and therapeutically as the one-airway concept.

Allergic rhinitis affects a large portion of the population. Patients are frequently sensitized to indoor allergens. The most important contributors are house dust mites, pets, and fungi. In very controlled environments where allergen exposure is significantly reduced, individuals have been shown to have clinical improvement in allergic rhinitis and/or asthma symptoms. Achieving sufficient exposure reduction in the home has proven difficult. Nonetheless, evidence exists that demonstrates exposure avoidance can be useful as an adjunct to other therapies, such as pharmacotherapy and immunotherapy, for the treatment of allergic rhinitis.

Antihistamines have long been a mainstay in the therapy for allergic rhinitis. Many different oral antihistamines are available for use, and they are classified as first generation or second generation based on their pharmacologic properties and side-effect profiles. The recent introduction of intranasal antihistamines has further expanded the role of antihistamines in the treatment of allergic rhinitis. Certain patient populations, such as children and pregnant or lactating women, require special consideration regarding antihistamine choice and dosing as part of rhinitis therapy.

Intranasal corticosteroids (INSs) are the first choice for rhinitis pharmacotherapy. This preference is because of their broad range of actions that result in reductions of proinflammatory mediators, cytokines, and cells. Over the past 30 years, INSs have been modified to improve their pharmacodynamic, pharmacokinetic, and delivery system properties, with attention to improving characteristics such as receptor binding affinity, lipophilicity, low systemic bioavailability, and patient preference. Clinically, they have been shown to be the most effective class of nasal medications for treating allergic rhinitis and nonallergic rhinopathy, with no clear evidence that any specific INS is superior to others.

Numerous controlled clinical trials have demonstrated the efficacy of specific allergen immunotherapy (SIT) in reducing the clinical symptoms and costs associated with allergic rhinitis. Compared with pharmacotherapy, SIT may provide persistent clinical benefits after treatment discontinuation. Subcutaneous and sublingual immunotherapy are the two most widely prescribed SIT routes worldwide. This review compares the efficacy, safety, preventive effect, immunologic mechanisms, and adherence rates associated with these two forms of SIT.

Clinical symptoms of allergic and nonallergic rhinitis are similar despite the significant difference in underlying mechanisms. Over-the-counter (OTC) treatments can be used as effective and affordable therapeutic modalities when recommended by a physician. Adjunct treatments, such as herbal medicine, acupuncture and homeopathy, have become increasingly popular. Most of the treatments reviewed in this article are available OTC and are a likely choice for patients suffering from acute or chronic rhinitis. This article provides an overview of treatment suggestions, benefits, and side effects for available OTC, prescription drug, and alternative choices in addition to the therapies described in other articles.

Whereas very mild rhinitis may be simply and successfully self-managed by patients using medications available over the counter, most patients with rhinitis who present to medical offices have more severe rhinitis that may need a more comprehensive diagnostic and therapeutic approach. Optimal care may require special diagnostic studies and combination therapies that are arrived at only after trying multiple different medication and therapeutic options. This article presents a systematic approach to office care of rhinitis from the perspective of an allergist-immunologist. More emphasis is given to discussion of dilemmas that face the specialist or more involved considerations that have been highlighted in recently published guidelines.

THE CLINICS ARE NOW AVAILABLE ONLINE!

Access your subscription at:
www.theclinics.com

Foreword

The Burden of Allergic Rhinitis Beyond Allergies

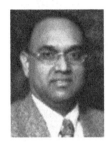

Rafeul Alam, MD, PhD
Consulting Editor

Nearly 25% of the U.S. population suffers from allergic rhinitis. This is clearly one of the most common human illnesses and is likely to impact the development of other illnesses. Another common pathologic process that affects all aging human beings is atherosclerosis. So, one interesting question is whether allergic rhinitis affects the development of atherosclerosis and, indirectly, cardiovascular illnesses and stroke. There is scientific rationale to take this issue seriously. It is well established that a low-grade inflammation involving macrophages is critical for the development of atherosclerosis. There is growing evidence that leukotrienes are involved in atherosclerosis. Genetic studies with mice have identified 5-lipoxygenase (5-LO) as an important contributor of atherosclerosis.[1] Certain variants of 5-LO promoters are associated with an increased risk for atherosclerosis as defined by increased carotid intimal thickness.[2,3] These variant promoters were predicted to increase the expression of leukotrienes. Family studies of early onset cardiovascular diseases have established a link between 5-LO and an increased risk for ischemic heart diseases.[4] Some epidemiological studies tend to lend support to these findings. In a 5-year prospective study of 826 subjects the patients with allergic disorders (allergic rhinitis and asthma) had a significantly increased risk (odds ratio, 2.5) for high intima-media thickness of carotid and femoral arteries.[5] Another study analyzed 9272 subjects and examined the incidence of stroke in patients with hay fever.[6] The odds ratio for stroke in allergic rhinitis patients was 1.87 after adjusting for age, sex, race, smoking status, body mass index, diabetes, hypertension, alcohol use, and hyperlipidemia. These findings are intriguing and, if confirmed, could have significant implications. One would like to see more rigorous and larger prospective studies to better define these correlations.

Supported by NIH Grants R56AI077535, PPG HL 36577, and N01 HHSN272200700048C.

Immunol Allergy Clin N Am 31 (2011) ix–x
doi:10.1016/j.iac.2011.05.013   immunology.theclinics.com

We are not addressing the link between allergic rhinitis and atherosclerosis in this particular issue. Nonetheless, a possible link with atherosclerosis makes it more important that we update our knowledge about allergic rhinitis. To do so, I have invited Dr Michael Kaliner, one of the most distinguished allergists and immunologists in the country. Dr Kaliner has brought together a group of experts who give succinct reviews on various forms of rhinitis, their pathogenesis, and relevance for other allergic conditions, clinical manifestations, prevention, pharmacotherapy, and immunotherapy. I am sure you will enjoy this issue.

Rafeul Alam, MD, PhD
Division of Allergy and Immunology
National Jewish Health and
University of Colorado Denver Health Sciences Center
1400 Jackson Street
Denver, CO 80206, USA

E-mail address:
alamr@njc.org

REFERENCES

1. Poeckel D, Funk CD. The 5-lipoxygenase/leukotriene pathway in preclinical models of cardiovascular disease. Cardiovasc Res 2010;86:243–53.
2. Dwyer JH, Allayee H, Dwyer KM, et al. Arachidonate 5-lipoxygenase promoter genotype, dietary arachidonic acid, and atherosclerosis. N Engl J Med 2004; 350:29–37.
3. De Caterina R, Zampolli A. From asthma to atherosclerosis—5-lipoxygenase, leukotrienes, and inflammation. N Engl J Med 2004;350:4–7.
4. Crosslin DR, Shah SH, Nelson SC, et al. Genetic effects in the leukotriene biosynthesis pathway and association with atherosclerosis. Hum Genet 2009;125: 217–29.
5. Knoflach M, Kiechl S, Mayr A, et al. Allergic rhinitis, asthma, and atherosclerosis in the Bruneck and ARMY studies. Arch Intern Med 2005;165:2521–6.
6. Matheson EM, Player MS, Mainous AG 3rd, et al. The association between hay fever and stroke in a cohort of middle aged and elderly adults. J Am Board Fam Med 2008;21:179–83.

Preface

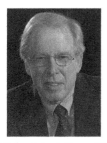

Michael A. Kaliner, MD
Guest Editor

I have always considered each issue of *Immunology and Allergy Clinics* to be a precious little gem. Thus, when asked to develop an issue on rhinitis, I immediately accepted, pleased to be able to contribute to this important series. It was easy to select both the topics and the authors. We looked at the clinical field of rhinitis and chose the most important epidemiologic, pathophysiologic, clinical, and treatment advances and asked those authors who had contributed the most to each area to write it up. Everyone accepted the offer. Thus, a star-studded group of investigators, clinicians, and academicians was easily assembled. The results are a pleasure to read.

"Rhinitis" is an up-to-date summary of the most important clinical fields in allergy and provides anything a clinician needs to know about these clinical entities. Lanny Rosenwasser has succinctly brought the pathophysiology of rhinitis into focus. Russ Settipane and I have separately discussed all the forms of rhinitis, what we know about their causes, and how to treat them. Gary Gross has explained how the various symptoms of rhinitis are caused, as a way to effectively manage them. Jon Corren has tied together the most important clinical expressions of allergic diseases and how they interact.

On the clinical treatment side, Bob Bush has addressed the topic of allergy avoidance. Hoyte and Katiel have summarized the knowledge of antihistamines. Eli Meltzer reviewed nasal corticosteroids. Dana Wallace and Linda Cox have compared SLIT and SCIT. Nataliya Kushnir has summarized all the other treatments, and Mark Dykowicz has put everything together in a review of the office treatment of rhinitis.

All in all, this is a satisfying little issue that will be useful for every allergy, ENT, or primary clinician who wants an update on rhinitis. I hope everyone agrees that this is a wonderful little text.

Michael A. Kaliner, MD
Institute for Asthma and Allergy
11002 Veirs Mill Road, Suite 414
Wheaton, MD 20902, USA

E-mail address:
makaliner@aol.com

Immunol Allergy Clin N Am 31 (2011) xi
doi:10.1016/j.iac.2011.05.012   **immunology.theclinics.com**
0889-8561/11/$ – see front matter © 2011 Elsevier Inc. All rights reserved.

Current Understanding of the Pathophysiology of Allergic Rhinitis

Lanny J. Rosenwasser, MD[a,b,]*

KEYWORDS

• Allergen • Allergic rhinitis • Immune response

The immune regulation related to the production of immunoglobulin E (IgE) is a critical factor in the allergic inflammatory process, and its expression is critical to diseases such as allergic rhinitis. The binding of allergens to IgE located on the cell surfaces of allergic effector cells such as mast cells, basophils, and on immune regulatory cells including dendritic cells (DCs), Langerhans cells, and macrophages trigger inflammatory cascades leading to activation of T cells and other factors such as cytokines that may be involved in the long-term inflammation and late-phase response associated with allergic rhinitis. The immediate response is generated by the allergic cells such as mast cells and basophils, and leads to some of the immediate symptoms associated with allergic rhinitis, although the immune response to allergens has a different timeframe for sensitization and expression and of age-mediated symptoms of allergic rhinitis. The pathophysiology of immune responses related to allergic rhinitis is critical for developing strategies that will be involved in the long-term control and prevention of allergic rhinitis.

CELLS OF THE IMMUNE RESPONSE IN THE PATHOPHYSIOLOGY OF ALLERGIC RHINITIS

In the allergic response, initial sensitization involves activation of allergen-specific T cells that orchestrate the production of allergen-specific IgE, which is the critical issue in allergic rhinitis. The modeling of the disease in this process in terms of allergic triggers involves an analysis on an experimental basis of an early phase response, which is mast cell- and basophil-dependent, and the late-phase, in which allergic inflammation and an influx of effector cells and immune cells take over in terms of

[a] Allergy-Immunology Division, Children's Mercy Hospital, 2401 Gillham Road, Kansas City, MO 64108, USA
[b] University of Missouri-Kansas City School of Medicine, 2401 Gillham Road, Kansas City, MO 64108, USA
* Allergy-Immunology Division, Children's Mercy Hospital, 2401 Gillham Road, Kansas City, MO 64108.
E-mail address: lrosenwasser@cmh.edu

Immunol Allergy Clin N Am 31 (2011) 433–439
doi:10.1016/j.iac.2011.05.009   immunology.theclinics.com
0889-8561/11/$ – see front matter © 2011 Elsevier Inc. All rights reserved.

the pathophysiology. Some of the same components that are involved in the sensitization process also may play a role after sensitization in terms of enhancing inflammation, especially with regard to the late-phase response. This article will review some of this in terms of what the potential mediators and mechanisms are and then will proceed to discuss some of the newer factors that might be playing a role in different aspects of allergic inflammation.

On the introduction of allergen into the body, antigen-presenting cells, which include macrophages and DCs similar to Langerhans cells in the skin, take up allergen by endocytosis, process it, and copresent it along with human leukocyte antigen class 2 molecules to CD4+ T cells (Th2 lymphocytes), which are the major regulators.[1] There are also newly recognized forms of these T cells that have become apparent in the last few months in terms of playing a role allergic responses, especially in asthma, as will be discussed later in this article.

In addition to interacting with the antigen-presenting cells during the activation process, CD4+ T cells undergo clonal expansion and can interact with B cells as well through the production of soluble products such as cytokines and by direct cellular interactions in the lymph nodes that lead to the secretion of IgE as the B cells are induced to differentiate into plasma cells. The subsequent binding of allergen-specific IgE to high-affinity receptors present on mast cells and basophils results in allergen priming.[1,2]

On re-exposure to the allergen, cross-linking of the IgE molecules on the cell surface leads to opening of calcium channels and activation of the cell. In the early phase response (the model for some of the immediate responses associated with allergic rhinitis), within 5 minutes the allergen causes deregulation predominantly of mast cells with the release of performed mediators,[1,3] including histamine, proteases, and some of the cytokines, including tumor necrosis factor (TNF). These mediators initiate some of the symptoms related to early phase responses that are the general symptoms associated with allergic rhinitis. Within 15 minutes, there is synthesis of the various produces of arachidonic and acid metabolism, including the cysteinyl leukotrienes, prostaglandins, and platelet-activating factor.[3,4] These processes contribute to the recruitment of other cells and the beginning of the late-phase response, and also bring into play other factors including cytokines and the blood vessels, nerves, and mucous glands in the upper airway; all play a role in the generation of congestion, rhinorrhea, pruritus, and sneezing. In the early phase response, I have already mentioned how histamine is a major player in terms of the preformed mediators affecting all of these symptoms,[5,6] but clearly, within 5 minutes these other materials including the leukotrienes and prostaglandins also can play a role in generating predominantly congestion and rhinorrhea,[6–8] although some of the other factors may play a role in pruritus and sneezing.

In the late response, these early mediators are involved in further recruitment of cells including the eosinophils, basophils, monocytes, macrophages, and lymphocytes into the inflammatory milieu.[9] There is even more mediator release and an increase in symptoms generally associated with congestion, but rhinorrhea and sneezing can be part of the late-phase responses as well. The allergic response is clearly modeled in this way, but the actual disease depends on ongoing development of the milieu that leads to the tissue being primed for these kinds of responses with a variety of triggers, even beyond allergens, that may play a role.[9] The mediators with both histamine and leukotrienes having that characteristic, but chemokines are generated also, including eotaxin and RANTES, which are strongly chemotactic. These all now have different nomenclature for chemokines and their receptor.

Proinflammatory cytokines such as TNF, interleukin (IL)-1, and IL-6, are all part of the nasal inflammatory milieu.[10] Leukotrienes play a role in this, not just through an increase in mucous production, but also through a variety of other factors such as tachykinins. The cysteinyl leukotrienes themselves affect blood vessel physiology so that transudation and edema are enhanced. Additionally, through an intermediate effect of neurokinins there also is sensitization of sensory C fibers, so there is an established role for leukotrienes in this process as well.[4] One of the things that becomes clear in the sensitization and elicitation phase is that T cells play a significant role. All IgE production and eosinophilia in mammals are thymus dependent and T cell dependent. The recognition of allergens by CD4$^+$ T-cell receptor (TCR) $\alpha\beta$ T cells in the nub or the crux of the sensitization and also the recall responses and the production of cytokines in a variety of ways is a critical part of this overall pathophysiological process. In the airways, both in the upper and the lower airways, the ability of accessory cells, antigen-presenting cells, to interact with T cells in eliciting these responses is critical. Therefore, the Langerhans cells in the skin, or the equivalent of those cells, the DCs in the airway, including the nose and sinuses, and macrophages, neutrophils, eosinophils, basophils, mast cells epithelium, endothelium, and even smooth muscle and fibroblasts, all under the right circumstances, can interact with lymphocytes, in particular T cells, to activate them. The DCs are some of the most organized of these antigen presenting cells. Their growth and development from bone marrow precursors depend on a variety of cytokines including granulocyte macrophage colony-stimulating factor, IL-3, IL-4, IL-3, IL-9, and TNF.[11] They can be divided into 1 subsets: the DCs type 1 (DC-1), which are capable of inducing Th1 type T cells and DC-2, which induce Th2 type of lymphocytes, CD4$^+$ lymphocytes (**Tables 1** and **2**).[11] These are the cells that are critically important for allergen recognition. They play a role predominantly in allergen or antigen capture and presentation to the T cells, and how they function in the tissues depends on the milieu in which they interact and develop. Therefore, in addition to the effects of cytokines mentioned previously, DC precursors develop into DC-1 cells if there is a milieu that is rich in IL-12. If the milieu is rich in the cytokine TSLP, then DC-2 type DCs are developed. If DC-2 interacts with T helper cell precursor in a milieu that includes IL-4, differentiation into Th2 cells occurs. If the DC-1 cell interacts with the T helper cell precursor in a milieu that is rich in IL-12, then the interferon γ-producing Th1 cells are produced.[11] So, it is clear that the milieu and the type of cytokines and inflammatory mediators that these cells interact and swim around are very important in terms of profiling the kind of response that will develop into an antigen or allergen. Among the T lymphocytes that are involved in responses that are CD8$^+$, TCR-$\alpha\beta$ type mature T cells that are restricted to class 1 MHC and allergen-derived peptides.[12] Generally, these are types of T cells that are active in cytotoxicity and it is generally not allergen that is the critical issue here but endogenous infections with viruses and other kind of potential targets for delayed-type hypersensitivity, including CD8$^+$ T cells. In the past, these were thought to be the suppressor cells, but new facts have become clear about this immunoregulatory cell that used to be known as a suppressor cell 10–20 years ago. There also is the Th1-type CD4$^+$ T cell that has a standard TCR and can be restricted to a peptide that could be derived from an allergen and that mediates generally delayed-type

Table 1		
Dentritic cells macrophages, APC in allergic responses		
	Cytokine Milieu	T cell Induction
DC-1	IL-12, INF2	Th$_1$
DC-2	TSLP, IL-4, IL-22	Th$_2$

Table 2 T cells subsets involved in allergic rhinitis		
Cells	Active Factor	Cytokines
TH_1	Tbet, STAT 4	INF2, IL-2
TH_2	GATA3, STAT6	IL-4, IL-5, IL-9, IL-13
TH_{17}	ROR2C, STAT3	TH_{17}, A-F
T reg	FoxP3, STAT 5	$TGF\beta$, IL-10

Others of importance in allergic responses, T gamma delta, innate NKT, CD8, $T_2\beta$.

hypersensitivity in host defense and not antibody synthesis.[12] The set of cytokines that is generally the product of these kinds of differentiated cells includes interferon γ, IL-2, lymphotoxin, and a variety of other cytokines. The Th2 CD4$^+$ T cells are the ones that are predominantly active in allergic rhinitis, allergic disease, and asthma, in which class 2 major histocompatibility complex and peptide derived from allergens activate these cells. They are critically important in antibody synthesis and, in particular, for IgE, and they make a set of cytokines that includes IL-4, IL-5, IL-9, and a variety of other cytokines that are active in this Th2 arm immunity.[12,13] There is a group of cells called TCR-$\gamma\delta$ cells that have neither CD4 nor CD8 on their surfaces and are involved in epithelial defense. They are present in the nose, but they also are present in the lungs and in the gastrointestinal tract. Additionally, they are restricted not to be MHC molecules but to a molecule on the surface of the macrophages called CD1.[14,15] Heat shock proteins, lipids, and glycolipids are the general targets for specificity of these $\gamma\delta$-cells, and they have a much more restricted range of potential interactions. However, various potential antigens have characteristics that might trigger these kinds of cells in allergic reaction.

The regulation naturally and via immune responses generated by allergen immunotherapy has now been shown to be significantly affected by a subpopulation of CD4 T cells termed T regulatory cells. These T-reg cells generated naturally in the thymus, and in the secondary lymphoid organs during development and sensitization, are an important initiation of the allergic immune response. However, over the past 10 to 15 years, these T regulatory cells have had their biochemical and functional as well as genetic programs defined. They express TGF-β and IL-10 as suppressive cytokines. Originally, it was thought that perhaps the secretion of these cytokines was critical for their suppressive effects, but in reality it is just their expression that may be a marker of how they act as suppressive cells. Additionally, the actual production of these cytokines does not seem to correlate with the potential inhibition or suppression of other cells directly interacting with target T cells, which would be the standard CD4$^+$ helper cells as discussed previously. These cells have not only CD4 on their surface but the T-cell activation antigen CD25. This is a protein that is part of the complex that interacts as a receptor for IL-2; therefore, it is a sign of activation. However, not all CD4$^+$ or CD25$^+$ T lymphocytes can be T regulatory cells. They have to express these cytokines, and they have to use a unique transcription factor called FoxP3 to have this regulatory effect. In regard to immunodeficiency, FoxP3 defects have been identified in certain groups of severe combined immune deficiency and other immune deficiencies.[16] So, not only is this an important factor for the regulation of IgE production, but it is also a potential marker of immunodeficiency.

Several studies in asthma have shown a certain variant of T cells called natural killer T (NKT) cells, which are highly expressed in asthma,[17] and the extension here is that similar NKT cells may be present at other sites of allergic inflammation including nose.

However, these are TCR restricted and invariant, so they have limited repertoires of the TCRs. CD4$^+$ T cells that react to allergens have a wide variety of specificities that interact with all of the potential allergens one may encounter, whereas these NKT cells have a very restricted repertoire to which they will react. Some of them, and in particular the NKT cells that are active in asthma, are CD4$^+$, and like the $\gamma\delta$-cells they are restricted to CD1b on the antigen-presenting cells, which means that probably the ligands that activate this are not the standard allergens; they are probably proteins or lipids that have affinity for CD1. This may mean that in some groups of patients with either nonallergic rhinitis or asthma these more unusual T cells may be in the dominant kind of inflammatory cells rather than the standard CD4$^+$ T cells.[18] These NKT cells that were reported by the group at Boston Children's Hospital have a greater proclivity and propensity to produce IL-4 and IL-13, and they produce much less interferon-γ, explaining how they potentially may play a role associated with allergic responses and allergic rhinitis. Therefore, although Allergies in America defined unmet needs on a clinical level, previously,[19] in this paper, some of the unmet needs in the field of pathophysiology are identified.

In addition, various of these ILs in the 20 series are a part of the IL-10 receptor that gives these variants in ligands that have been identified. Almost all of these, from IL-19 to IL-29, seem to have less activity than IL-10 in terms of the ability to fight viral infections or suppress other cytokines, which were some of the basic things that IL-10 did, but then there are a couple of other ILs that are of importance as well. Another group of cytokines that is of interest is the IL-17 family.[20] There are actually 6 of these cytokines, IL-17 A, B, C, D, E, and F. IL-17E is actually the same as II-25, and that is the one that is associated with Th2 cell activation and is involved with eosinophilia and airway responsiveness both in animal models in the mouse and in people. The genetics of the IL-17 family have been linked to asthma and allergic proclivities in family studies done in a variety of settings and populations ranging from Japan to here in the United States.[21,22] There is another group of cytokines that is part of the extended IL-1 family that seems to be very interesting and is called IL-33. Of particular interest is the possible contribution to the pruritus of allergic rhinitis of IL-31 (**Table 3**).This is a major mediator of atopic dermatitis in both people and mice, which indicates this unique cytokine seems to be the mediator of pruritus in both animal models and in patients with atopic dermatitis. It is produced by CD3$^+$ cutaneous lymphocyte antigen-positive T lymphocytes, and it would be interesting to see if some of the pruritus one gets in the nose might be due to the same cytokine.[23–30]

In terms of allergic rhinitis, the symptoms listed are associated with mediators, both common preformed mediators and short-term mediators that get generated during allergen exposure. One can see the relative contribution of some of these mediators to some of these symptoms based on some of the ways in which one could put this together. The source of information was the *Allergy Report* (*The Allergy Report* is

Table 3
Families of newer cytokines active in allergic responses

IL-10 Family	IL-19, 20, 22, 24, 26, 28, 29
IL-17 Family	IL-17A-F, IL-25, (IL-17-E)
IL-1 Family	IL-18, IL-32, IL-33
T regulatory cells	IL-34, IL-35
Skin-pruritus	IL-31
IL-2 Family	IL-15, IL-17, IL-21, IL-23, IL-27

a component of the American Academy of Allergy, Asthma and Immunology's *Allergic Disorders*: Promoting Best Practice initiative: at www.theallergyreport.com; Sept. 5, 2006), and there is some limitation as to how strong the data are regarding how much of this is due to which mediator.

The burden of response related to allergic rhinitis and the intervention of treatment protocols have been identified in a variety of guidelines published by international and national professional organizations over the past 3 or 4 years. This includes the initial area guidelines and the most recent 2010 revision, and in addition various other guidelines that have been identified.

Figuring out a way to interrupt this process will be a critical issue. Allergen responses trigger upper airway responses through IgE-mediated mast cell activation as the initial phase, and a complex cascade related to this 2-phase response results in a variety of different cells and mediators being recruited. Repeated allergen exposure leads to persistent hyper-responsiveness and inflammation in the upper airway. Despite how much is known, there still are unknown pathophysiological factors that need to be defined.

REFERENCES

1. Young MC. Rhinitis, sinusitis, and polyposis. Allergy Asthma Proc 1998;19:211–8.
2. Naclerio RM. Allergic rhinitis. N Engl J Med 1991;325:860–9.
3. Frieri M. Inflammatory issues in allergic rhinitis and asthma. Allergy Asthma Proc 2005;26:163–9.
4. Jordan TR, Rasp G, Pfrogner E, et al. An approach of immunoneurological aspects in nasal allergic late phase. Allergy Asthma Proc 2005;26:382.
5. Mygind N, Dahl R. Challenge tests in nose and bronchi: pharmocological modulation of rhinitis and asthma. Clin Exp Allergy 1996;26:S39–43.
6. Bisgaard H, Olsson P, Bende M. Effect of leukotriene D4 on nasal mucosal blood flow, nasal airway resistance, and nasas secretion in humans. Clin Allergy 1986; 16:289–97.
7. Donnelly AL, Glass M, Minkwitz MC, et al. The leukotriene D4-receptor antagonist, ICI 204, 219, relieves symptoms of acute seasonal allergic rhinitis. Am J Respir Crit Care Med 1995;151:1734–9.
8. Howarth PH. Mediators of nasal blockage in allergic rhinitis. Allergy 1997;52: S12–8.
9. White M. Mediators of inflammation and the inflammatory process. J Allergy Clin Immunol 1999;103:S378–81.
10. Steinke JW, Borish L. Cytokines and chemokines. J Allergy Clin Immunol 2006; 117:S441–5.
11. Akbari O, Umetsu DT. Role of regulatory dendritic cells in allergy and asthma. Curr Allergy Asthma Rep 2005;5:56–61.
12. Chaplin DD. Overview of the human immune response. J Allergy Clin Immunol 2006;117:S430–5.
13. Bellanti JA. Cytokines and allergic diseases: clinical aspects. Allergy Asthma Pro 1998;19:337–41.
14. Gigal LH. Basic science for the clinician 35: CKI, invariant NKT (iNKT) cells, and gamma delta T-cells. J Clin Rheumatol 2005;11:336–9.
15. Jutel M, Akdis M, Blaser K, et al. Are regulatory T cells the target of venom immunotherapy? Curr Opin Allergy Clin Immunol 2005;5:365–9.
16. Chatila TA. Role of regulatory T cells in human diseases. J Allergy Clin Immunol 2005;116:949–59.

17. Akbari O, Faul JL, Hoyte EG, et al. CD4+ invariant T-cell receptors + natural killer T calls and asthma. N Engl J Med 2006;345:1117–29.
18. Kay AB. Natural killer T cells and asthma. N Engl J Med 2006;354:1186–8.
19. Nathan RA. The burden of allergic rhinitis. Allergy Asthma Proc 2007;28:3–9.
20. Huang SH, Frydas S, Kempuraj D, et al. Interleukin-17 and the interleukin-17. Family member network. Allergy Asthma Proc 2004;25:17–21.
21. Kawaguchi M, Takahashi D, Hizawa N, et al. IL-17F sequence variant (His161Arg) is associated with protection against asthma and antoganizes wild-type IL-17 activity. J Allergy Clin Immunol 2006;117:795–801.
22. Schmitz J, Owyang A, Oldham E. IL-33, an interleukin-1-like cytokine that signals via the IL-1 receptor-related protein ST2 and induces T helper type 2- associated cytokines. Immunity 2005;23:479–90.
23. Bilsborough J, Luenh DY, Maurer M, et al. IL-31 is associated with cautaneous lymphocyte antigen-positive skin homing T cells in patients with atopic dermatitis. J Allergy Clin Immunol 2005;117:418–25.
24. Finegold I. Allergen immunotherapy: present and future. Allergy Asthma Proc 2007;28:44–9.
25. Rosenwasser LJ. New insights into the pathophysiology of allergic rhinitis. Allergy Asthma Proc 2007;28:10–5.
26. Brozek JL, Bousquet J, Baena-Cagnani CE, et al. Allergic rhinitis and its impact on asthma (ARIA) guidelines: 2010 revision. J Allergy Clin Immunol 2010;126:3.
27. Bousquet J, Khaltaenv N, Cruz AA, et al. Allergic rhinitis and its impact on asthma (ARIA) 2008 update (in collaboration with the World Health Organization, GA(2) Len and AllerGen). Allergy 2008;63(Suppl 86):8–160.
28. Ait-Khaled N, Pearce N, Anderson HR, et al. Global map of the prevalence of snyptoms of rhinoconjuctivitis in children: the International Study of Asthma and Allergies in Childhood (ISAAC) phase three. Allergy 2009;64:123–48.
29. Scadding GK, Durham SR, Mirakian R, et al. BSACI guidelines for the management of allergic and nonallergic rhinitis. Clin Exp Allergy 2008;38:19–42.
30. Wallace DV, Dykewicz MS, Bernstein DI, et al. The diagnosis and management of rhinitis: an updated practice parameter. J Allergy Clin Immunol 2008;122:S1–84.

Nonallergic Rhinopathy (Formerly Known as Vasomotor Rhinitis)

Michael A. Kaliner, MD[a,b,c],*

KEYWORDS

- Nonallergic rhinopathy • Vasomotor rhinitis • Allergic rhinitis
- Nasal corticosteroids • Nasal antihistamines

This review focuses on the poorly understood condition of nonallergic rhinopathy (NAR) at a clinical level, with an eye on current optimal treatment. The pathophysiology of this disease is not well understood, and the reader is referred to more comprehensive books and reviews for an extensive discussion of pathophysiology.[1,2] Nonallergic vasomotor rhinitis (VMR; also referred to as nonallergic rhinitis and/or idiopathic rhinitis) is a term that has been used to describe a common nasal condition of unclear pathophysiology. The term NAR is recommended to replace nonallergic VMR.[3] VMR suggests that intrinsic nasal vascular and glandular abnormalities are the principle physiologic causes of inflammation of the nasal mucous membrane. However, current information suggests that NAR is probably caused by neurosensory abnormalities and does not include inflammation as an important component.[1,2] Thus, it is believed that it is more accurate to term this condition a rhinopathy (a disorder of the nose) rather than a form of rhinitis (inflammation of the nose). The single unequivocal criterion for these patients is that they are not allergic; NAR is a more appropriate term for this disorder.[3]

DEFINITION OF NAR

NAR is a chronic nasal condition with symptoms that may be perennial, persistent, intermittent, or seasonal and/or elicited by recognized triggers. There is a well-recognized set of clinical exposures that lead to the symptoms, predominantly congestion and rhinorrhea. The clinical characteristics as outlined provide well-defined inclusion and exclusion criteria that should permit precise identification of patients for accurate diagnosis and participation in clinical trials. NAR is defined by

[a] Institute for Asthma and Allergy, Chevy Chase, MD 20815, USA
[b] Institute for Asthma and Allergy, Wheaton, MD 20902, USA
[c] George Washington University School of Medicine, Washington, DC 20037, USA
* 6515 Hillmead Road, Bethesda, MD 20817.
E-mail address: makaliner@aol.com

Immunol Allergy Clin N Am 31 (2011) 441–455
doi:10.1016/j.iac.2011.05.007   immunology.theclinics.com

clinical characteristics, which are summarized below and described in detail in the following sections of this review.[3]

1. NAR is a chronic disease with some, but not necessarily all, of the following symptoms:
   - Primary symptoms
     - Nasal congestion
     - Rhinorrhea
   - Other associated symptoms
     - Postnasal drip in the absence of a pharyngeal cause of mucous hypersecretion or acid reflux disease
     - Throat clearing
     - Cough
     - Eustachian tube dysfunction (ear pressure/popping/pain)
     - Sneezing
     - Hyposmia
     - Facial pressure/headache
     - Generally no nasal, pharyngeal, or ocular itching.
2. Symptoms of NAR may be perennial, persistent, or seasonal (ie, climatic, see later) and/or elicited by defined triggers. These triggers may include the following:
   - Cold air
   - Changes in climate (such as temperature, humidity, and/or barometric pressure)
   - Strong smells (such as perfume, cooking smells, flowers, and chemical odors)
   - Environmental tobacco smoke
   - Changes in sexual hormone levels
   - Pollutants and chemicals (eg, volatile organics)
   - Exercise
   - Alcohol ingestion.
3. Explanatory details of NAR:
   - Symptoms may be described as perennial, persistent, intermittent, or seasonal
   - Seasonal symptoms occur in response to seasonal climatic shifts in temperature, humidity, and barometric pressure
   - Symptoms may be brought on by 1 or more of the defined precipitants
   - Patients responsive to environmental climate changes as a trigger are not different from those triggered by perfumes or strong smells
   - There is no current information suggesting that patients for whom no specific triggers are identified differ from patients with clearly defined triggers. Thus, NAR may be the clinical diagnosis regardless of the presence or the absence of defined triggers
   - There is a female-to-male incidence ratio for NAR of 2:1 to 3:1
   - NAR presents predominantly with adult onset
   - The nasal mucosa in NAR usually looks normal
   - NAR is associated with negative or irrelevant skin prick tests or antigen-specific IgE tests
   - NAR may present with concomitant conditions, such as the following
     - Food-related rhinorrhea
     - Eustachian tube dysfunction (ear pressure/popping/pain)
     - Senile rhinitis.
4. NAR symptoms are not caused by other known etiologic factors for rhinopathy, such as the following:
   - Chronic rhinosinusitis or nasal polyposis

- Nonallergic rhinitis with eosinophilia syndrome (NARES), with nasal eosinophilia greater than 5%
- Aspirin-related chronic rhinosinusitis, nasal polyps, and asthma, although NAR is one of the clinical characteristics of aspirin-exacerbated respiratory disease
- Infectious rhinitis or rhinosinusitis (eg, viral upper respiratory infections, bacterial/fungal rhinosinusitis, and bacterial rhinitis)
- Anatomic abnormalities
- Adverse reactions to drug usage (eg, adverse effects of systemic medications and/or excess use of topical decongestants)
- Cerebrospinal fluid leak
- Pregnancy.

CHARACTERISTICS OF NAR

Before the extensive and precise identification of the characteristics of NAR summarized herein and elsewhere,[3] the diagnosis of this condition was made by exclusion. To establish a definitive diagnosis of NAR as well as NARES, all other nonallergic rhinitis syndromes had to be properly considered and excluded.[4] A diagnosis of NAR required negative specific IgE responses by skin, serologic, or entopy testing. Differentiation of the nonallergic conditions, NAR and NARES, is defined by the presence or absence of eosinophils in the nasal passages. Therefore, NAR is truly a noninflammatory nonallergic condition, whereas NARES is an inflammatory nonallergic condition. It should be emphasized that symptoms and physical findings alone are not diagnostic of allergic rhinitis (AR) compared with NAR because patients with NAR often manifest similar features.[5,6] On the other hand, it is now recognized that if patients experience characteristic nasal symptoms in response to environmental triggers as defined earlier, then there is a degree of NAR present, even if allergic testing should prove positive (mixed rhinitis [MR][5]). Therefore, an accurate history taking and proper diagnostic testing are essential to precisely classify these disorders (see later).

As a way to characterize the clinical symptoms and triggers of patients with rhinitis, Bernstein and coworkers[7,8] developed a questionnaire survey designed to recognize differences between AR and NAR subtypes. Results from this questionnaire indicate that patients who develop symptoms later in life (older than 35 years); who have no family history of allergies, no seasonal allergy symptoms, or no perennial symptoms induced by cats or other furry pets; and who have symptoms induced by perfumes and fragrances have a likelihood of 95% of having a physician diagnosis of NAR.[5] Of note, clinical symptoms are not generally sufficiently useful for differentiating chronic rhinitis subtypes.[7] Data indicate that both AR and NAR have an equally high incidence of congestion and postnasal drip, with AR having slightly more rhinorrhea.[7]

In questioning a group of patients selected to participate in a seasonal AR (SAR) study, symptoms were triggered in 85% (116/136) of patients while outdoors during the spring, summer, or fall; 45% (61/136) by cats; 29% (39/136) by dogs; and 21% (29/136) by furry pets. Also, 54% (74/136) of patients had symptoms triggered by cigarette smoke, 72% (98/136) by weather changes, 49% (67/136) by perfumes, 35% (47/136) by incense, and 40% (54/136) by cleaning products. Thus, most patients enrolled in this SAR study also experienced irritant-induced symptoms in response to perfumes, cleaning products, incense, and smoke, suggesting that they also met diagnostic criteria for a nonallergic component to their chronic rhinitis diagnosis (ie, MR[7]).

Subsequently, the rhinitis questionnaire was distributed to subjects in 2 additional AR studies at baseline. It was found that more than 88% of enrolled subjects in both studies indicated that they experienced significant symptoms in response to a spectrum of irritant triggers.[9] Therefore, most patients enrolled in these SAR studies who also experienced irritant-induced symptoms in response to perfumes, cleaning products, incense, and smoke met diagnostic criteria for MR. MR is the condition in which patients have a mixture of allergic and nonallergic rhinitis. The frequency of MR in the population of patients with chronic rhinitis ranges from 22% to 34% depending on the study, with NAR recognized as the causative condition in 23% to 27%.[10]

EPIDEMIOLOGY OF NAR

The Task Force on Practice Parameters defines VMR (idiopathic rhinitis) as a "heterogeneous group of patients with chronic nasal symptoms that are not immunologic or infectious in origin and are usually not associated with nasal eosinophilia."[11]

Although no studies specifically designed to examine the epidemiology of NAR or VMR have been reported, 9 epidemiologic studies report data regarding the relative prevalence of NAR in comparison with that of AR (**Table 1**).[12–20] Of the 9 studies, 7 used skin testing with variable techniques (prick, intradermal, or both or undefined) to distinguish nonallergic rhinitis from AR. These 9 studies, when added in total, are heavily influenced by the enormity of the data from Schatz and colleagues,[20] but when analyzed independently of the Schatz data, they reveal a relative prevalence rate of 76% for AR and 24% for nonallergic rhinitis, closely approximating a ratio of 3:1.

ESTIMATED PREVALENCE OF NAR IN THE UNITED STATES AND WORLDWIDE

The data from rhinitis epidemiology studies suggest that the ratio of AR prevalence (pure and mixed combined) to that of pure NAR is 3:1. This ratio can be extrapolated to determine a conservative estimate of the prevalence of NAR in the United States based on established prevalence rates of AR. If the assumption is made that 20% of the population suffers from AR,[21] then on the basis of current population estimates for the United States of just more than 300 million, the US prevalence of AR is 60 million people. Applying the 3:1 (AR/NAR) ratio, approximately 20 million Americans would be expected to suffer from NAR (or approximately 7% of the total population). Given a current world population of 6.75 billion, similar extrapolation suggests that approximately 450 million people suffer from NAR worldwide. It is not known whether NAR is equally prevalent throughout the world and whether local weather (humidity), climate, air pollution, or genetic factors affect NAR prevalence.

Table 1
Relative rhinitis prevalence: allergic versus nonallergic

Author	Year	N	AR%	NAR%
Mullarkey et al[12]	1980	142	48	52
Enberg[13]	1989	128	64	36
Togias[14]	1990	362	83	17
Leynaert et al[15]	1999	1142	75	25
Mercer et al[17]	2002	278	78	22
Settipane[16]	2003	975	77	23
Bachert et al[18]	2006	743	75	24
Mølgaard et al[19]	2007	1186	77	23
Schatz et al[20]	2008	47,894	71	29
—		Total 52,850	71	29

Subtotal without Schatz et al: 76% AR; 24% NAR.

FURTHER CHARACTERIZATION OF NAR

NAR is often described as being characterized by nonallergic symptom triggers, including weather (changes in temperature or relative humidity); alcohol; tobacco smoke; dusts; automotive emission fumes; nonspecific irritant stimuli, such as chlorine; and odors, such as bleach, perfume, or solvents.[3] However, no epidemiologic data exist to further categorize NAR based on trigger type. Sex and age demographic data can be extrapolated from NAR data, suggesting a female predominance and an older population for NAR than for AR.[22,23]

CLASSIFICATION OF NONALLERGIC RHINITIS SYNDROMES

The generally accepted universal clinical characteristics of the diseases classified within the category of chronic nonallergic rhinitis syndromes include only the following[1]: nasal symptoms and[2] no evidence of concomitant allergic disease as determined by negative skin prick testing results for relevant allergens and/or negative allergen-specific antibody test results.[11] This classification automatically excludes infectious rhinitis, rhinosinusitis, and mechanical/anatomic abnormalities as causes of the chronic symptoms. There are at least 8 separate clinical entities that can be classified among the disorders that make up the nonallergic rhinitis syndromes (**Box 1**), with NAR being the clinically most common and important one.[3,23] The cost of care for AR in the United States is estimated at more than $5 billion to $6 billion annually.[24,25] It is estimated that NAR accounts for $2 billion to $3 billion. Hard data on the incidence and frequency of rhinitis subtypes are limited. However, it is recognized that NAR is the most prevalent, affecting an estimated 37% to 61% of patients diagnosed with rhinitis.[26,27] In a survey of US medical practices, a prospective classification of 2500 patients with rhinitis was performed, and it was found that 43% of the patients had pure AR, 23% had pure VMR, and 34% had rhinitis with features of both AR and NAR (sometimes known as MR).[26,27] These data suggest that at least 57% of patients with rhinitis have some contributions from NAR causing their rhinitis symptoms. Similar European studies have found that approximately 1 in 4 patients complaining of nasal symptoms has pure NAR.[28] Recent estimates suggest that 50 million Europeans have NAR, with a total prevalence of more than 200 million worldwide.[28]

Box 1
Recognized nonallergic rhinitis subtypes

1. Drug-induced rhinitis

2. Gustatory rhinitis (rhinorrhea associated with eating, especially hot and spicy foods)

3. Hormonally induced rhinitis

4. NARES

5. Senile rhinitis

6. Atrophic rhinitis

7. Cerebrospinal fluid leak

8. NAR (formerly known as VMR)

Data from Refs.[3,11,29]

There have been several recent attempts at classifying the chronic nasal syndromes not associated with allergic disease.[11,29,30] The reader is referred to these references for additional approaches to this problem and for a more complete bibliography. The approach taken herein combines the overall recommendations from these 3 sources, combined with input from other experts at a consensus conference held in 2009 and from which several recent references were published in the World Allergy Organization Journal in 2009 and are extensively cited herein. There are at least 8 subtypes that fill the criteria for nonallergic rhinitis (see **Box 1**).[31]

The 2 nonallergic processes, infectious rhinitis (including bacterial rhinitis and chronic rhinosinusitis) and mechanical/anatomic abnormalities, are excluded from this classification. Hormonally induced rhinitis reflects responses to endogenous female hormones. The rhinitis of pregnancy is an extremely common condition, affecting up to 20% to 30% of pregnancies, and is particularly notable during the last trimester. This rhinitis typically resolves spontaneously within 2 weeks of delivery. It is usually assumed that the rhinitis of pregnancy reflects the mucosal engorgement found in the last trimester as a consequence of progesterone stimulation. Thus, the nasal mucosa becomes engorged and congestion ensues because all mucous membranes are affected by the hormonal changes of pregnancy.[32] Some patients develop similar symptoms premenstrually on a cyclical basis.[32]

Drug-induced rhinitis includes rhinitis medicamentosa, which is the descriptive name for the nasal congestion and rebound rhinitis caused by repeated administration of topical nasal decongestants. The most common cause of rhinitis medicamentosa is the overuse of topical nasal decongestants such as oxymetazoline or phenylephrine. When used briefly (<3–5 days consecutively), these medications provide significant relief of nasal congestion. However, with chronic use, rebound nasal congestion can occur and can be quite severe. The exact mechanism is poorly understood, but theories suggest involvement of recurrent nasal tissue hypoxia and negative neural feedback with chronic decreased α_2-receptor responsiveness.[33]

More broadly, other medications[11] can cause chronic nasal symptoms through a host of different mechanisms. Antihypertensive medications, including β-blockers, angiotensin-converting enzyme inhibitors, reserpine, calcium channel blockers, and methyldopa, cause nasal congestion. A very bothersome side effect seen with α-receptor antagonists used for benign prostatic hyperplasia and phosphodiesterase 5 inhibitors for erectile dysfunction is nasal congestion. Aspirin and nonsteroidal anti-inflammatory drugs also may contribute to congestion, especially in patients with a history of nasal polyposis. Oral contraceptive pills also can cause congestion in some women. Personal observations suggest that topical eye drops, such as β-blockers for glaucoma, may also cause nasal symptoms.

Chronic nasal symptoms are found associated with a variety of other medical conditions, the full range of which is beyond the scope of this article. For example, nasal congestion can be seen in distinct diseases such as hypothyroidism and chronic fatigue syndrome. Baraniuk and colleagues[34] found that 46% of patients with chronic fatigue syndrome also have NAR and that 76% of these patients have ongoing nasal complaints.

Anatomic anomalies can also contribute to NAR. Adenoid hypertrophy, nasal septal deviation, and idiopathic turbinate hypertrophy or other structural abnormalities can cause chronic nasal obstruction with little relief from medications. Surgical intervention can be curative.

Senile rhinitis is a clinically defined condition most common in the elderly and can lead to persistent watery rhinorrhea that may be worsened by food or environmental irritants. Gustatory rhinitis is the condition that causes anterior rhinorrhea and/or postnasal drip after eating, especially hot or spicy foods.[35] Gustatory rhinitis is more frequent in older individuals and overlaps with senile rhinitis. Both gustatory and senile rhinitis involve excessive secretions and are effectively treated with topical anticholinergic agents.[35] These rhinitis can occur concomitantly with NAR.

Atrophic rhinitis may occur as a primary idiopathic syndrome with mucous gland atrophy or as a secondary syndrome after overzealous surgeries, with too many mucus-secreting tissues removed. Because mucus is required to restrict bacterial growth in mucous membranes, these patients have dry mucosa and often contract ozena. A few bacterial diseases (*Pseudomonas ozena* and *Klebsiella rhinoscleromatis*) also can cause atrophic rhinitis.[11] Cerebrospinal fluid (CSF) leak in patients with a history of craniofacial trauma or past facial/sinus surgeries must be considered when evaluating persistent rhinorrhea. Increased intracranial pressure can increase the risk of spontaneous CSF leak.

Historically, NAR variants have been divided into 2 groups based on nasal cytology: NARES and non-NARES. However, in this era, nasal cytologic examination is rarely performed in clinical practice. When NARES was described,[12] 20 patients had the same spectrum of symptoms as seen in AR and were noted to have eosinophilia in nasal secretions. However, the results of skin testing and radioallergosorbent testing were negative. Thus, these patients with eosinophilia had the hallmarks of AR except for specific IgE antibodies. Patients with NARES characteristically respond well to topical nasal corticosteroids (NCCS). However, most clinicians no longer do nasal smears, and the relationship of NARES with the other forms of NAR is not known.

Occupational rhinitis is not a separate category but simply designates the location where exposure to nasal triggers is encountered. In practice, many patients complain of occupational rhinitis. Rhinitis from occupation exposures can be caused by irritants and/or allergens. Noxious fumes, odors, and environmental irritants are classic provocateurs of occupational rhinitis, whereas colophony (solder fumes), chemicals, enzymes, and countless other manufacturing by-products can act as allergens to some exposed people.[11,36] At present, with cleaner more-controlled environments, one might expect fewer occupational diseases, but patients often believe that work-related exposures are still a common cause of rhinitis. A good history taking, combined with inventive provocations (such as exposure to soldering fumes or detergent powder), helps define what condition or exposure is responsible for the patient's problems.[36]

Chronic rhinosinusitis, with or without nasal polyps, is another cause of chronic rhinitis. The symptoms of nasal congestion, postnasal drip with throat clearing and cough, facial pressure, headache, purulent drainage, and anosmia should lead the astute clinician to examine suspected sinus involvement. Because the inflammation in sinusitis may be infectious or immunologically mediated, these syndromes are usually not considered part of the nonallergic rhinitis syndromes. Bacterial rhinitis refers to a localized nasal infection with *Staphylococcus* or *Streptococcus* species in the anterior portion of the nose. Such patients have recurrent purulent drainage, nasal congestion, and local crusting but retain a normal sense of smell and have normal radiographic study results of the sinuses. Thus, this is a local bacterial infection of the nose, for example, bacterial rhinitis. This condition is effectively treated with topical antibiotics such a mupirocin.

Aspirin-exacerbated respiratory disease usually includes NAR as one of the clinical characteristics, along with sinusitis, nasal polyposis, asthma, and eosinophilia worsened with aspirin or nonsteroidal antiinflammatory drug exposure.[11] The NAR seen in aspirin sensitivity is usually a form of NARES and may precede the development of other manifestations of the syndrome.

SOME ADDITIONAL DETAILS ABOUT NAR

The most frequent form of nonallergic rhinitis observed clinically is NAR characterized by persistent or intermittent nasal symptoms that can be triggered by environmental conditions that do not bother normal individuals. The diagnosis can now be made by clinical history taking and exclusion of other known causes. If a patient has appropriate nasal symptoms (usually rhinorrhea, congestion, postnasal drip, headaches, facial pressure, throat clearing, and/or coughing) worsened or triggered by 1 or more of the environmental conditions noted earlier, then NAR is present. Concomitant ocular symptoms tend to be minimal, and the symptoms of nasal and palatal itches and also sneezing spells are not common. Some patients with NAR have persistent nasal symptoms and no other recognized cause. These patients may or may not respond to the environmental conditions that trigger other symptoms in other patients. The clinical characteristics of these patients (predominantly female sex, adult onset, clinical symptoms, and response to treatment) are indistinguishable from those of patients with NAR with recognized triggers. It is proposed that these patients also have NAR.

Unlike AR, NAR is usually adult onset and is not worsened by exposure to classic allergens such as pollen, house dust mite, dogs, or cats. A validated questionnaire has been created to help identify patients with NAR.[6] Because NAR may be caused by shifts in temperature, humidity, and/or barometric pressure, patients may experience seasonal symptoms associated with changes in these climatic conditions experienced during the spring and fall. Seasonal NAR can, therefore, be confused with SAR.[37]

The diagnosis of NAR is based solely on the patient's history of symptoms and their triggers, whereas the diagnosis of AR requires an appropriate history taking and confirmatory allergy testing, either positive relevant skin prick test results or allergen-specific IgE test results. These 2 diseases are not mutually exclusive, and at least 60% of patients with AR develop nasal symptoms in response to nonallergic environmental triggers. To have pure NAR, however, the patient must have negative relevant skin test results or in vitro allergen-specific antibody test results.

There are some limited data that histamine can be released from the nasal mucosa after inhaling cold dry air, which elicits cold air–induced rhinitis in some sensitive patients. In a set of cold dry air challenges, in vivo histamine release was observed with cold air–induced rhinitis but not with other forms of NAR.[38] The importance of the histamine release in the development of the rhinitis symptoms was considered to be unrelated.

The epidemiologic predominance of women with VMR suggests that female hormones might play some role, but there are little supporting data. One study reported that 71% of patients with VMR were women compared with 62% of those with MR and 55% of those with AR.[6]

TREATMENT OF NAR

Although each form of nonallergic rhinitis should be treated individually, NAR is the most well-studied and clinically important form and the only type for which clinical studies have led to approved treatments. In the following discussion, treatment of nonallergic rhinitis focuses on NAR, but some mention is made of other forms of rhinitis where appropriate. The medications used for treating NAR have been studied less extensively than those for AR, but there are still multiple therapeutic options available.

NCCS

NCCS treat inflammatory conditions regardless of cause. There is substantial evidence that corticosteroids benefit AR; some forms of nonallergic rhinitis, including NAR[39]; and chronic rhinosinusitis. In a study of 983 patients with NARES and non-NARES, fluticasone propionate (FP) at both 200 and 400 μg significantly improved total nasal symptoms scores when compared with placebo, and no difference was noted between the 2 concentrations.[40] In the United States, of all the NCCS approved by the Food and Drug Administration (FDA) available at present, only FP is approved for the treatment of both allergic and nonallergic rhinitis.

Although none of the other current NCCS have received the US FDA approval for use in NAR, there are some supportive data for the efficacy of intranasal budesonide and mometasone in some patients with perennial rhinitis.[41,42] There is also one published study demonstrating that there was no benefit from FP in NAR. In that study, patients with NAR receiving 200 μg of daily FP showed a reduction in inflammatory mediators but no improvement in symptoms as compared with placebo.[43] By contrast, clinical experience suggests that all NCCS have some effectiveness in treating NAR. As a class, NCCS treats the broadest spectrum of NAR symptoms and seems to have at least some degree of efficacy in all NAR variants. Thus, for the treatment of NAR, NCCS are considered a first-line therapy.

Antihistamines

It is quite likely that all patients with NAR have tried oral antihistamines, either in the form of over-the-counter medications or as prescribed by physicians who assume that the symptoms are caused by allergies. Histamine release has not been seen in NAR, other than cold air–induced rhinitis.[38] Thus, the use of oral antihistamines makes little sense, and these medications have rarely been studied in NAR. A 1982 study does show that first-generation antihistamines can improve NAR symptoms when combined with a decongestant.[44] It is predictable that first-generation antihistamines might reduce rhinorrhea through anticholinergic actions, whereas second-generation nonsedating antihistamines have minimal anticholinergic activity. Typically, second-generation antihistamines are of no benefit in NAR. Oral antihistamines are generally ineffective in reducing congestion in AR and thus are not expected to work in NAR either. The combination of an antihistamine and a decongestant might help reduce the congestion seen in NAR, but no such indication has been approved by the US FDA. Clinical experience suggests that antihistamine/decongestant combinations are somewhat effective in NAR.

By contrast, intranasal antihistamines are very effective in treating AR (both azelastine and olopatadine are approved for treating SAR). Azelastine is also approved by the FDA for treatment of NAR. Although azelastine is primarily a second-generation antihistamine, it is unlikely that its efficacy in NAR is because of histamine receptor blockade. Instead, it is probably azelastine's actions as an antiinflammatory and neuroinflammatory blocker that makes this medication useful in treating VMR/NAR.[45] Azelastine has been shown to deplete inflammatory neuropeptides in the nasal mucosa; reduce levels of proinflammatory cytokines, leukotrienes, and cell adhesion molecules; and inhibit mast cell degranulation.[46]

In 2 multicenter, randomized, double-blind, placebo-controlled, parallel-group clinical trials, azelastine showed considerable efficacy in the treatment of each of the symptoms of NAR, including congestion.[47] Treatment for more than 21 days caused a significant reduction in the total VMR symptom score from baseline when compared with placebo ($P = .002$), and every nasal symptom was effectively reduced. Symptom improvement was rapid with most patients experiencing relief within 1 week. There were no serious adverse events, although a bitter taste was experienced by some in the azelastine group. In studies of AR, onset of effect with nasal azelastine is seen in 15 to 30 minutes.[46] Based on these clinical studies and extensive clinical experience, nasal antihistamines are considered a first-line therapy for NAR.[11,45]

A meta-analysis has suggested that NCCS are slightly more effective than nasal antihistamines in the treatment of AR, but no such analyses exist comparing these products in treating NAR. The data from the study by Yanez and Rodrigo[48] are often quoted to substantiate a claim that NCCS are superior to nasal antihistamines in treating rhinitis, but the data cited do not use the products approved in the United States and involve multiple products used at widely varying doses and using no consistent dose schedule. Thus, the data from Yanez and Rodrigo do not apply to the products used in the United States and should be viewed skeptically unless they are extended to studies with US products.[49] Several recent studies comparing olopatadine[50] or azelastine[51] with FP showed equivalence in treating rhinitis.

Olopatadine was recently compared with fluticasone.[50] In this study, 130 patients were randomized to 2 sprays per nostril per day for a 2-week course of treatment of SAR with olopatadine (0.6%) or fluticasone (50 μg). Both the treatments significantly reduced both reflective and instantaneous assessments of nasal and ocular symptoms over the 2-week study ($P<.05$) and were safe and well tolerated. Both olopatadine and fluticasone nasal sprays reduced SAR symptoms (ocular and nasal) by the same amount, with the only significant difference being that olopatadine provided a greater and faster onset of action.[50] These current data indicate that both nasal antihistamines are noninferior to NCCS and support their role as a first-line treatment option.

When NCCS and azelastine were combined in the treatment of AR, the effects of the combination were additive. In a randomized double-blind trial comparing FP alone versus azelastine alone versus the 2 in combination for the treatment of AR, the combination produced a further reduction of 40% in total nasal symptom scores as compared with either FP or azelastine alone. The combination of FP and azelastine reduced congestion by 48% compared with the individual components.[52] Additional studies with azelastine and FP[53] as well as olopatadine and FP[54] support these suggestions. The combination has yet to be studied in NAR, but extensive clinical experience suggests that this combination is highly effective in NAR as well. Based on both published clinical studies and extensive clinical experience, the use of azelastine (and olopatadine) alone and in combination with NCCS is a preferred first-line treatment of NAR as well as AR.[45,46,49]

Anticholinergics

Ipratropium bromide (IB) is a potent intranasal anticholinergic with utility in the treatment of rhinorrhea in AR and NAR. It has been studied in both adults and children. IB specifically treats rhinorrhea and does little to improve congestion. Intranasal anticholinergics work best for rhinorrhea-predominant NAR variants, such as cold air–induced rhinitis (skier's nose)[55] and gustatory and senile rhinitis.[35] In 28 patients with cold air–induced rhinitis, IB reduced symptoms and the number of tissues required during and after cold exposure ($P = .0007$ and $P = .0023$, respectively).[56] In children with perennial AR or NAR, the effect of IB was superior to placebo and equivocal to beclomethasone dipropionate (BD) for the treatment of both rhinorrhea and congestion. However, IB was less effective than BD for controlling sneezing.[57]

Similar to the nasal antihistamines, there seems to be an additive effect when IB is used in conjunction with NCCS.[58] In a study comparing beclomethasone versus IB versus the 2 combined, the combination group had better symptom control of rhinorrhea. Beclomethasone monotherapy was found to treat sneezing and congestion better than IB monotherapy. Both medications were well tolerated. No study combining IB and nasal antihistamines for the treatment of NAR has been reported, but clinical experience indicates that this combination works well with patients who primarily experience rhinorrhea and postnasal drip.

Oral anticholinergics such as methscopolamine have not been studied in NAR but likely improve symptoms particularly in patients with rhinorrhea as a predominant symptom or in patients with significant postnasal drainage. Many first-generation antihistamines and decongestants also have strong anticholinergic properties. However, side effects such as dry mouth, sedation, and urinary hesitancy limit the usefulness of these drugs. Clinical experience suggests that oral methscopolamine combined with an oral first-generation antihistamine is helpful in treating patients with postnasal drip and that adding this combination to nasal IB, nasal antihistamines, or NCCS is useful.

Decongestants

Both oral and topical decongestants effectively treat congestion regardless of cause; however, none have been studied for NAR. Oral pseudoephedrine is an effective decongestant and can be considered for chronic use. However, side effects such as neurogenic and cardiac stimulations, palpitations, and insomnia affect a significant number of patients. Furthermore, the medication is relatively contraindicated in patients with hypertension. Thus, pseudoephedrine must be used cautiously. Phenylephrine is also an oral decongestant. It has been studied far less than pseudoephedrine and is considered a generally less-potent medication.

Topical decongestants, such as oxymetazoline and phenylephrine, are fast-acting potent local decongestants. These medications cannot be used chronically because continual use for more than 3 to 10 days leads to rhinitis medicamentosa. For patients with NAR with intermittent nasal congestion, a topical decongestant can be used for short-term relief of congestion.

Other NAR Therapies

Even though NAR affects many patients, very few medications have been adequately studied for the treatment of this condition. In patients who do not adequately respond to NCCS, intranasal antihistamines, or IB, other agents can be considered. There are a few limited studies examining intranasal capsaicin in NAR. In theory, repetitive capsaicin application depletes certain neuroinflammatory chemicals. Van Rijswijk and colleagues[59] did demonstrate decreased nasal symptoms in patients with NAR treated with capsaicin. Similarly, botulinum toxin A injected into the inferior and middle turbinates of patients with NAR has been shown to decrease congestion, sneezing, rhinorrhea, and nasal itch.[60] In patients with congestion as the predominant nasal symptom who have clinical evidence of turbinate hypertrophy, surgical reduction of the inferior turbinates may be of some benefit.[61] Nasal washing with isotonic or hypertonic saline has a demonstrated benefit particularly in chronic rhinosinusitis and seems to benefit some patients with NAR.[62] Antileukotrienes have not been studied in NAR, but there is at least some theoretical benefit in patients with aspirin sensitivity and/or nasal polyposis.

SUMMARY

NAR is the new designation for the conditions formerly referred to as VMR or nonallergic idiopathic rhinitis. The clinical characteristics and differential diagnosis are provided in detail in this review, and the disease should now be characterized suffi-ciently for clinical studies. The development of acceptable inclusion and exclusion criteria for NAR[23] should facilitate new and much needed clinical studies for this disease to define which medications might be useful in treatment. Moreover, with these precise characteristics, the diagnosis of NAR can be made on clinical grounds rather than as a diagnosis of exclusion. The current treatment of NAR is generally successful and uses nasal antihistamines and NCCS either individually or in combina-tion. As there are a substantial number of patients for whom nonallergic triggers play an important role in their disease, both the recognition and effective treatment of NAR should have a positive effect on their lives.

REFERENCES

1. Baraniuk JN, Shusterman D. Nonallergic rhinitis. New York: Informa Healthcare; 2007.
2. Baraniuk JN. Pathogenic mechanisms of idiopathic nonallergic rhinitis. World Allergy Organiz J 2009;2:106–14.
3. Kaliner MA, Baraniuk JN, Benninger M, et al. Consensus definition of nonallergic rhinopathy (NAR), previously referred to as vasomotor rhinitis (VMR), nonallergic rhinitis, and/or idiopathic rhinitis. WAO J 2009;2(6):119–20.
4. Nassef M, Shapiro G, Casale TB, et al. Identifying and managing rhinitis and its subtypes: allergic and nonallergic components—a consensus report and mate-rials from the Respiratory and Allergic Disease Foundation. Curr Med Res Opin 2006;22:2541–8.
5. Bernstein JA, Rezvani M. Mixed rhinitis: a new subclass of chronic rhinitis?. In: Kaliner M, editor. Current review of rhinitis. 2nd edition. Philadelphia: Current Medicine; 2006. p. 69–78.
6. Brandt D, Bernstein JA. Questionnaire evaluation and risk factor identification for nonallergic vasomotor rhinitis. Ann Allergy Asthma Immunol 2006;96:526–32.
7. Brandt D, Bernstein JA. Questionnaire diagnosis of non-allergic rhinitis. In: Baraniuk JN, Shusterman D, editors. Nonallergic rhinitis. New York: Marcel Dekker, Inc; 2008. p. 55–68.
8. Bernstein JA, Brandt D, Ratner P, et al. Assessment of a rhinitis questionnaire in a seasonal allergic rhinitis population. Ann Allergy Asthma Immunol 2008;100: 512–3.
9. Bernstein JA, Brandt DM, Martin V. Differentiation of chronic rhinitis subtypes using an Irritant Index Scale. Presented at the American College of Allergy, Asthma and Immunology Annual Meeting. Dallas (TX), November 8–13, 2007.
10. Settipane RA, Lieberman P. Update on nonallergic rhinitis. Ann Allergy Asthma Immunol 2001;86:494–508.
11. Wallace DV, Dykewicz MS, Bernstein DI, et al, Joint Task Force on Practice; Amer-ican Academy of Allergy, Asthma & Immunology; American College of Allergy, Asthma and Immunology; Joint Council of Allergy, Asthma and Immunology. The diagnosis and management of rhinitis: an updated practice parameter. J Allergy Clin Immunol 2008;122(Suppl 2):S1–84.
12. Mullarkey MF, Hill JS, Webb DR. Allergic and nonallergic rhinitis: their character-ization with attention to the meaning of nasal eosinophilia. J Allergy Clin Immunol 1980;65:122–6.
13. Enberg RN. Perennial nonallergic rhinitis: a retrospective review. Ann Allergy Asthma Immunol 1989;63:513–6.

14. Togias A. Age relationships and clinical features of nonallergic rhinitis. J Allergy Clin Immunol 1990;85:182.
15. Leynaert B, Bousquet J, Neukirch C, et al. Perennial rhinitis: an independent risk factor for asthma in nonatopic subjects. Results from the European Community Respiratory Health Survey. J Allergy Clin Immunol 1999;104:301–4.
16. Settipane RA. Rhinitis: a dose of epidemiological reality. Allergy Asthma Proc 2003;24:147–54.
17. Mercer MJ, van der Linde GP, Joubert G. Rhinitis (allergic and nonallergic) in an atopic pediatric referral population in the grasslands of inland South Africa. Ann Allergy Asthma Immunol 2002;89:503–12.
18. Bachert C, van Cauwenberge P, Olbrecht J, et al. Prevalence, classification and perception of allergic and nonallergic rhinitis in Belgium. Allergy 2006;61:693–8.
19. Mølgaard E, Thomsen SF, Lund T, et al. Differences between allergic and nonallergic rhinitis in a large sample of adolescents and adults. Allergy 2007;62: 1033–7.
20. Schatz M, Zeiger RS, Chen W, et al. The burden of rhinitis in a managed care organization. Ann Allergy Asthma Immunol 2008;101:240–7.
21. Settipane RA, Charnock DR. Epidemiology of rhinitis: allergic and nonallergic. Clin Allergy Immunol 2007;19:23–34.
22. Bernstein IL, Li JT, Bernstein DI, et al, American Academy of Allergy, Asthma and Immunology; American College of Allergy, Asthma and Immunology. Allergy diagnostic testing: an updated practice parameter. Ann Allergy Asthma Immunol 2008;100(3 Suppl 3):S1–148.
23. Kaliner M, Baraniuk JN, Benninger MS, et al. Consensus description of inclusion and exclusion criteria for clinical studies of nonallergic rhinopathy, previously referred to as vasomotor rhinitis (VMR) nonallergic rhinitis or idiopathic rhinitis. World Allergy Organiz J 2009;2:180–4.
24. Ray NF, Baraniuk JN, Thamer M, et al. Direct expenditures for the treatment of allergic rhinoconjunctivitis in the United States in 1996, including contributions of related airway illnesses. J Allergy Clin Immunol 1999;103:401–7.
25. Reed SD, Lee TA, McCrory DC. The economic burden of allergic rhinitis: a critical evaluation of the literature. Pharmacoeconomics 2004;22:345–61.
26. Settipane RA, Settipane GA. Nonallergic rhinitis. In: Kaliner MA, editor. Current review of rhinitis. 2nd edition. Philadelphia: Current Medicine; 2006. p. 55–68.
27. Kaliner M, Lieberman P. Incidence of allergic, nonallergic and mixed rhinitis in clinical practice. Presented at the Annual Meeting of the American Academy of Otolaryngology Head and Neck Surgery (AAO-HNS) Foundation. Washington, DC, September 24–27, 2000; Poster PO75.
28. Bousquet J, Fokkens W, Burney P, et al. Important research questions in allergy and related diseases: nonallergic rhinitis: a GALEN paper. Allergy 2008;63: 842–53.
29. Scarupa MD, Kaliner MA. Nonallergic rhinitis, with a focus on vasomotor rhinitis: clinical importance, differential diagnosis, and effective treatment recommendations. World Allergy Organiz J 2009;2:20–5.
30. Greiner AN, Meltzer EO. Pharmacologic rationale for treating allergic and nonallergic rhinitis. J Allergy Clin Immunol 2006;118:985–96.
31. Kaliner MA. Classification of nonallergic rhinitis syndromes with a focus on vasomotor rhinitis, proposed to be known henceforth as nonallergic rhinopathy. World Allergy Organiz J 2009;2:98–101.
32. Kaliner MA. Recognizing and treating nonallergic rhinitis. Female Patient 2002; 27:20–32.

33. Graf PM. Rhinitis medicamentosa. In: Baraniuk JN, Shusterman D, editors. Nonallergic rhinitis. New York: Informa; 2007. p. 295–304.
34. Baraniuk JN, Clauw DJ, Gaumond E. Rhinitis symptoms in chronic fatigue syndrome. Ann Allergy Asthma Immunol 1998;81:359–65.
35. Raphael G, Raphael MH, Kaliner M. Gustatory rhinitis: a syndrome of food-induced rhinorrhea. J Allergy Clin Immunol 1989;83:110–5.
36. Hellgren J, Toren K. Nonallergic occupational rhinitis. In: Baraniuk JN, Shusterman D, editors. Nonallergic rhinitis. New York: Informa; 2007. p. 241–8.
37. Wedback A, Enbom H, Eriksson NE, et al. Seasonal nonallergic rhinitis (SNAR)—a new disease entity? A clinical and immunological comparison between SNAR, seasonal allergic rhinitis and persistent non-allergic rhinitis. Rhinology 2005;43: 86–92.
38. Togias A, Lykens K, Kagey-Sobotka A, et al. Studies on the relationships between sensitivity to cold, dry air, hyperosmolal solutions, and histamine in the adult nose. Am Rev Respir Dis 1990;141:1428–33.
39. Meltzer EO. The treatment of vasomotor rhinitis with intranasal corticosteroids. World Allergy Organiz J 2009;2:166–79.
40. Webb DR, Meltzer EO, Finn AF, et al. Intranasal fluticasone is effective for perennial nonallergic rhinitis with or without eosinophilia. Ann Allergy Asthma Immunol 2002;88:385–90.
41. Day JH, Andersson CB, Briscoe MP. Efficacy and safety of intranasal budesonide in the treatment of perennial rhinitis in adults and children. Ann Allergy Asthma Immunol 1990;64(5):445–50.
42. Lundblad L, Sipila P, Farstad T, et al. Mometasone furoate nasal spray in the treatment of perennial non-allergic rhinitis: a Nordic, multicenter, randomized, double-blind, placebo-controlled study. Acta Otolaryngol 2001;121(4):505–9.
43. Blom HM, Godthelp T, Fokkens WJ, et al. The effect of nasal steroid aqueous spray on nasal complaint scores and cellular infiltrates in the nasal mucosa of patients with nonallergic, noninfectious perennial rhinitis. J Allergy Clin Immunol 1997;100:739–47.
44. Broms P, Malm L. Oral vasoconstrictors in perennial non-allergic rhinitis. Allergy 1982;37:67–74.
45. Kaliner MA. Azelastine and olopatadine in the treatment of allergic rhinitis. Ann Allergy Asthma Immunol 2009;103:373–80.
46. Kaliner MA. A novel and effective approach to treating rhinitis with nasal antihistamines. Ann Allergy Asthma Immunol 2007;99:383–91.
47. Banov CH, Lieberman P, Vasomotor Rhinitis Study Groups. Efficacy of azelastine nasal spray in the treatment of vasomotor (perennial nonallergic) rhinitis. Ann Allergy Asthma Immunol 2001;86(1):28–35.
48. Yanez A, Rodrigo GJ. Intranasal corticosteroids versus topical H1 receptor antagonists for the treatment of allergic rhinitis: a systematic review with meta-analysis. Ann Allergy Asthma Immunol 2002;89:479–84.
49. Kaliner MA, Berger WE, Ratner RH, et al. The role of intranasal antihistamines in the treatment of allergic rhinitis, IV: efficacy of intranasal antihistamines. Ann Allergy Asthma Immunol 2011;106(Suppl):S6–11.
50. Kaliner MA, Storms W, Tilles S, et al. Comparison of olopatadine 0.6% nasal spray versus fluticasone propionate 50 microg in the treatment of seasonal allergic rhinitis. Allergy Asthma Proc 2009;30:255–62.
51. Data on file, Meda Pharmaceuticals Inc, Somerset.
52. Ratner PH, Hampel F, Van Bavel J, et al. Combination therapy with azelastine hydrochloride nasal spray and fluticasone propionate nasal spray in the

treatment of patients with seasonal allergic rhinitis. Ann Allergy Asthma Immunol 2008;100:74–81.

53. Hampel FC, Ratner PH, Van Bavel J, et al. Double-blind, placebo-controlled study of azelastine and fluticasone in a single nasal spray delivery device. Ann Allergy Asthma Immunol 2010;105:168–73.

54. LaForce CF, Carr W, Tilles SA, et al. Evaluation of olopatadine hydrochloride nasal spray, 0.6%, used in combination with an intranasal corticosteroid in seasonal allergic rhinitis. Allergy Asthma Proc 2010;31:132–40.

55. Silvers WS. The skier's nose: a model of cold-induced rhinorrhea. Ann Allergy Asthma Immunol 1991;67:32–6.

56. Bonadonna P, Senna G, Zanon P, et al. Cold-induced rhinitis in skiers-clinical aspects and treatment with ipratropium bromide nasal spray: a randomized controlled trial. Am J Rhinol 2001;15:297–301.

57. Milgrom H, Biondi R, Georgitis JW, et al. Comparison of ipratropium bromide 0.03% with beclomethasone dipropionate in the treatment of perennial rhinitis in children. Ann Allergy Asthma Immunol 1999;83(2):105–11.

58. Dockhorn R, Aaronson D, Bronsky E, et al. Ipratropium bromide nasal spray 0.03% and beclomethasone nasal spray alone and in combination for the treatment of rhinorrhea in perennial rhinitis. Ann Allergy Asthma Immunol 1999; 82(4):349–59.

59. Van Rijswijk JB, Boeke EL, Keizer JM, et al. Intranasal capsaicin reduces nasal hyperreactivity in idiopathic rhinitis: a double-blind randomized application regimen study. Allergy 2003;58:754–61.

60. Ozcan C, Vayisoglu Y, Dogu O, et al. The effect of intranasal injection of botulinum toxin A on the symptoms of vasomotor rhinitis. Am J Otolaryngol 2006;27(5): 314–8.

61. Ikeda K, Oshima T, Suzuki M, et al. Functional inferior turbinosurgery (FITS) for the treatment of resistant chronic rhinitis. Acta Otolaryngol 2006;126:739–45.

62. Scarupa MD, Kaliner MA. Adjuvant therapies in the treatment of acute and chronic rhinosinusitis. In: Hamilos D, Baroody F, editors. Chronic rhinosinusitis. New York: Marcel Dekker; 2007. p. 251–63.

Other Causes of Rhinitis: Mixed Rhinitis, Rhinitis Medicamentosa, Hormonal Rhinitis, Rhinitis of the Elderly, and Gustatory Rhinitis

Russell A. Settipane, MD

KEYWORDS

- Rhinitis • Rhinitis medicamentosa • Hormonal rhinitis
- Gustatory rhinitis • Mixed rhinitis • Geriatric

Although other articles in this issue discuss 2 major classifications of rhinitis, allergic and nonallergic rhinitis (see the articles by Michael A. Kaliner and Lanny J. Rosenwasser elsewhere in this issue for further exploration of this topic), it is important to consider a more comprehensive differential of possible rhinitis types when considering the diagnosis of chronic rhinitis (**Box 1**), including at least 9 subtypes of nonallergic rhinitis (**Box 2**): drug-induced rhinitis, gustatory rhinitis, hormonal-induced rhinitis, infectious rhinitis, nonallergic rhinitis with eosinophilia syndrome (NARES), occupational rhinitis, senile rhinitis (rhinitis of the elderly), atrophic rhinitis, and nonallergic rhinopathy, formerly referred to as vasomotor rhinitis.[1–3] This article focuses on some of the most common types of chronic rhinitis, including mixed rhinitis (allergic and nonallergic overlap), rhinitis medicamentosa, hormonal rhinitis, rhinitis of the elderly, and gustatory rhinitis.

MIXED RHINITIS

Mixed rhinitis is defined as the coexistence of both allergic and nonallergic rhinitis.[1,4] It has been reported to occur in approximately 44% to 87% of patients with allergic

Conflicts of interest: Dr Settipane is a speaker, and/or research grant recipient for Merck, Alcon, Meda, Teva, Sunovion, and Astra-Zeneca.
Brown University, Alpert Medical School, Providence, RI, USA
E-mail address: setti5@aol.com

Immunol Allergy Clin N Am 31 (2011) 457–467
doi:10.1016/j.iac.2011.05.011
0889-8561/11/$ – see front matter © 2011 Published by Elsevier Inc.

Box 1
Types of rhinitis

1. Allergic rhinitis
   a. Seasonal
   b. Perennial
   c. Episodic
2. Nonallergic rhinitis
   a. Vasomotor rhinitis
      i. Irritant triggered (eg, chlorine)
      ii. Cold air
      iii. Exercise (eg, running)
      iv. Undetermined or poorly defined triggers
   b. Gustatory rhinitis
   c. Infectious
      i. Acute
      ii. Chronic
   d. NARES
3. Occupational rhinitis
   a. Caused by protein and chemical allergens, immunoglobulin E (IgE)–mediated
   b. Caused by chemical respiratory sensitizers, immune mechanism uncertain
   c. Work-aggravated rhinitis
4. Other rhinitis syndromes
   a. Hormonally induced
      i. Pregnancy rhinitis
      ii. Menstrual cycle related
   b. Drug induced
      i. Rhinitis medicamentosa
      ii. Oral contraceptives
      iii. Antihypertensives and cardiovascular agents
      iv. Aspirin/nonsteroidal antiinflammatory drugs
      v. Other drugs
   c. Atrophic rhinitis
   d. Rhinitis associated with inflammatory-immunologic disorders
      i. Granulomatous infections
      ii. Wegener granulomatosis
      iii. Sarcoidosis
      iv. Midline granuloma
      v. Churg-Strauss
      vi. Relapsing polychondritis
      vii. Amyloidosis

Data from Wallace DV, Dykewicz MS, Bernstein DI, et al. The diagnosis and management of rhinitis, an updated practice parameter. J Allergy Clin Immunol 2008;122(Suppl):S1–84.

Box 2
Chronic nonallergic rhinitis syndromes

Drug-induced rhinitis, including rhinitis medicamentosa

Gustatory rhinitis

Hormonal-induced rhinitis, including the rhinitis of pregnancy

Infectious rhinitis, including both bacterial rhinitis and rhinosinusitis

NARES

Occupational rhinitis

Senile rhinitis

Atrophic rhinitis

Cerebrospinal fluid leak

Vasomotor rhinitis, also called idiopathic nonallergic rhinitis and nonallergic rhinopathy

Data from Refs.[1–3]

---

rhinitis and may be more common than either pure allergic rhinitis or nonallergic rhinitis.[1,5–7] Although allergic rhinitis has been estimated to affect 30 to 60 million individuals in the United States,[1] the number of individuals with mixed rhinitis in the United States is estimated to range somewhere between 13 million and 52 million, with the cost being substantial.[8]

The pathophysiology of mixed rhinitis involves all the features of pure allergic rhinitis,[9] but is also characterized by the nonspecific nasal hyperreactivity that is characteristic of nonallergic rhinopathy.[10–12]

The clinical presentation of mixed rhinitis is variable and is characterized by a historical presence of rhinitis symptoms that are not fully explained by specific IgE sensitization. An example may be a patient who is monosensitized to ragweed pollen, but who manifests perennial rhinitis symptoms of nonallergic, noninfectious cause that are exacerbated during the ragweed season. Further complicating the diagnosis of mixed rhinitis are recent reports showing that some patients with rhinitis with negative skin tests may manifest localized IgE-mediated mucosal allergy.[13]

It may be important to make a distinction between chronic rhinitis phenotypes because symptom triggers, response to treatment, and prevalence of comorbidities such as sinusitis may be significantly different.[14] For example, in a recent study, allergy immunotherapy (AIT) was found to be effective in treating both allergic rhinitis and mixed rhinitis, but patients with mixed rhinitis required significantly more medication after completing a full course of AIT, presumably to control nonallergic-induced symptoms.[15] In another example, investigators showed reduced effectiveness of an oral antihistamine alone in patients with localized mucosal allergy compared with allergic rhinitis.[16]

Currently, no treatment is specifically approved by the US Food and Drug Administration (FDA) for the treatment of mixed rhinitis. The standard approach has been to treat patients with this condition similarly to other patients with allergic[17] or nonallergic rhinitis,[18–20] as outlined by Nataliya M. Kushnir; Hoyte and Katial; Eli O. Meltzer; and Mark S. Dykewicz elsewhere in this issue. The specific type of treatment that the patient is prescribed depends in large part on how physicians perceive the severity of symptoms, and correlates with the physician's ability to differentiate between the symptoms of allergic and nonallergic rhinitis.[21] It is hoped that the future development of patient-centric questionnaires that can reliably characterize and differentiate allergic rhinitis, mixed rhinitis, and nonallergic rhinitis phenotypes will result in improved clinical ability to further investigate the natural history/epidemiology, mechanisms, and development of novel therapies for mixed rhinitis.[14]

RHINITIS MEDICAMENTOSA

Rhinitis medicamentosa is a syndrome of rebound nasal congestion that results from the overuse of intranasal α-adrenergic decongestants (containing oxymetazoline or phenylephrine) or from abuse of cocaine.[1] The prevalence of this condition is unknown.

An underlying rhinitis disorder often leads to this form of self-treatment. When used briefly (<3–5 days consecutively), α-adrenergic decongestants provide fast and effective relief of nasal congestion. However, with chronic use, rebound nasal congestion can occur and can be severe. In the United States, topical decongestant preparations are labeled with a warning to discontinue use after 3 days of treatment because of the risk of this condition developing. The cumulative dose of nasal decongestant, or the treatment duration required to initiate this condition, has not been conclusively determined. Therefore, these medications should only be used for the shortest period of time required.

The exact mechanism is poorly understood, but theories suggest involvement of recurrent nasal tissue hypoxia and negative neural feedback with chronic decreased α-2 receptor responsiveness.[22] The pathophysiology resulting from prolonged usage of α-adrenergic decongestants may lead to a hypertrophy of the nasal mucosa. Patients develop tachyphylaxis at the level of the vascular α receptors, as reflected by a reduction in both the decongestive effect of the α-adrenergic agents and a reduction of drug duration reflected by their need for more frequent doses to provide adequate decongestion.

Rhinitis medicamentosa results in drug-induced damage of the nasal mucosa characterized by the following histologic changes: nasociliary loss, squamous cell metaplasia, epithelial edema, epithelial cell denudation, goblet cell hyperplasia, increased expression of the epidermal growth factor receptor, and inflammatory cell infiltration.[23] Functionally, the loss and destruction of ciliated epithelial cells explain the reduced mucociliary clearance.[24] In addition, the vascular endothelium reveals ultrastructural changes, possibly resulting from increased vascular permeability and interstitial edema.[24] Rebound swelling seems to be caused by interstitial edema rather than by vasodilatation.[25] Benzalkonium chloride, an ingredient in some vasoconstrictor spray products, may augment local pathologic effects.[26]

Classically, the physical examination reveals erythematous nasal mucosa (often described as beefy red) that is congested, granular, and with areas of punctate bleeding caused by tissue friability. Nasal septal perforation is a rare complication.[27]

The diagnosis of rhinitis medicamentosa is dependent on a careful history. Every patient presenting with the complaint of nasal congestion should be questioned as to the extent of use of topical decongestant nasal sprays. Because a similar presentation may occur with prolonged use of other vasoconstrictor agents such as cocaine, the use of this illicit drug should be questioned as well.

Successful treatment of rhinitis medicamentosa is dependant on withdrawal from topical decongestant use as well as treatment of the underlying rhinitis disorder. Stopping the topical decongestant is the first line of treatment. Although different therapeutic approaches exist, ranging from intraturbinate corticosteroid injections[28] to oral or topical corticosteroids[29–33] and diode laser inferior turbinate reduction in therapy-refractory cases,[34] there is no comparative evidence to suggest which approach is best. On successful discontinuation of the topical decongestant, the patient should be followed for recurrence and evaluated for an underlying cause.

HORMONAL RHINITIS

Causes of hormonal rhinitis include pregnancy and menstrual cycle–related rhinitis.[1] Although hormonal disorders such as hypothyroidism and acromegaly have been suggested to cause or contribute to rhinitis, the evidence for this association remains largely anecdotal.[35,36] The development of a type of rhinitis unique to the pregnant patient has been referred to as vasomotor rhinitis (nonallergic rhinopathy) of pregnancy or pregnancy rhinitis.[1] It affects 1 in 5 pregnant women, with onset in any stage of gestation.[37] It has been proposed that pregnancy rhinitis should be defined as rhinitis without an infectious, allergic, or medication-related cause that starts before the last 6 weeks of pregnancy, persists until delivery, and typically resolves completely and spontaneously within 2 weeks after delivery.[38]

Rhinitis symptoms, particularly nasal congestion, are common during pregnancy.[1] However, the rhinitis that occurs during most pregnancies often has been present before the onset of the pregnancy and often is secondary to common types of rhinitis that are unrelated to pregnancy.[39] Therefore, the exact extent to which pregnancy is a causal factor is unknown; it may play more of an aggravating role. Preexisting allergic rhinitis worsens in approximately one-third of pregnant patients.[40] In addition, episodes of bacterial rhinosinusitis have been noted to be 6 times more common during pregnancy.[41]

It has been suggested that the hormones of pregnancy, oral contraceptives, other estrogens, and even cyclical premenstrual hormones can contribute to rhinitis symptoms.[42] During pregnancy, physiologic changes may contribute to increased nasal congestion/obstruction. Increased progesterone, estrogen, prolactin, vasoactive intestinal peptide, and/or placental growth hormone levels during pregnancy have been associated with several secondary phenomena.[38] Among these changes are vasodilatation combined with a massive expansion of circulating blood volume, contributing to an increase in nasal vascular pooling and possible progesterone-induced vascular smooth muscle relaxation.[43] Thus, the nasal mucosa becomes engorged and congestion ensues as the mucous membranes are affected by the hormonal changes of pregnancy.[42] In addition, pregnancy-associated hormones may directly induce nasal mucous gland hyperactivity, resulting in increased nasal secretions/rhinorrhea.[43] However, there is no convincing evidence that any of these hormones contribute directly to pregnancy rhinitis.[38] Furthermore, although oral contraceptives have been implicated as causes of nasal symptoms, a recent study found no nasal physiologic effects on female patients receiving oral contraceptive treatment.[44]

A complete discussion of the treatment of rhinitis during pregnancy is beyond the scope of this article and is reviewed elsewhere.[1] It is sufficient to note that the main issue in treating rhinitis during pregnancy is caution with medication use. First-line treatment should include a reliance on the safest forms of treatment, such as exercise, head of bed elevation, nasal alar dilatation, saline rinses, and an avoidance of irritants. Regarding medication, topical medical therapy is generally preferred to systemic therapy. Although there is no research on the safety of short-term topical decongestants combined with intranasal corticosteroids in pregnancy, these treatment options have been suggested for management of pregnancy rhinitis when nonpharmacologic approaches are not effective.[38,45] When weighing medical treatment options for rhinitis in pregnancy, the FDA risk categorization of medications can provide some guidance; however, the value of these recommendations is limited because they are based largely on animal data and very limited human data. Therefore, as part of the decision making process, it is also beneficial to review the most recent human cohort and case-control studies, as well as birth registry data.

RHINITIS IN THE ELDERLY

For the purposes of this discussion, rhinitis in the elderly is defined as rhinitis occurring in a population more than 65 years of age. Although several specific age-related changes in the nose have been identified,[46] including the development of hyposmia,[47] formal epidemiologic data regarding rhinitis in the elderly are limited. Allergic rhinitis has been estimated to occur in up to 12% of patients older than 65 years[48] and is becoming increasingly recognized as common in the elderly.[49] However nonallergic causes may be more prevalent with advancing age.[50]

Rhinitis in the elderly may be influenced by age-related physiologic alterations such as cholinergic hyperactivity and anatomic changes.[1] Among these anatomic changes are atrophic structural changes in the connective tissue, mucosal glands, and vasculature of the nose. These anatomic changes can result in drying and increased nasal congestion, often magnifying or complicating other causes of rhinitis. Decreased nasal blood flow to the mucosa may contribute to the development of local atrophy, with consequent symptoms of atrophic rhinitis, congestion, crusting, and fetor.[51] Both primary and secondary atrophic rhinitis have been reported to be more prevalent in senior populations, with reported mean occurrence ages of 52 and 56 years, respectively.[52] Treatment of primary and secondary atrophic rhinitis involves reducing crusting and alleviating the foul odor by instituting a regimen of nasal hygiene, such as nasal lavage and crust debridement, and the use of topical and/or systemic antibiotics when purulent secretions or an acute infection is present.[1,53]

Rhinitis in the elderly may be caused by the same types of rhinitis that are common in other age populations; however, the prevalence of the various types may differ. For example, because the elderly are more likely to be receiving prescription medications for a wide variety of medical conditions, drugs may be a more prevalent cause or contributor to chronic rhinitis in this age group. Drug-induced rhinitis may be caused by host of different mechanisms and medications, including angiotensin-converting enzyme inhibitors, phosphodiesterase-5–selective inhibitors, phentolamine, and α-receptor antagonists.[1]

In addition to causing rhinitis, drugs taken by the elderly can interfere with skin test sensitivity, which is a concern because of the higher prevalence of medication use in this age group.[54] The usefulness of diagnostic testing for allergic sensitivities may also be affected by the aging process. Age has been shown to be an important predictor of skin test reactivity, with peak reactivity occurring between 12 and 24 years of age.[55] In addition, because age-related changes in the skin suppress the response to skin-prick tests, allergic rhinitis may be underdiagnosed in the elderly.[56] When applying skin tests in this population, if the area of skin where allergen skin tests are to be placed is atrophic or severely sun damaged, an alternative site should be sought. If no suitable area of skin can be identified, in vitro allergen testing should be considered.[57] Because the performance characteristics of serum-specific IgE, compared with prick skin testing, varies among different allergens, in vitro specific IgE measurement, should be considered as complementary rather than equivalent to skin testing.[58] Evidence supporting in vitro allergen testing in the elderly has recently been reported.[59] When the skin-prick test and in vitro tests for specific IgE are performed simultaneously, differences in allergic test results to dust mite have been found to vary according to age group. For patients more than 50 years of age, in vitro testing for specific IgE was found to be the preferred method for detecting allergy to house-dust mites; whereas for patients less than 30 years old, skin-prick testing was preferred.[59] However, positive allergy testing in the elderly may not correlate with true allergic rhinitis, which may be confirmed by nasal provocation.[60] Although skin-prick test and specific IgE have good negative predictive value in elderly patients with rhinitis, a recent study that used nasal allergen challenge as a diagnostic comparator showed that the positive predictive value of these tests may be limited in the elderly population and, therefore, require more careful interpretation.[61]

Treatment recommendations for allergic and nonallergic rhinitis in the elderly are limited by the paucity of clinical trials targeting treatment of older populations, and is complicated by the potential for drug interactions and adverse effects. The selection of pharmacologic treatments for elderly patients requires approaches empirically tailored to the specific age-dependent physiologic factors (such as metabolic alterations, changes in the nasal mucosa, difficulty swallowing, and visual or motor problems) that may affect responses to therapy.[49] Although oral antihistamines are associated with a higher incidence of adverse events and drug interactions in older, compared with younger individuals, topical antihistamines may be better tolerated.[62–69] The sympathomimetic effects of oral decongestants are of concern in the presence of comorbidities that are known to be more common in the elderly. Leukotriene receptor antagonists have the potential for interactions with a wide range of drugs. Intranasal corticosteroids improve congestion and olfactory function[70,71] and seem to have favorable safety and efficacy profiles in older individuals with allergic rhinitis, similar to a younger population.[49,72] Comparative studies have helped to elucidate the symptom relief provided and the associated cost with these different classes of medications.[73–75]

Rhinitis sicca is a condition that may occur secondary to Sjögren syndrome, atrophic rhinitis, or as a normal part of aging. Although rhinitis in the elderly may present with dryness of the mucosa, elderly patients with rhinitis more frequently experience pronounced, clear rhinorrhea resulting from cholinergic hyperactivity associated with the aging process. Although for rhinitis sicca, treatment with the liberal use of nasal saline sprays is appropriate, the watery rhinorrhea resulting from nonallergic rhinopathy of elderly patients has been shown to respond to intranasal ipratropium bromide, as shown by double-blind, placebo-controlled trials performed in subjects more than 60 years of age.[76] However, because of the potential for unwanted anticholinergic effects, ipratropium bromide should be used with caution in patients with preexisting glaucoma or prostatic hypertrophy.[77]

GUSTATORY RHINITIS

The syndrome of watery rhinorrhea occurring immediately after ingestion of foods, particularly hot and spicy foods, has been termed gustatory rhinitis; however, almost any foods can be implicated. It is a nonallergic condition that is vagally mediated.[78] Although the prevalence of this condition is unknown, based on clinical observations, it is believed to be more common amongst the elderly and frequently overlaps with rhinitis of the elderly.

Foods can provoke rhinitis symptoms by a variety of different mechanisms; these include nasal vasodilatation, food allergy, and/or other undefined mechanisms.[1] However, the pathophysiology of gustatory rhinitis has been shown to result from vagally mediated mechanisms. Studies with spicy food ingestion have shown that the pathophysiology involves a purely neurogenic reflex mechanism, with the efferent pathway being parasympathetic nerve fibers.[79,80] Why some patients may have a more exaggerated reflex mechanism is unknown. Food allergy is rarely the cause of rhinitis except in the setting of anaphylaxis, at which time there are usually other associated symptoms resulting from gastrointestinal, dermatologic, or other systemic manifestations.[81]

Effective treatment of this gustatory rhinitis is pretreatment with topical ipratropium bromide before ingestion of spicy food.[78,79]

REFERENCES

1. Wallace DV, Dykewicz MS, Bernstein DI, et al. The diagnosis and management of rhinitis, an updated practice parameter. J Allergy Clin Immunol 2008;122(Suppl): S1–84.
2. Scarupa MD, Kaliner MA. Nonallergic rhinitis, with a focus on vasomotor rhinitis: clinical importance, differential diagnosis and effective treatment recommendations. World Allergy Organiz J 2009;2:20–5.
3. Kaliner A. Classification of nonallergic rhinitis syndromes with a focus on vasomotor rhinitis, proposed to be known henceforth as nonallergic rhinopathy. World Allergy Organiz J 2009;2:98–101.
4. Settipane RA, Lieberman P. Update on nonallergic rhinitis. Ann Allergy Asthma Immunol 2001;86:494–507.
5. Settipane RA. Rhinitis: a dose of epidemiological reality. Allergy Asthma Proc 2003;24:147–54.
6. Settipane RA, Charnock DR. Epidemiology of rhinitis: allergic and nonallergic. Clin Allergy Immunol 2007;19:23–34.
7. Settipane RA. Epidemiology of vasomotor rhinitis. World Allergy Organiz J 2009; 2:115–8.
8. Blaiss MS. Allergic rhinitis: direct and indirect costs. Allergy Asthma Proc 2010; 31:375–80.
9. Broide DH. Allergic rhinitis: pathophysiology. Allergy Asthma Proc 2010;31: 370–4.
10. Kim YH, Oh YS, Kim KJ, et al. Use of cold dry air provocation with acoustic rhinometry in detecting nonspecific nasal hyperreactivity. Am J Rhinol Allergy 2010; 24:260–2.
11. Shusterman DJ, Tilles SA. Nasal physiological reactivity of subjects with nonallergic rhinitis to cold air provocation: a pilot comparison of subgroups. Am J Rhinol Allergy 2009;23:475–9.
12. Baraniuk J. Pathogenic mechanisms of idiopathic nonallergic rhinitis. World Allergy Organiz J 2009;2:106–14.
13. Khan DA. Allergic rhinitis with negative skin tests: does it exist? Allergy Asthma Proc 2009;30:465–9.
14. Bernstein JA. Allergic and mixed rhinitis: epidemiology and natural history. Allergy Asthma Proc 2010;31:365–9.
15. Smith AW, Rezvani M, Bernstein JA. Is response to allergen immunotherapy a good phenotypic marker for differentiating between allergic and mixed rhinitis? Allergy Asthma Proc 2011;32:49–54.
16. Kim YH, Jang TY. Clinical characteristics and therapeutic outcomes of patients with localized mucosal allergy. Am J Rhinol Allergy 2010;24:e89–92.
17. Wallace DV. Pet dander and perennial allergic rhinitis: therapeutic options. Allergy Asthma Proc 2009;30:573–83.
18. Lieberman P. The role of antihistamines in the treatment of vasomotor rhinitis. World Allergy Organiz J 2009;2:156–61.

19. Naclerio R. Anticholinergic drugs in nonallergic rhinitis. World Allergy Organiz J 2009;2:162–5.
20. Meltzer E. The treatment of vasomotor rhinitis with intranasal corticosteroids. World Allergy Organiz J 2009;2:166–79.
21. Meltzer EO, Nathan RA, Derebery J, et al. Physician perceptions of the treatment and management of allergic and nonallergic rhinitis. Allergy Asthma Proc 2009; 30:75–83.
22. Graf PM. Rhinitis medicamentosa. In: Baraniuk JN, Shusterman D, editors. Nonallergic rhinitis. New York: Informa; 2007. p. 295–304.
23. Ramey JT, Bailen E, Lockey RF. Rhinitis medicamentosa. J Investig Allergol Clin Immunol 2006;16:148–55.
24. Knipping S, Holzhausen HJ, Goetze G, et al. Rhinitis medicamentosa: electron microscopic changes of human nasal mucosa. Otolaryngol Head Neck Surg 2007;136:57–61.
25. Graf P, Hallén H, Juto JE. The pathophysiology and treatment of rhinitis medicamentosa. Clin Otolaryngol Allied Sci 1995;20:224–9.
26. Graf P. Adverse effects of benzalkonium chloride on the nasal mucosa: allergic rhinitis and rhinitis medicamentosa. Clin Ther 1999;21:1749–55.
27. Keyserling HF, Grimme JD, Camacho DL, et al. Nasal septal perforation secondary to rhinitis medicamentosa. Ear Nose Throat J 2006;85:376 378–9.
28. Mabry RL. Intraturbinal steroid injection: indications, results, and complications. South Med J 1978;71:789–91, 794.
29. Lekas MD. Rhinitis during pregnancy and rhinitis medicamentosa. Otolaryngol Head Neck Surg 1992;107:845–8 [discussion: 849].
30. Ferguson BJ, Paramaesvaran S, Rubinstein E. A study of the effect of nasal steroid sprays in perennial allergic rhinitis patients with rhinitis medicamentosa. Otolaryngol Head Neck Surg 2001;125:253–60.
31. Hallén H, Enerdal J, Graf P. Fluticasone propionate nasal spray is more effective and has a faster onset of action than placebo in treatment of rhinitis medicamentosa. Clin Exp Allergy 1997;27:552–8.
32. Graf PM, Hallén H. Changes in nasal reactivity in patients with rhinitis medicamentosa after treatment with fluticasone propionate and placebo nasal spray. ORL J Otorhinolaryngol Relat Spec 1998;60:334–8.
33. Graf P. Rhinitis medicamentosa: a review of causes and treatment. Treat Respir Med 2005;4:21–9.
34. Caffier PP, Frieler K, Scherer H, et al. Rhinitis medicamentosa: therapeutic effect of diode laser inferior turbinate reduction on nasal obstruction and decongestant abuse. Am J Rhinol 2008;22:433–9.
35. Settipane GA, Klein DE. Non allergic rhinitis: demography of eosinophils in nasal smear, blood total eosinophil counts and IgE levels. N Engl Reg Allergy Proc 1985;6:363–6.
36. Ellegård EK, Karlsson NG, Ellegård LH. Rhinitis in the menstrual cycle, pregnancy, and some endocrine disorders. Clin Allergy Immunol 2007;19:305–21.
37. Ellegård EK. Clinical and pathogenetic characteristics of pregnancy rhinitis. Clin Rev Allergy Immunol 2004;26:149–59.
38. Ellegard E, Karlsson G. Nasal congestion during pregnancy. Clin Otolaryngol Allied Sci 1999;24:307–11.
39. Incaudo GA, Schatz M. Rhinosinusitis associated with endocrine conditions: hypothyroidism and pregnancy. In: Schatz M, Zeiger RS, Settipane GA, editors. Nasal manifestations of systemic diseases. Providence (RI): OceanSide Publications; 1991. p. 53–62.

40. Schatz M, Zeiger RS. Diagnosis and management of rhinitis during pregnancy. Allergy Proc 1988;9:545–54.
41. Sorri M, Bortikanen-Sorri AL, Kanja J. Rhinitis during pregnancy. Rhinology 1980; 18:83–6.
42. Kaliner MA. Recognizing and treating nonallergic rhinitis. Female Patient 2002; 27:20–32.
43. Toppozada H, Michaels L, Toppazada M, et al. The human respiratory nasal mucosa in pregnancy. J Larynol Otol 1982;96:613–26.
44. Wolstenholme CR, Philpott CM, Oloto EJ, et al. Does the use of the combined oral contraceptive pill cause changes in the nasal physiology in young women? Am J Rhinol 2006;20:238–40.
45. National Heart, Lung, and Blood Institute, National Asthma Education and Prevention Program Asthma and Pregnancy Working Group. NAEPP expert panel report. Managing asthma during pregnancy: recommendations for pharmacologic treatment-2004 update. J Allergy Clin Immunol 2005;115:34–46.
46. Edelstein DR. Aging of the normal nose in adults. Laryngoscope 1996;106:1–25.
47. Gaines AD. Anosmia and hyposmia. Allergy Asthma Proc 2010;31:185–9.
48. Enright PL, Kronmal RA, Higgins MW, et al. Prevalence and correlates of respiratory symptoms and disease in the elderly. Cardiovascular Health Study. Chest 1994;106:827–34.
49. Slavin RG. Special considerations in treatment of allergic rhinitis in the elderly: role of intranasal corticosteroids. Allergy Asthma Proc 2010;31:179–84.
50. Crawford WW, Gowda VC, Klaustermeyer WB. Age effects on objective measures of atopy in adult asthma and rhinitis. Allergy Asthma Proc 2004;25:175–9.
51. Busse PJ, Kilaru K. Complexities of diagnosis and treatment of allergic respiratory disease in the elderly. Drugs Aging 2009;26:1–22.
52. Moore EJ, Kern EB. Atrophic rhinitis: a review of 242 cases. Am J Rhinol 2001;15: 355–61.
53. Leonard DW, Bolger WE. Topical antibiotic therapy for recalcitrant sinusitis. Laryngoscope 1999;109:668–70.
54. Shah KM, Rank MA, Davé SA, et al. Predicting which medication classes interfere with allergy skin testing. Allergy Asthma Proc 2010;31:477–82.
55. Gergen PJ, Turkeltaub PC, Kovar MG. The prevalence of allergic skin test reactivity to eight common aeroallergens in the U.S. population: results from the second National Health and Nutrition Examination Survey. J Allergy Clin Immunol 1987;80:669–79.
56. Skassa-Brociek W, Manderscheid JC, Michel FB, et al. Skin test reactivity to histamine from infancy to old age. J Allergy Clin Immunol 1987;80:711–6.
57. King MJ, Lockey RF. Allergen prick-puncture skin testing in the elderly. Drugs Aging 2003;20:1011–7.
58. Calabria CW, Dietrich J, Hagan L. Comparison of serum-specific IgE (Immuno-CAP) and skin-prick test results for 53 inhalant allergens in patients with chronic rhinitis. Allergy Asthma Proc 2009;30:386–96.
59. Jung YG, Cho HJ, Park GY, et al. Comparison of the skin-prick test and Phadia ImmunoCAP as tools to diagnose house-dust mite allergy. Am J Rhinol Allergy 2010;24:226–9.
60. Chusakul S, Phannaso C, Sangsarsri S, et al. House-dust mite nasal provocation: a diagnostic tool in perennial rhinitis. Am J Rhinol Allergy 2010;24:133–6.
61. King MJ, Tamulis T, Lockey RF. Prick puncture skin tests and serum specific IgE as predictors of nasal challenge response to *Dermatophagoides pteronyssinus* in older adults. Ann Allergy Asthma Immunol 2008;101:12–7.

62. Kaliner MA, Oppenheimer J, Farrar JR. Comprehensive review of olopatadine: the molecule and its clinical entities. Allergy Asthma Proc 2010;31:112–9.
63. LaForce CF, Carr W, Tilles SA, et al. Evaluation of olopatadine hydrochloride nasal spray, 0.6%, used in combination with an intranasal corticosteroid in seasonal allergic rhinitis. Allergy Asthma Proc 2010;31:132–40.
64. Shah S, Berger W, Lumry W, et al. Efficacy and safety of azelastine 0.15% nasal spray and azelastine 0.10% nasal spray in patients with seasonal allergic rhinitis. Allergy Asthma Proc 2009;30:628–33.
65. Bernstein JA, Prenner B, Ferguson BJ, et al. Double-blind, placebo-controlled trial of reformulated azelastine nasal spray in patients with seasonal allergic rhinitis. Am J Rhinol Allergy 2009;23:512–7.
66. Chipps BE, Harder JM. Antihistamine treatment for allergic rhinitis: different routes, different outcomes? Allergy Asthma Proc 2009;30:589–94.
67. Hernandez-Trujillo V. Antihistamines treatment for allergic rhinitis: different routes, different mechanisms? Allergy Asthma Proc 2009;30:584–8.
68. Lieberman P. Histamine, antihistamines, and the central nervous system. Allergy Asthma Proc 2009;30:482–6.
69. Cassell HR, Katial RK. Intranasal antihistamines for allergic rhinitis: examining the clinical impact. Allergy Asthma Proc 2009;30:349–57.
70. Salapatek A, Patel P, Gopalan G, et al. Mometasone furoate nasal spray provides early, continuing relief of nasal congestion and improves nasal patency in allergic patients. Am J Rhinol Allergy 2010;24:433–8.
71. Sivam A, Jeswani S, Reder L, et al. Olfactory cleft inflammation is present in seasonal allergic rhinitis and is reduced with intranasal steroids. Am J Rhinol Allergy 2010;24:286–90.
72. Given JT, Cheema AS, Dreykluft T, et al. Fluticasone furoate nasal spray is effective and well tolerated for perennial allergic rhinitis in adolescents and adults. Am J Rhinol Allergy 2010;24:444–50.
73. Sardana N, Santos C, Lehman E, et al. A comparison of intranasal corticosteroid, leukotriene receptor antagonist, and topical antihistamine in reducing symptoms of perennial allergic rhinitis as assessed through the Rhinitis Severity Score. Allergy Asthma Proc 2010;31:5–9.
74. Hay J, Jhaveri M, Tangirala M, et al. Cost and resource utilization comparisons of second-generation antihistamines vs. montelukast for allergic rhinitis treatment. Allergy Asthma Proc 2009;30:634–42.
75. Kalpaklioglu AF, Kavut AB. Comparison of azelastine versus triamcinolone nasal spray in allergic and nonallergic rhinitis. Am J Rhinol Allergy 2010;24:29–33.
76. Malmberg H, Grahne B, Holopainen E, et al. Ipratropium (Atrovent) in the treatment of vasomotor rhinitis of elderly patients. Clin Otolaryngol Allied Sci 1983; 8:273–6.
77. Bronsky EA, Druce H, Findlay SR, et al. A clinical trial of ipratropium bromide nasal spray in patients with perennial nonallergic rhinitis. J Allergy Clin Immunol 1995;95:1117–22.
78. Waibel KH, Chang C. Prevalence and food avoidance behaviors for gustatory rhinitis. Ann Allergy Asthma Immunol 2008;100:200–5.
79. Raphael G, Raphael MH, Kaliner MA. Gustatory rhinitis: a syndrome of food induced rhinorrhea. J Allergy Clin Immunol 1989;83:110–5.
80. Raphael GD, Hauptschein-Raphael M, Kaliner MA. Gustatory rhinitis. Am J Rhinol 1989;3:145–9.
81. Lieberman J, Sicherer SH. The diagnosis of food allergy. Am J Rhinol Allergy 2010;24:439–43.

What are the Primary Clinical Symptoms of Rhinitis and What Causes Them?

Gary N. Gross, MD[a,b,*]

KEYWORDS

- Rhinitis • Symptoms • Neuropeptides

The nose has a limited repertoire of responses regardless of the triggers. These responses primarily serve as a protective mechanism for the lower respiratory tract.[1] Although the nasal reactions to pollens, particles, and pollution may have a beneficial effect for the lower airway, they create symptoms in some individuals that lead to significant morbidity. In large surveys of patients, the typical nasal symptoms include nasal congestion, nasal drainage (including postnasal drainage), sneezing, and itching.[2–4] Ocular symptoms include itchy/red eyes and watery eyes. Other symptoms that may be secondary include cough (often related to postnasal drainage or to stimulation of nasal sensory nerves[5]) and headache and sinus pressure (related to congestion).[6] Rhinitis has been associated with sleep-disordered breathing, which could be the basis for the fatigue, irritability, and difficulty concentrating.[7–9] The symptoms of allergic rhinitis extend far beyond the nose, and the morbidity associated with rhinitis is significant. The nasal symptoms of rhinitis and their causes are the focus of this review.

Patients may have immunologic sensitivities to specific allergens, or they may have a heightened response to what would be benign exposures (irritants) in others. The many different permutations of triggers and responses have made it difficult to determine the exact mechanisms in the groups of patients studied. Some studies have focused on isolated triggers and mediators, whereas a real-life clinical situation often involves multiple triggers and many mediators. The inflammatory mechanism in allergic rhinitis involves immunoglobulin (Ig)E-activating mast cells and the consequent early and then late-phase reactions that have been well described previously.

[a] Division of Allergy and Immunology, University of Texas Southwestern Medical School, 5323 Harry Hines Boulevard, Dallas, TX 75390, USA
[b] Dallas Allergy & Asthma Center, 5499 Glen Lakes Drive, Dallas, TX 75231, USA
* Dallas Allergy & Asthma Center, 5499 Glen Lakes Drive, Dallas, TX 75231.
E-mail address: garyngross@gmail.com

Immunol Allergy Clin N Am 31 (2011) 469–480
doi:10.1016/j.iac.2011.05.006 immunology.theclinics.com
0889-8561/11/$ – see front matter © 2011 Elsevier Inc. All rights reserved.

Mediators, such as histamine, leukotrienes, prostaglandins, bradykinin, and platelet-activating factor, are released. Lymphocytes are activated and release cytokines that enhance the cellular inflammatory response and lead to the late-phase reaction.[10,11] Neuropeptides and nasal secretions have been extensively reviewed.[12] Recent investigations have studied the neuropeptides substance P and secretoneurin, which are increased in nasal mucosa and nasal lavage fluid in patients with allergic rhinitis. In vitro studies indicate these neuropeptides are potent chemoattractants for basophils, providing yet another interaction of the nervous system and inflammatory cells.[13] These inflammatory mediators and neuropeptides have a high degree of interconnectedness.

Furthermore, the various types of rhinitis are determined mainly by clinical descriptions and definitions, and, therefore, study populations may exhibit overlap, further confounding the data. For instance, in one study of idiopathic rhinitis, patients with vasomotor rhinitis were excluded.[14] Other reports use the two terms, idiopathic and vasomotor, synonymously. The literature varies as to the initiating features of these diseases, partly because of the differences in the definitions. Idiopathic rhinitis has been suggested to have an inflammatory basis by some investigators,[14] whereas others think hyperactive neuronal pathways are more likely responsible.[15,16] The understanding of causal factors in the symptoms of rhinitis depends, in part, on the clear definition of the population being studied. Efforts to clarify these various clinical entities may lead to a better understanding of both possible causes and a potential therapy.[17]

The inflammatory response in rhinitis triggered by allergens, whether systemic or local, is the initiating feature of symptoms. Recent studies have demonstrated that some patients who previously would have been classified as having idiopathic rhinitis may instead have a local allergic rhinitis.[18–20] Nasal challenge studies have attempted to elucidate the mediators and mechanisms responsible for symptoms of rhinitis.[21,22] These mediators have been studied in various models to better understand the cause of rhinitis symptoms. Nasal-allergen challenge studies have evaluated both symptoms and mediators in an attempt to attribute certain symptoms to specific mediators.[23,24] Wang and colleagues[24] found that itch and sneeze started within 20 to 30 seconds and abated about 5 minutes after the antigen challenge. Rhinorrhea and nasal congestion started a few minutes after the challenge and lasted more than 1 hour. When evaluating histamine, tryptase, and leukotriene C4, the investigators were unable to find any significant correlation between the concentration and dynamics of the mediators in nasal secretions and the specific nasal symptoms. This lack of correlation to specific symptoms is reflective of the complex nature of the underlying pathophysiology. The two unique aspects of nasal anatomy and physiology that interact to produce the typical symptoms of rhinitis are the vascular (**Fig. 1**) and the neurologic (**Fig. 2**) systems.

These systems have recently been reviewed.[25,26] The allergic response and mast cell activation produces mediators, such as histamine, tryptase, leukotrienes, and prostaglandins. Although histamine nasal challenge can produce all the symptoms of allergic rhinitis, it is clear that other mediators are also responsible for the clinical symptoms in patients.[27] Investigators have used specific mediators, such as histamine or serotonin, applied to the nasal mucosa to identify the subsequent symptoms these substances produce.[28] These investigators found that in normal volunteers serotonin produced itch, sneeze, and drainage similar to histamine, but produced less congestion than histamine. Histamine-related symptoms may be mediated directly via the histamine receptors on vessels or through activation of neuronal H1 receptors. Other histamine receptors, H2 and H3, may play a role in nasal

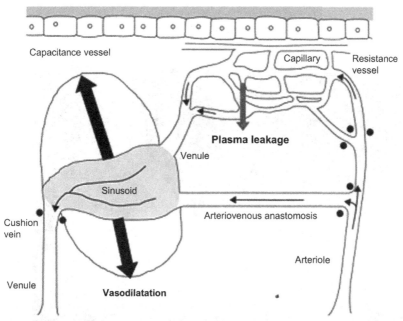

Fig. 1. Vascular mechanism of nasal congestion. (*From* Ichimura K. Mechanism of nasal obstruction in patients with allergic rhinitis. Clin Exp Allergy Rev 2010;10:21; with permission.)

congestion.[29] Such studies help differentiate the direct effect on neuronal reflex initiation of symptoms from those effects of mediators on the vascular bed in causing rhinitis symptoms.

Other investigators have attempted to differentiate between the cause of symptoms in nonallergic and allergic rhinitis by using nasal challenge models. Capsaicin selectively stimulates a subpopulation of sensory fibers. These fibers (unmyelinated C fibers and some Aδ fibers) provide stimulus to the central nervous system through their sensory function and also have an efferent arch through antidromic release of neuropeptides.[30] The capsaicin challenge has been used to further differentiate the mechanisms causing symptoms in allergic and nonallergic rhinitis. In a study of nonallergic rhinitis (defined by negative skin tests) compared with allergic subjects (with both rhinitis groups having perennial symptoms of nasal congestion or rhinorrhea), capsaicin challenge was used to compare nasal responses.[31] These investigators found that all subjects developed burning, lacrimation, and rhinorrhea after the capsaicin challenge. Although rhinorrhea was present in all groups, the composition of nasal lavage fluids was different between the groups. Lactoferrin (a marker of submucosal gland secretion), albumin (a marker of vascular effect through plasma extravasation), and total protein were measured. Only the patients with allergic rhinitis had a significant increase in albumin secretion compared with nonallergic and nonrhinitic subjects, suggesting that in allergic rhinitis there is a hyperresponsiveness to neuronal stimulation. Increased neuronal responsiveness in patients with symptomatic allergic rhinitis has been shown in other studies. Nasal challenge with bradykinin produced greater symptom scores in patients with symptomatic allergy than in those challenged out of their season or in nonallergic control subjects.[32] There were significantly greater symptoms of rhinorrhea and congestion in allergic subjects tested in season versus

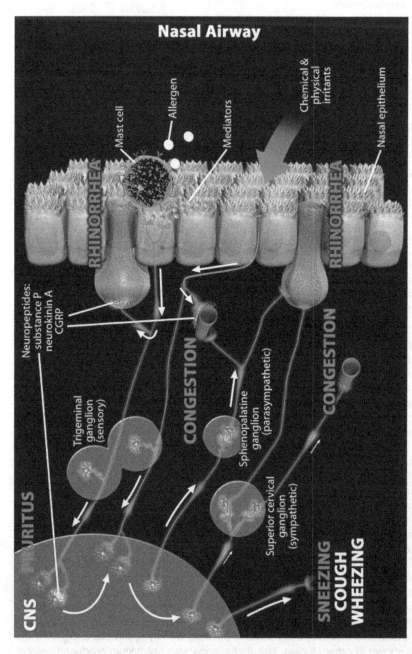

Fig. 2. Neuronal mechanisms of rhinitis symptoms. CNS, central nervous system. (*From* Sarim S, Undem B, Sanico A, et al. The role of the nervous system in rhinitis. J Allergy ClinI Immunol 2006;118:1001; with permission.)

out of season, and there were a greater number of sneezes noted (although not statistically significant). This enhanced responsiveness in patients during their allergy season has been attributed to the increased sensitivity of the inflamed nasal mucosa in allergic rhinitis. Recent studies have demonstrated significant increases of neuropeptides (substance P, vasoactive intestinal peptide, and neuropeptide Y) in the mucosal nerve fibers of patients with seasonal allergic rhinitis compared with controls.[33]

It now appears that the nerve hypersensitivity and growth may change in patients with allergic rhinitis. Studying inferior turbinate biopsy specimens from subjects with allergic rhinitis, nonallergic rhinitis, and controls, Keh and colleagues[34] showed differences in voltage-gated sodium channels. These sodium channels (Nav1.7, Nav1.8, and Nav1.9) were increased in tissues of allergic and nonallergic rhinitis subjects compared with controls. The channels are thought to play a role in the neuronal hypersensitivity seen in patients with rhinitis. Neurotrophins also contribute to hyperresponsiveness seen in patients with allergic rhinitis. Nerve growth factor (NGF) and brain-derived neurotrophic factor (BDNF) have been demonstrated in nasal mucosa.[35] Increased BDNF expression positively correlates with the maximum increase in total nasal symptom scores.[36] These neurotrophins are released from activated eosinophils. The increased symptoms and hyperresponsiveness to nonspecific stimuli may be partly caused by these neurotrophins released during the allergic response. The fact that there are also neurotrophin receptors on eosinophils in patients who have allergic rhinitis suggests a possible positive feedback loop amplifying this hyperresponsiveness.

Symptoms of vasomotor rhinitis may be primarily neurogenic, although inflammation and mast cell mediator release can occur secondary to this neurogenic activation.[37] The similarity between the causal factors in allergic and nonallergic rhinitis symptoms may account for some of the shared therapeutic effectiveness of the same drugs for both clinical entities.

THE CARDINAL SYMPTOMS OF RHINITIS

Nasal congestion is recognized in most patient surveys as the most bothersome symptom identified by sufferers of allergic rhinitis. Nasal obstruction is defined as discomfort manifested as a feeling of insufficient airflow through the nose.[38] Because nasal congestion is a subjective symptom, it is not always recognized in patients, especially those who have had the disease for many years and accept a degree of obstruction as normal. Observations of obstruction recognized on examination or by airflow measurement do not always correlate with a patient's perception of symptoms.[39] When severe nasal obstruction exists, patients may be bothered by their lack of sense of smell or taste but may not recognize the obstruction.

Nasal congestion in allergic rhinitis results mainly from tissue edema and vasodilatation in the nasal mucosa. The microvascular anatomy of the nose has been recently reviewed and consists of precapillary resistance vessels, capillaries, veins and venous erectile tissue, and capacitance vessels, as well as numerous arteriovenous anastomoses .[25] This vascular system (with arteriovenous anastomosis and with capacitance vessels in the nasal turbinates) differs from other areas of the respiratory tract. As these vessels become engorged and distended, the turbinates may block the airway lumen. This swelling may have a teleologic purpose and occur alternately from side to side in a normal state to enhance filtration and respiratory defense.[40] The enlarged turbinate in a confined space also produces symptoms of nasal congestion and obstruction. Ichimura[41] recently reviewed the mechanisms of nasal obstruction. The autonomic nervous system is primarily responsible for the control of blood flow in the nose, with sympathetic tone maintaining contraction of the cavernous sinusoids. If the sympathetic tone is reduced by inhibition of noradrenaline release, then direct vasodilatation occurs. This inhibition is thought to be mediated partly on presynaptic nerve endings by the H_3 histamine receptor and prostaglandin E_2 receptor.

Histamine plays an essential role in causing nasal congestion. Histamine challenge, as well as specific H2 and H3 agonist challenge, can cause nasal congestion.[29] Using H1 and H2 antagonists, these investigators were not able to totally block the congestion after the histamine challenge, thus suggesting that the H3 receptor might play a role in reducing vascular sympathetic tone by inhibiting norepinephrine release.

Nasal challenge studies have demonstrated the presence of several mediators in addition to histamine that may contribute to nasal congestion. These mediators include bradykinin, platelet-activating factor, prostaglandin D2 (PGD2), leukotrienes C4 and D4, substance P, and calcitonin-gene related protein (CGRP).[42] These mediators will be explored more thoroughly regarding their roles in nasal congestion. Bradykinin and platelet-activating factor may cause vasodilatation by direct action on vessel walls or through vasodilatory substances, such as nitric oxide (NO).[43] Maniscalco and colleagues[43] used platelet-activating factor and bradykinin nasal challenges to produce nasal congestion measured by anterior rhinomanometry. They confirmed that NO was important in the nasal response to bradykinin, but was not involved in the increased nasal resistance after the platelet-activating factor challenge. Nasal congestion may thus be mediated through NO or caused directly depending on the mediator involved. Substance P can be released from sensory neurons by a variety of stimuli, including allergens and other mediators. Substance P has been shown to increase nasal blood flow and microvascular leakage.[44] Hanf and colleagues[45] studied nasal tissue from subjects with allergic rhinitis and nonallergic controls who had surgery for nasal obstruction. Although substance P stimulated histamine release from tissue of both allergic and nonallergic subjects, there was increased histamine release in nasal tissues from subjects with allergic rhinitis. The amplification of the vascular response in rhinitis by this interplay of a neurotransmitter having a positive feedback on mast cell histamine release further illustrates the complex nature of the congestion seen in rhinitis.

Of the mediators released by mast cells in response to allergens, prostaglandin D_2 is regarded as the most potent inducer of nasal congestion. Nasal challenge with PGD2 produces nasal congestion in both normal subjects and in those with rhinitis.[46,47] A specific PGD2 receptor antagonist has recently been shown to reduce such congestion in PGD2 nasal challenge studies.[48] These studies suggest that PGD2 is a primary mediator enhancing congestion in patients with rhinitis.

The role of leukotrienes in rhinitis has been the subject of recent reviews.[49,50] Early studies delineated the effect of leukotriene D4 in producing nasal congestion. Several studies have looked at the clinical benefit of blocking this pathway either with 5-lipoxygynase inhibitors or with leukotriene receptor blockers.[51,52] These studies and reviews have shown efficacy of these two classes of leukotriene modifiers compared with placebo treatments, indicating that leukotrienes are partially responsible for some of the symptoms in allergic rhinitis.[53]

The rhinorrhea associated with rhinitis may be associated with a variety of stimulants, including the ingestion of food and the exposure to cold air.[54,55] The mechanisms causing symptoms in rhinitis were the subject of investigation over several years at the National Institutes of Health (NIH), and these results regarding rhinitis were reviewed several years ago.[56] Since that time, other investigations of rhinorrhea have evaluated the differences in idiopathic (nonallergic) and allergic rhinitis, as well as differences between patients with active, symptomatic, and asymptomatic allergic rhinitis. Comparing the effects of bradykinin stimulation in normal, nonallergic subjects to patients with either perennial or seasonal allergic rhinitis, investigators have shown increased secretions containing increased lactoferrin levels in patients with perennial allergic rhinitis.[32] They also demonstrated that in seasonal allergic rhinitis, bradykinin stimulation produced greater secretions with higher lactoferrin and albumin levels during the pollen season. The increases in lactoferrin suggest there is enhanced glandular secretion in patients with allergic rhinitis compared with normal control subjects. Increased lactoferrin and albumin secretions noted seasonally suggest that there is increase vascular leakage and glandular secretion during the pollen season. Further studies show that patients with idiopathic rhinitis compared with those with allergic rhinitis or no rhinitis have increased secretions following cold stimulation of the feet as well as cold, dry air nasal challenge.[16] Aberrant neurologic responses appear to be the most likely cause of this nasal secretory response. Using natural environmental factor variations in a study of nonallergic and noninfectious patients with perennial allergic rhinitis, Braat and colleagues[57] showed a correlation between nasal secretions and environmental NO and ozone levels. Symptom scores also related to minimum daytime temperature. These investigators did not evaluate possible mechanisms for these findings. Using nasal mucosa tissue samples from allergic and nonallergic patients, Schierhorn and colleagues[58] demonstrated an increase in both neurokinin A and substance P following tissue exposure to ozone. The tissue from allergic patients released more of both neuropeptides than the tissue of the nonallergic patients. These experiments suggest that nasal mucosa may respond to increased ozone exposure in a manner similar to bronchial mucosa with an increased release of neuropeptides. In summary, neurogenic mechanisms stimulating cholinergic efferent pathways with enhancement from allergic inflammation seem to be the primary causes of rhinorrhea in rhinitis.

Nasal itch is considered one of the diagnostic symptoms of rhinitis, although it appears to be more common in seasonal allergic rhinitis than in other types of rhinitis. In one study, nasal itching and sneezing were the most common presenting symptoms in both seasonal allergic rhinitis and in perennial allergic rhinitis with seasonal exacerbations.[59] This finding is consistent with IgE-mediated rhinitis involving histamine release from mast cells. Nasal itch is produced by histamine nasal challenge and blocked by H1-receptor antagonists. The itch is thought to be completely mediated by nasal sensory nerves through the activation of neuronal H1 receptors.[60] These nasal sensory neurons are also capsaicin sensitive. The capsaicin receptor, transient receptor potential vanilloid-1 (TRPV1), has been identified on both nasal neuronal cells and nonneuronal cells in human nasal mucosa.[61] This receptor is in a family of transient receptor potential (TRP) ion channel activators that have been identified. They may play a role in the nasal response to temperature as well as aroma (**Fig. 3**).[35]

In studying patients with seasonal allergic rhinitis, Alenmyr[62] demonstrated a significant sensation of itch following the capsaicin challenge during the pollen season but not before the season. Another TRPV1 stimulant, olvanil, also produced the itch sensation during, but not before, the pollen season. Activation of other TRP receptors (TRPA1 and TRPM8) did not produce the itch sensation either before or during the pollen season in these 10 patients with seasonal allergic rhinitis. This study and others showing increased neuronal markers in patients with allergic rhinitis may help explain the enhanced ability for nonspecific stimuli to produce symptoms in patients with allergic rhinitis.[63]

Sternutation (sneezing) is also induced by the application of capsaicin to the nasal mucosa.[64] Although the sneeze reflex is a common symptom of allergic and nonallergic rhinitis, it can also occur after such nonspecific events as exposure to bright

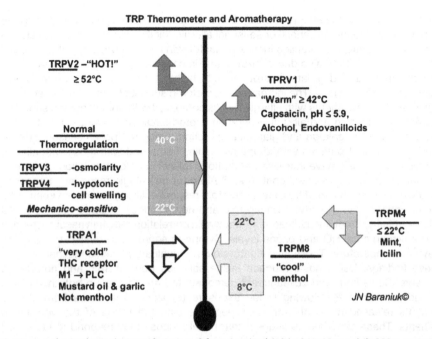

Fig. 3. Ion channel regulation of neuronal function in rhinitis. M1, Muscarinic M1 receptor; PLC, phospholipase C; THC, tetrahydrocannibinol. (*From* Baraniuk JN. Neural regulation of mucosal function. Pulm Pharmacol Ther 2008;21:447; with permission.)

light.[65] Baraniuk and Kim[66] recently described the complex constellation of consequences that occurs when the sneeze reflex is invoked. These investigators review multiple states of sneeze induction in addition to the classical pathway of histamine-induced activation of type C trigeminal neurons. Complications of the sneeze reflex may also occur, adding further morbidity to the symptoms of allergic rhinitis.[67] The sneezing reflex was evaluated in patients with allergic rhinitis and in healthy volunteers using histamine to induce the sneeze.[68] The investigators found a significantly greater percentage of responders in patients with allergic rhinitis at all dosing levels of histamine provocation. They also showed that nerve growth factor levels in nasal lavage fluids from patients with allergic rhinitis were significantly increased compared with the healthy controls, suggesting a possible role of this factor in the hyperresponsiveness of patients who are allergic.

As more is learned about the complex neurologic inflammation and vascular responsiveness associated with rhinitis and the induction of neurons and increased neuronal sensitivity in rhinitis, more effective interventions to control the symptoms of allergic and idiopathic rhinitis should emerge. The similarities in the mechanisms causing the symptoms in allergic and idiopathic rhinitis provide a rationale for the current treatment of the two clinical entities.

REFERENCES

1. Tai CF, Baraniuk JN. Upper airway neurogenic mechanisms. Curr Opin Allergy Clin Immunol 2002;2(1):11–9.
2. Elizabeth FJ, Elisabeth S, Richard LD, et al. Clinical outcomes and adverse effect monitoring in allergic rhinitis. J Allergy Clin Immunol 2005;115(3):S390–413.

3. Canonica GW, Bousquet J, Mullol J, et al. A survey of the burden of allergic rhinitis in Europe. Allergy 2007;62(Suppl 85):17–25.
4. Meltzer EO, Blaiss MS, Derebery MJ, et al. Burden of allergic rhinitis: results from the pediatric allergies in America survey. J Allergy Clin Immunol 2009;124(3): S43–70.
5. Tatar M, Plevkova J, Brozmanova M, et al. Mechanisms of the cough associated with rhinosinusitis. Pulm Pharmacol Ther 2009;22(2):121–6.
6. LaForce C, Gentile DA, Skoner DP. A randomized, double-blind, parallel-group, multicenter, placebo-controlled study of the safety and efficacy of extended-release guaifenesin/pseudoephedrine hydrochloride for symptom relief as an adjunctive therapy to antibiotic treatment of acute respiratory infections. Postgrad Med 2008;120(2):53–9.
7. Meltzer EO. Does rhinitis compromise night-time sleep and daytime productivity? Clin Exp Allergy Rev 2002;2(2):67–72.
8. Juniper EF, Rohrbaugh T, Meltzer EO. A questionnaire to measure quality of life in adults with nocturnal allergic rhinoconjunctivitis. J Allergy Clin Immunol 2003; 111(3):484–90.
9. Meltzer EO, Nathan R, Derebery J, et al. Sleep, quality of life, and productivity impact of nasal symptoms in the United States: findings from the Burden of Rhinitis in America survey. Allergy Asthma Proc 2009;30(3):244–54.
10. Durham SR. The inflammatory nature of allergic disease. Clin Exp Allergy 1998; 28(Suppl 6):20–4.
11. Gelfand E. Inflammatory mediators in allergic rhinitis. J Allergy Clin Immunol 2004;114:S135–8.
12. Baraniuk JN, Kaliner M. Neuropeptides and nasal secretion. Am J Physiol 1991; 261(4 Pt 1):L223–35.
13. Cima K, Vogelsinger H, Kahler CM. Sensory neuropeptides are potent chemoattractants for human basophils in vitro. Regul Pept 2010;160(1–3):42–8.
14. Powe DG, Huskisson RS, Carney AS, et al. Evidence for an inflammatory pathophysiology in idiopathic rhinitis. Clin Exp Allergy 2001;31(6):864–72.
15. van Rijswijk JB, Blom HM, Fokkens WJ. Idiopathic rhinitis, the ongoing quest. Allergy 2005;60(12):1471–81.
16. Numata T, Konno A, Hasegawa S, et al. Pathophysiological features of the nasal mucosa in patients with idiopathic rhinitis compared to allergic rhinitis. Int Arch Allergy Immunol 1999;119(4):304–13.
17. Kaliner MA, Baraniuk JN, Benninger MS, et al. Consensus description of inclusion and exclusion criteria for clinical studies of nonallergic rhinopathy (NAR), previously referred to as vasomotor rhinitis (VMR), nonallergic rhinitis, and/or idiopathic rhinitis. World Allergy Organiz J 2009;2(8):180–4.
18. Powe DG, Jones NS. Local mucosal immunoglobulin E production: does allergy exist in non-allergic rhinitis? Clin Exp Allergy 2006;36(11):1367–72.
19. Smurthwaite L, Walker SN, Wilson DR, et al. Persistent IgE synthesis in the nasal mucosa of hay fever patients. Eur J Immunol 2001;31(12):3422–31.
20. Rondon C, Fernandez J, Lopez S, et al. Nasal inflammatory mediators and specific IgE production after nasal challenge with grass pollen in local allergic rhinitis. J Allergy Clin Immunol 2009;124(5):1005–11.e1001.
21. Naclerio RM, Meier HL, Kagey-Sobotka A, et al. Mediator release after nasal airway challenge with allergen. Am Rev Respir Dis 1983;128(4):597–602.
22. Proud D, Togias A, Naclerio RM, et al. Kinins are generated in vivo following nasal airway challenge of allergic individuals with allergen. J Clin Invest 1983;72(5): 1678–85.

23. White MV, Kaliner MA. Mediators of allergic rhinitis. J Allergy Clin Immunol 1992; 90(4 Pt 2):699–704.
24. Wang D, Smitz J, Waterschoot S, et al. An approach to the understanding of the nasal early-phase reaction induced by nasal allergen challenge. Allergy 1997; 52(2):162–7.
25. Widdicombe J. Microvascular anatomy of the nose. Allergy 1997;52(Suppl 40): 7–11.
26. Sarin S, Undem B, Sanico A, et al. The role of the nervous system in rhinitis. J Allergy Clin Immunol 2006;118(5):999–1014.
27. Howarth PH, Salagean M, Dokic D. Allergic rhinitis: not purely a histamine-related disease. Allergy 2000;55(Suppl 64):7–16.
28. Tønnesen P, Mygind N. Nasal challenge with serotonin and histamine in normal persons. Allergy 1985;40(5):350–3.
29. Taylor-Clark T, Sodha R, Warner B, et al. Histamine receptors that influence blockage of the normal human nasal airway. Br J Pharmacol 2005;144(6): 867–74.
30. Philip G, Baroody FM, Proud D, et al. The human nasal response to capsaicin. J Allergy Clin Immunol 1994;94(6 Pt 1):1035–45.
31. Sanico AM, Philip G, Proud D, et al. Comparison of nasal mucosal responsiveness to neuronal stimulation in non-allergic and allergic rhinitis: effects of capsaicin nasal challenge. Clin Exp Allergy 1998;28(1):92–100.
32. Riccio MM, Proud D. Evidence that enhanced nasal reactivity to bradykinin in patients with symptomatic allergy is mediated by neural reflexes. J Allergy Clin Immunol 1996;97(6):1252–63.
33. Heppt W, Thai Dinh Q, Cryer A, et al. Phenotypic alteration of neuropeptide-containing nerve fibres in seasonal intermittent allergic rhinitis. Clin Exp Allergy 2004;34(7):1105–10.
34. Keh SM, Facer P, Simpson KD, et al. Increased nerve fiber expression of sensory sodium channels Nav1.7, Nav1.8, And Nav1.9 in rhinitis. Laryngoscope 2008; 118(4):573–9.
35. Baraniuk JN. Neural regulation of mucosal function. Pulm Pharmacol Ther 2008; 21(3):442–8.
36. Raap U, Braunstahl G-J. The role of neurotrophins in the pathophysiology of allergic rhinitis. Curr Opin Allergy Clin Immunol 2010;10(1):8–13.
37. Garay R. Mechanisms of vasomotor rhinitis. Allergy 2004;59(Suppl 76):4–9 [discussion: 9–10].
38. Jessen M, Malm L. Definition, prevalence and development of nasal obstruction. Allergy 1997;52(Suppl 40):3–6.
39. Sipila J, Suonpaa J, Silvoniemi P, et al. Correlations between subjective sensation of nasal patency and rhinomanometry in both unilateral and total nasal assessment. ORL J Otorhinolaryngol Relat Spec 1995;57(5):260–3.
40. Eccles R. A role for the nasal cycle in respiratory defence. Eur Respir J 1996;9(2): 371–6.
41. Ichimura K. Mechanism of nasal obstruction in patients with allergic rhinitis. Clin Exp Allergy Rev 2010;10:20–7.
42. Howarth PH. Mediators of nasal blockage in allergic rhinitis. Allergy 1997; 52(Suppl 40):12–8.
43. Maniscalco M, Sofia M, Faraone S, et al. The effect of platelet-activating factor (PAF) on nasal airway resistance in healthy subjects is not mediated by nitric oxide. Allergy 2000;55(8):757–61.

44. Lundblad L. Protective reflexes and vascular effects in the nasal mucosa elicited by activation of capsaicin-sensitive substance P-immunoreactive trigeminal neurons. Acta Physiol Scand Suppl 1984;529:1–42.
45. Hanf G, Schierhorn K, Brunnee T, et al. Substance P induced histamine release from nasal mucosa of subjects with and without allergic rhinitis. Inflamm Res 2000;49(10):520–3.
46. Doyle WJ, Boehm S, Skoner DP. Physiologic responses to intranasal dose-response challenges with histamine, methacholine, bradykinin, and prostaglandin in adult volunteers with and without nasal allergy. J Allergy Clin Immunol 1990;86(6 Pt 1):924–35.
47. Leroux J, Khemici E, Haasz M, et al. Nasal congestive responses to prostaglandin D2 (PGD2) are enhanced in rhinitic subjects. J Allergy Clin Immunol 2003;111(1):S80–1.
48. Van Hecken A, Depre M, De Lepeleire I, et al. The effect of MK-0524, a prostaglandin D(2) receptor antagonist, on prostaglandin D (2)-induced nasal airway obstruction in healthy volunteers. Eur J Clin Pharmacol 2007;63(2):135–41.
49. Peters-Golden M, Henderson WR Jr. The role of leukotrienes in allergic rhinitis. Ann Allergy Asthma Immunol 2005;94(6):609–18.
50. Haberal I, Corey JP. The role of leukotrienes in nasal allergy. Otolaryngol Head Neck Surg 2003;129(3):274–9.
51. Knapp HR. Reduced allergen-induced nasal congestion and leukotriene synthesis with an orally active 5-lipoxygenase inhibitor. N Engl J Med 1990; 323(25):1745–8.
52. Li JT. Review: leukotriene-receptor antagonists are less effective than intranasal corticosteroids for allergic rhinitis. ACP J Club 2004;141(2):45.
53. Wilson AM, O'Byrne PM, Parameswaran K. Leukotriene receptor antagonists for allergic rhinitis: a systematic review and meta-analysis. Am J Med 2004;116(5): 338–44.
54. Raphael G, Raphael MH, Kaliner M. Gustatory rhinitis: a syndrome of food-induced rhinorrhea. J Allergy Clin Immunol 1989;83(1):110–5.
55. Silvers WS. The skier's nose: a model of cold-induced rhinorrhea. Ann Allergy 1991;67(1):32–6.
56. Raphael GD, Baraniuk JN, Kaliner MA. How and why the nose runs. J Allergy Clin Immunol 1991;87(2):457–67.
57. Braat JP, Mulder PG, Duivenvoorden HJ, et al. Pollutional and meteorological factors are closely related to complaints of non-allergic, non-infectious perennial rhinitis patients: a time series model. Clin Exp Allergy 2002;32(5):690–7.
58. Schierhorn K, Hanf G, Fischer A, et al. Ozone-induced release of neuropeptides from human nasal mucosa cells. Int Arch Allergy Immunol 2002;129(2):145–51.
59. Sibbald B, Rink E. Epidemiology of seasonal and perennial rhinitis: clinical presentation and medical history. Thorax 1991;46(12):895–901.
60. Taylor-Clark TE. Insights into the mechanisms of histamine-induced inflammation in the nasal mucosa. Pulm Pharmacol Ther 2008;21(3):455–60.
61. Seki N, Shirasaki H, Kikuchi M, et al. Expression and localization of TRPV1 in human nasal mucosa. Rhinology 2006;44(2):128–34.
62. Alenmyr L, Hogestatt ED, Zygmunt PM, et al. TRPV1-mediated itch in seasonal allergic rhinitis. Allergy 2009;64(5):807–10.
63. O'Hanlon S, Facer P, Simpson KD, et al. Neuronal markers in allergic rhinitis: expression and correlation with sensory testing. Laryngoscope 2007;117(9): 1519–27.

64. Geppetti P, Fusco BM, Marabini S, et al. Secretion, pain and sneezing induced by the application of capsaicin to the nasal mucosa in man. Br J Pharmacol 1988; 93(3):509–14.
65. Whitman BW, Packer RJ. The photic sneeze reflex: literature review and discussion. Neurology 1993;43(5):868–71.
66. Baraniuk JN, Kim D. Nasonasal reflexes, the nasal cycle, and sneeze. Curr Allergy Asthma Rep 2007;7(2):105–11.
67. Songu M, Cingi C. Sneeze reflex: facts and fiction. Therap 2009;3(3):131–41.
68. Sanico AM, Koliatsos VE, Stanisz AM, et al. Neural hyperresponsiveness and nerve growth factor in allergic rhinitis. Int Arch Allergy Immunol 1999;118(2–4): 154–8.

The Relationship of Rhinitis and Asthma, Sinusitis, Food Allergy, and Eczema

Ricardo A. Tan, MD[a], Jonathan Corren, MD[b],*

KEYWORDS

• Rhinitis • Asthma • Food allergy • Eczema

Atopy, the predisposition for immunoglobulin E (IgE)–mediated responses to stimuli, is the common thread linking allergic rhinitis, asthma, food allergy, and eczema or atopic dermatitis. The exact nature of the relationship between these conditions continues to be the subject of active research. In this article, rhinitis refers to allergic rhinitis. Sinusitis or inflammation in the paranasal sinuses can be an extension of nasal allergic inflammation or an infectious complication of uncontrolled rhinitis.

Research into the epidemiology, genetics, natural history, risk factors, and treatment of these conditions continues to reveal strong and close associations. Allergic rhinitis, asthma, atopic dermatitis, and food allergy share a common mechanism involving specific IgE triggering the release of inflammatory mediators into the nose, lungs, gastrointestinal tract, and skin. The concept of the atopic march suggests that these conditions are manifestations in a continuum that starts with atopic dermatitis and progresses to allergic rhinitis, asthma, and food allergy.

The most exciting aspect of the relationship between these conditions may lie in potential preventive strategies to halt the atopic march and in therapeutic modalities that target several or all of these conditions at the same time.

ALLERGIC RHINITIS AND ASTHMA

Allergic rhinitis is associated with asthma in 40% of patients, whereas 80% to 95% of patients with allergic asthma also have rhinitis.[1,2] Allergic rhinitis is considered a risk factor for development of asthma.[3,4] In a 23-year follow-up study of 1836 college freshmen initially evaluated for the presence of asthma, allergic rhinitis, and positive allergen skin tests to a pollen, animal extracts, and mold, participants with allergic

[a] California Allergy and Asthma Medical Group, 11645 Wilshire Boulevard, Suite 1155, Los Angeles, CA 90025, USA
[b] Allergy Medical Clinic, 10780 Santa Monica Boulevard, Suite 280, Los Angeles, CA 90025, USA
* Corresponding author.
E-mail address: jcorren@ucla.edu

Immunol Allergy Clin N Am 31 (2011) 481–491
doi:10.1016/j.iac.2011.05.010
0889-8561/11/$ – see front matter © 2011 Elsevier Inc. All rights reserved.

rhinitis and positive skin tests were 3 times more likely to develop asthma.[4] Rhinitis may be a risk factor even in nonatopic subjects, as shown in a study from the longitudinal cohort of the Tucson Epidemiologic Study of Obstructive Lung Diseases. After adjustment for atopic status, age, sex, smoking status, and presence of chronic obstructive pulmonary disease, rhinitis still significantly increased risk for asthma 3 times in atopic and nonatopic patients.[3]

Numerous studies of the genetics, epidemiology and natural history of these conditions have shown the link between allergic rhinitis and asthma.[1,2,5–7] In the Copenhagen Allergy Study, a prospective population-based study, subjects evaluated 8 years after initial screening showed that all patients who developed allergic asthma to pollen, animals, and dust mites also had allergic rhinitis to these allergens, leading the investigators to state that allergic rhinitis and allergic asthma are manifestations of the same disease entity.[5]

The Allergic Rhinitis and its Impact on Asthma (ARIA) guidelines, first developed in 1999 by the World Health Organization and an international panel of experts and updated in 2008, recognizes the importance of this relationship.[8]

Clinically, allergic rhinitis and asthma symptoms are both triggered by the allergic cascade resulting in IgE cross-linking on mast cells and basophils and the release of inflammatory mediators including histamine, leukotrienes, and prostaglandins. Both allergic rhinitis and asthma can manifest in an early-phase reaction occurring within 15 minutes to an hour after allergen exposure and a late-phase reaction occurring 4 to 6 hour later.

The one-airway or unified airway concept linking the upper and lower airways is well recognized and accepted.[9–11] Proposed mechanisms for the close association between the nasal and bronchial airways include (1) the nasobronchial neural reflex, (2) drainage of inflammatory material from the nose to the lungs, (3) loss of protective function of the nose, and (4) systemic propagation of nasal inflammation.

A nasobronchial reflex has long been suggested by studies showing bronchial constriction after nasal exposure to dry, cold air.[12] Nasal allergen provocation has been shown to increase bronchial responsiveness.[13,14] Changes in lower airway resistance have also been found with nasal methacholine provocation.[15] However, studies to confirm this reflex have not shown consistent results.[16]

Direct drainage of inflammatory or infected material from the nasal passages into the lungs had been considered a straightforward mechanism for inflammatory interaction between the 2 areas. Aspiration of nasal secretions can occur, especially during sleep and in impaired individuals. However, studies using radiolabeled substances have not shown nasal material draining into the bronchial airways in patients with increased bronchial responsiveness.[17]

The nose warms and humidifies, and filters irritants and allergens from, inhaled air. Loss of this protective function from nasal congestion and subsequent mouth breathing leads to increased bronchial responsiveness from cold and dry air as well as increased exposure to allergens and irritants.[18,19]

Systemic inflammation induced first in the upper or lower airways and affecting both is currently believed to be a major mechanism at work in this relationship. Increase in peripheral eosinophils and leukocyte cytokine expression are seen after nasal allergen provocation.[20] Allergen inhalation is also associated with increased eosinophil and basophil progenitors, as well as interleukin (IL)-5 levels, in bone marrow 24 hours after allergen inhalation.[21]

Evidence of inflammation in the lower airway can be seen after local nasal allergen provocation. Nasal allergen provocation was performed in subjects with seasonal allergic rhinitis out of season with bronchial and nasal biopsy specimens obtained before and 24 hours after the provocation. Eosinophils and expression of intercellular adhesion molecule (ICAM)-1, vascular cell adhesion molecule (VCAM)-1, and E–selectin were increased in bronchial epithelium 24 hours after nasal provocation, suggesting that the airway inflammation occurs through upregulation of adhesion molecules.[13] In another study, exhaled nitric oxide (eNO) was measured in children with allergic rhinitis and asthma after allergen-specific nasal challenge and found to be significantly higher than in control groups.[22]

Conversely, segmental bronchial provocation has been shown to affect the nasal mucosa. Bronchial and nasal biopsies obtained before and 24 hours after segmental bronchial provocation in nonasthmatics with allergic rhinitis showed increased basophils in both nasal and bronchial mucosa at 24 hours.[23]

Studies have shown improvement in asthma with treatment of allergic rhinitis. In an early study to determine the clinical relevance of the one-airway concept, subjects with ragweed-sensitive seasonal allergic rhinitis and asthma and bronchial hyperresponsiveness to methacholine were randomized to receive either intranasal beclomethasone (336 μg/d) or placebo for the entire ragweed season. After 6 weeks of treatment, intranasal beclomethasone therapy prevented the expected increase in bronchial hyperresponsiveness that was seen in the placebo group.[24] This beneficial effect of intranasal beclomethasone on bronchial hyperresponsiveness has been confirmed in another study with subjects with perennial allergic rhinitis and asthma.[25] Intranasal fluticasone propionate has been studied in subjects with grass pollen and *Parietaria*-sensitive allergic rhinitis and asthma and been found to prevent increase in bronchial hyperresponsiveness during the pollen season.[26]

Allergen immunotherapy for allergic rhinitis may decrease the development of asthma in children and adults. In one study, patients with seasonal allergic rhinitis but no asthma were randomized to receive either *Parietaria*-specific immunotherapy or placebo and followed for 3 years. Although sputum eosinophils and bronchial hyperresponsiveness to methacholine did not change, immunotherapy appeared to prevent progression to asthma (14% in immunotherapy group vs 47% in placebo group).[27] The Preventive Allergy Treatment (PAT) study followed children between 6 and 14 years of age who received specific immunotherapy for grass and/or birch pollen or no immunotherapy for 3 years. A follow-up 2 years after termination of immunotherapy showed significantly less asthma in the immunotherapy group.[28]

Treatment of allergic rhinitis in asthmatic patients has also been shown to decrease asthma-related emergency room visits and hospitalizations. A large, retrospective cohort study involving 4944 subjects with allergic asthma showed that asthma-related events requiring emergency room visits or hospitalizations occurred more often in those with untreated allergic rhinitis compared with those receiving regular treatment (6.6% vs 1.3%).[29]

Patients with allergic rhinitis should be evaluated for asthma periodically by good history taking, physical examination, and pulmonary function testing so early intervention can be started when asthma is detected. However, all patients with asthma should always be examined and aggressively treated for concomitant allergic rhinitis. A systemic approach using medications that treat both rhinitis and asthma, including corticosteroids (intranasal and inhaled), leukotriene receptor antagonists, immunotherapy, and immunomodulation, is advocated by many practitioners.[8,30]

ALLERGIC RHINITIS AND SINUSITIS

Nasal inflammation in rhinitis often extends into the paranasal sinuses and patients suffering exacerbations complain of both nasal obstruction and sinus pressure or blockage. The accepted use of the term rhinosinusitis recognizes the common pathophysiology and clinical presentation often shared by these anatomic areas.[31]

The nose and paranasal sinuses have a functional and anatomic interdependence. Normal sinus function requires patent sinus ostia and normal ciliary beating of mucus through the ostia into the nasal cavity. The sinuses are air cavities within the facial and skull bones with small openings or ostia that, when obstructed, cause changes in oxygenation and acidity that lead to bacterial growth and infection. The sinuses drain either into the osteomeatal complex (maxillary, frontal, anterior ethmoid) or sphenoethmoidal recess (sphenoid, posterior ethmoid) of the nose. The osteomeatal complex opens into the middle meatus, between the inferior and middle turbinates. Visualization of purulent drainage from these ostia confirms the presence and location of sinusitis. The most important factors in the development of sinusitis are (1) the function of the cilia, (2) the patency of the ostia, and (3) the nature of the sinus secretions.

Allergic, nonallergic, and viral rhinitis can all lead to sinus ostia obstruction. Immotile cilia syndrome and other disorders of ciliary movement, immune deficiencies, mechanical obstruction (eg, nasal polyps, septal deviation), and cystic fibrosis can also predispose to sinusitis.

Most bacterial sinusitis is preceded by a viral respiratory illness of up to 7 days. Symptoms persisting beyond 7 days are likely to be caused by the onset of an acute bacterial sinusitis. Acute sinusitis is defined by a duration of up to 4 weeks, subacute sinusitis by between 4 to 8 weeks, and chronic sinusitis by persistent infection beyond 8 to 12 weeks.

Acute bacterial sinusitis presents with nasal obstruction, facial pressure or pain sometimes radiating to the upper teeth, or purulent nasal discharge. Fever may be present. Chronic bacterial sinusitis is often missed because it may present with only 1 symptoms such as persistent postnasal drip, coughing, headache, halitosis, or nasal obstruction with no other associated symptoms. Chronic sinusitis should be a differential diagnosis in patients with persistent nasal congestion refractory to allergic rhinitis treatment.

In both acute and chronic bacterial sinusitis, the organisms most commonly responsible are *Streptococcus pneumoniae*, *Hemophilus influenzae* and *Moraxella catarrhalis*. In chronic sinusitis, infection may also commonly be caused by *Staphylococcus aureus*, group A streptococcus, *Pseudomonas aeruginosa*, and anaerobic bacteria such as *Fusobacterium* and *Bacteroides*. In cystic fibrosis, the most common organism is *P aeruginosa*.[32] Although less common than bacterial sinusitis, fungal sinusitis is no longer seen only in immunocompromised individuals.[33,34]

Allergic rhinitis is usually perennial, and is present in about 60% of patients with chronic sinusitis.[35] The exact mechanism by which allergy predisposes to sinusitis is not clear. In one study, 40 subjects with perennial allergic rhinitis underwent computed tomography scans of the paranasal sinuses, rhinomanometry, nasal endoscopy, and nasal swab. Compared with a control group, sinusitis was increased in the allergic rhinitis group (67.5% vs 33.4%). The investigators concluded that factors aside from pathogens and mechanical obstruction may contribute to this association between allergic rhinitis and sinusitis.[35] Th2 cytokines, including IL-4 and IL-13, are found in the mucosal tissue of patients with chronic sinusitis, suggesting an allergic component to chronic inflammation.[36,37] The role of mucosal IgE, mast cells, and non–IgE-mediated hypersensitivity are also being studied to clarify the association between rhinitis and sinusitis.[38]

Treatment of concomitant rhinitis can often overlap with therapy for acute and chronic bacterial sinusitis. Topical intranasal steroids are first-line antiinflammatory therapy for rhinitis and have also been found to be beneficial in providing symptomatic improvement of nasal and sinus obstruction in acute and chronic sinusitis.[39–41] Although frequently used in clinical practice, a meta-analysis found insufficient evidence to show a clear overall benefit for topical steroids in chronic rhinosinusitis without polyps, but their use was found to be safe and may show some symptomatic benefit.[42]

Short bursts of systemic steroids (eg, prednisone 30–40 mg/d for 5–7 days) are often used as adjunctive therapy to antibiotics to ensure that sinus ostia are open to allow drainage of purulent material.[32] Studies have shown efficacy of systemic steroids in chronic sinusitis with nasal polyps.[41]

ALLERGIC RHINITIS AND ECZEMA

Eczema, or atopic dermatitis, is a chronic relapsing inflammatory skin disease that is closely associated with allergic rhinitis and asthma. Up to 75% of patients with atopic dermatitis develop allergic rhinitis, whereas approximately 50% develop asthma.[43] The pathophysiology of atopic dermatitis, like allergic rhinitis, involves Th2 cytokines including IL-4, IL-5, and IL-13.

Current research is focused on the role of atopic dermatitis as a precursor of the future appearance of allergic rhinitis and asthma. The sequence of atopic disease manifestations, usually starting from atopic dermatitis and progressing to allergic rhinitis, asthma, or food allergy, has been termed the atopic march.[44] Epidemiologic evidence from prospective studies following children with atopic dermatitis for many years support this concept.[45–48] In a German prospective birth cohort study that followed 1314 newborns for 7 years, 50% of children with atopic dermatitis had allergic airway disease by the age of 5 years.[46] In another prospective study that followed 94 children aged 4 to 35 months with atopic dermatitis for 7 years, 45% developed allergic rhinitis and 43% developed asthma.[48]

Impairment of the epidermal barrier predisposing to atopic dermatitis is suggested to be the initiating event for the atopic march. Epidermal barrier dysfunction in combination with genetic and environmental factors is proposed to be a mechanism for the development of atopic dermatitis. Biopsy studies show that the skin barrier is damaged both in acute eczematous lesions and in clinically unaffected skin. The epidermal barrier breakdown is likely caused by increased levels of stratum corneum chymotryptic enzyme, a protease enzyme that causes premature breakdown of corneodesmosomes. Environmental irritants and factors such as soap, detergents, and topical corticosteroids can further increase production of stratum corneum chymotryptic enzyme. Exogenous proteases from house dust mites and S aureus may also contribute to barrier dysfunction. Inflammation from these multifactorial causes produces further impairment of the barrier.[49]

Mutations in the filaggrin gene have been implicated as major genetic defects that lead to disruption of the epidermal barrier. Filaggrin polymorphisms are now considered a major risk factor for atopic dermatitis.[50] The loss-of-function null mutations R501X and 2282del4 in the filaggrin gene have been found in atopic dermatitis and ichthyosis vulgaris.[51] The filaggrin protein aggregates keratin filaments in the skin. Reduced or absent filaggrin leads to defective keratinization and poor formation and hydration of the skin barrier.[52] The epidermal barrier does not seem to be seriously compromised in the nasal and bronchial epithelium in the same way as in the skin. Filaggrin is expressed in the cornified nasal epithelium but not in the transitional or respiratory epithelium. Although filaggrin mutations have not shown direct effects on the human upper and lower airways, they have been associated with increased risk for allergic rhinitis alone as well as asthma in the presence of atopic dermatitis.[53]

It is still unclear how the progression of the atopic march occurs. The current hypothesis is that the epidermal pathophysiology producing atopic dermatitis leads to introduction of environmental allergens and irritants that subsequently cause systemic sensitization involving IL-17 and shifting to the Th2 pathway. There is evidence in animal studies that the skin can be the entry point for triggering systemic allergic inflammation that affects the nose and the lungs. Epicutaneous skin exposure to allergen may produce a systemic Th2 cytokine response leading to nasal and lower airway inflammation.[54–56] Thymic stromal lymphopoietin (TSLP) may also play a role, because mice studies show that deletion from the skin of sensitized mice can prevent the atopic march.[57]

A reverse atopic march has been proposed, with patients developing asthma first with later appearance of atopic dermatitis. A prospective study followed almost 700 children aged 6 to 9 years with asthma alone for 9 years. Twenty percent of the children developed atopic dermatitis at the end of 9 years. The children who developed atopic dermatitis did not differ in family history and other demographic characteristics from those who did not.[58]

Efforts are being made to determine whether early intervention in infants or children with atopic dermatitis might be able to halt or slow the atopic march. Most studies have focused on the effect on future development of asthma caused by its more serious morbidity. Successful intervention strategies might also decrease the progression to allergic rhinitis. However, studies have been inconclusive.

In the Early Treatment of the Atopic Child (ETAC) study, 795 infants with atopic dermatitis, aged 1 to 2 years, were given cetirizine or placebo and followed for 18 months. The investigators found that cetirizine delays or prevents development of asthma in a subgroup of infants with atopic dermatitis sensitized to grass pollen and dust mite.[59] The Early Prevention of Asthma in Atopic Children (EPAAC) study followed infants aged 1 to 2 years with known grass and dust mite sensitivity who were given levocetirizine or placebo for 18 months but did not show significant delay or prevention of asthma.[60] The ongoing 6-year Study of Atopic March (SAM) study is following 1100 infants aged 3 to 18 months with atopic dermatitis and who are receiving pimecrolimus cream or placebo to determine whether this treatment affects the development of asthma. Clinical trials of probiotics, beneficial bacterial cultures, have shown promising results when given to infants at high risk for atopy, and are being investigated for potential intervention in the atopic march.[61,62]

Many patients experience concomitant flare-ups of both conditions, especially after dust mite exposure. Antihistamines are used to treat both nasal symptoms in allergic rhinitis and skin itching from atopic dermatitis. Although patients may experience improvement in both rhinitis and eczema with antihistamine treatment, there are no studies indicating that short-term or long-term specific treatment of allergic rhinitis (eg, intranasal steroids) produces improvement in atopic dermatitis.

ALLERGIC RHINITIS AND FOOD ALLERGY

Food allergies are more common in children than in adults. Food allergies occur in about 1% to 2% of adults in the general population.[63] In the United States, about 3.9% of children less than 18 years of age have food allergy.[64] There is a close association and a much higher incidence of food allergy in individuals with other atopic disorders than in the general population. Food allergy is present in 35% of children with moderate to severe atopic dermatitis.[65] In children with asthma, 6% had food-induced reactions.[66]

In a study in France, 6672 schoolchildren aged 9 to 11 years were evaluated for food allergy, asthma, and allergic rhinitis, through skin prick testing and parent-completed questionnaires.[67] There was a statistically significant association between food allergy and asthma and allergic rhinitis even in those who did not report respiratory symptoms with food reactions. The association was significant even after adjustment for aeroallergen sensitization in the children with food allergy.

In a retrospective cross-sectional study, 283 adults with allergic rhinitis were tested for 9 inhalants and 3 foods (peanut, shrimp, milk), and total IgE.[68] A high prevalence of food allergy was found with peanut (23.4% prevalence) and shrimp (22.2% prevalence), which are the most common food allergens. The presence of peanut allergy was best in predicting other food allergies.

In the atopic march, atopic dermatitis is usually the first clinical event typically followed by food allergy, allergic rhinitis, and asthma. Sensitization to food allergens seems to precede sensitization to inhalant allergens. In a prospective birth cohort study (the Multicenter Allergy Study [MAS]), the annual incidence of sensitization to food allergens was 10% at 1 year of age, and decreased to 3% at 6 years of age. However, the incidence of sensitization to inhalant allergen started at 1.5% at 1 year and increased to 8% at 6 years.[46] A large Japanese study analyzing questionnaires completed by the parents of more than 13,000 schoolchildren found that 5.4% had allergy to eggs, milk, and wheat in infancy, but 80% became tolerant by school age. However, the food-allergic infants had significantly higher risk of developing atopic dermatitis, allergic rhinitis, asthma as well as allergy to other foods.[69] An implication of these studies is that food allergy may predict the appearance of allergic rhinitis, but more studies are needed to clarify this hypothesis.

Many patients report that certain foods, such as milk or wheat, trigger acute rhinitis or worsen chronic rhinitis. However, true isolated rhinitis as the sole symptom of food allergy is not common. Gustatory rhinitis or increased mucus production caused by vasomotor stimulation from chewing likely accounts for many of these cases. The Practice Parameters from the Joint Council of Allergy, Asthma and Immunology states that food allergy is a rare cause of rhinitis without associated gastrointestinal, dermatologic, or systemic manifestation.[70]

Avoidance is the primary management measure for food allergies. Desensitization for food allergy and the use of anti-IgE agents such as omalizumab are still investigational.[71] At this time, treatment and improvement of either allergic rhinitis or food allergy is not known to affect the course or prognosis of the other condition.

SUMMARY

The relationship between allergic rhinitis and sinusitis, asthma, atopic dermatitis, and food allergy is strongly supported by genetic, epidemiologic, pathophysiologic, and clinical evidence. The mechanism for atopic manifestations all involve IgE-mediated responses leading to release of inflammatory mediators into the nasal, bronchial, gastrointestinal, and dermatologic systems.

The one-airway approach recognizes the close interaction between the upper and lower airways. Most patients with asthma have allergic rhinitis. Exacerbations of allergic rhinitis contribute to worsening of asthma. Nasal provocation has been shown in many studies to cause bronchial hyperresponsiveness. Systemic inflammation induced from the upper or lower airways is believed to be responsible for involvement of both areas. Treatment of allergic rhinitis seems to delay or prevent development of asthma in children.

The nose and paranasal sinuses function closely anatomically and functionally. Infectious sinusitis is a common complication of uncontrolled rhinitis. Control of underlying rhinitis is an important component of management of chronic sinusitis.

The atopic march links atopic dermatitis as the usual initial manifestation of atopy to later progression to allergic rhinitis, asthma, and food allergy. Epidermal barrier dysfunction associated with filaggrin gene mutations seems to lead to the appearance of atopic dermatitis. Ongoing studies are attempting to determine whether preventive strategies can delay the appearance of allergic rhinitis and asthma in infants and children with atopic dermatitis.

In patients with rhinitis, it is essential to evaluate for asthma, sinusitis, atopic dermatitis, and food allergy as early as the first office visit so that avoidance, diagnostic, and management approaches can be coordinated in a comprehensive manner.

REFERENCES

1. Greisner WA 3rd, Settipane RJ, Settipane GA. Co-existence of asthma and allergic rhinitis: a 23-year follow-up study of college students. Allergy Asthma Proc 1998;19(4):185–8.
2. Danielsson J, Jessen M. The natural course of allergic rhinitis during 12 years of follow-up. Allergy 1997;52(3):331–4.
3. Guerra S, Sherrill DL, Martinez FD, et al. Rhinitis as an independent risk factor for adult-onset asthma. J Allergy Clin Immunol 2002;109(3):419–25.
4. Settipane RJ, Hagy GW, Settipane GA. Long-term risk factors for developing asthma and allergic rhinitis: a 23-year follow-up study of college students. Allergy Proc 1994;15(1):21–5.
5. Linneberg A, Henrik Nielsen N, Frølund L, et al. The link between allergic rhinitis and allergic asthma: a prospective population-based study. The Copenhagen Allergy Study. Allergy 2002;57(11):1048–52.
6. Leynaert B, Neukirch F, Demoly P, et al. Epidemiologic evidence for asthma and rhinitis comorbidity. J Allergy Clin Immunol 2000;106(5 Suppl):S201–5.
7. Bousquet J, Van Cauwenberge P, Khaltaev N. Allergic rhinitis and its impact on asthma. J Allergy Clin Immunol 2001;108(5 Suppl):S147–334.
8. Bousquet J, Khaltaev N, Cruz AA, et al. Allergic Rhinitis and its Impact on Asthma (ARIA) 2008 update (in collaboration with the World Health Organization, GA(2) LEN and AllerGen). Allergy 2008;63(Suppl 86):8–160.
9. Braunstahl GJ. The unified immune system: respiratory tract-nasobronchial interaction mechanisms in allergic airway disease. J Allergy Clin Immunol 2005; 115(1):142–8.
10. Togias A. Rhinitis and asthma: evidence for respiratory system integration. J Allergy Clin Immunol 2003;111(6):1171–83 [quiz: 1184].
11. Dixon AE. Rhinosinusitis and asthma: the missing link. Curr Opin Pulm Med 2009; 15(1):19–24.
12. Fontanari P, Zattara-Hartmann MC, Burnet H, et al. Nasal eupnoeic inhalation of cold, dry air increases airway resistance in asthmatic patients. Eur Respir J 1997; 10(10):2250–4.
13. Braunstahl GJ, Overbeek SE, Kleinjan A, et al. Nasal allergen provocation induces adhesion molecule expression and tissue eosinophilia in upper and lower airways. J Allergy Clin Immunol 2001;107(3):469–76.
14. Corren J, Adinoff AD, Irvin CG. Changes in bronchial responsiveness following nasal provocation with allergen. J Allergy Clin Immunol 1992;89(2):611–8.

15. Littell NT, Carlisle CC, Millman RP, et al. Changes in airway resistance following nasal provocation. Am Rev Respir Dis 1990;141(3):580–3.
16. Schumacher MJ, Cota KA, Taussig LM. Pulmonary response to nasal-challenge testing of atopic subjects with stable asthma. J Allergy Clin Immunol 1986; 78(1 Pt 1):30–5.
17. Bardin PG, Van Heerden BB, Joubert JR. Absence of pulmonary aspiration of sinus contents in patients with asthma and sinusitis. J Allergy Clin Immunol 1990;86(1):82–8.
18. Assanasen P, Baroody FM, Naureckas E, et al. The nasal passage of subjects with asthma has a decreased ability to warm and humidify inspired air. Am J Respir Crit Care Med 2001;164(9):1640–6.
19. Bousquet J, Boushey HA, Busse WW, et al. Characteristics of patients with seasonal allergic rhinitis and concomitant asthma. Clin Exp Allergy 2004;34(6): 897–903.
20. Togias AG. Systemic immunologic and inflammatory aspects of allergic rhinitis. J Allergy Clin Immunol 2000;106(5 Suppl):S247–50.
21. Dorman SC, Sehmi R, Gauvreau GM, et al. Kinetics of bone marrow eosinophilo-poiesis and associated cytokines after allergen inhalation. Am J Respir Crit Care Med 2004;169(5):565–72.
22. Marcucci F, Passalacqua G, Canonica GW, et al. Lower airway inflammation before and after house dust mite nasal challenge: an age and allergen exposure-related phenomenon. Respir Med 2007;101(7):1600–8.
23. Braunstahl GJ, Overbeek SE, Fokkens WJ, et al. Segmental bronchoprovocation in allergic rhinitis patients affects mast cell and basophil numbers in nasal and bronchial mucosa. Am J Respir Crit Care Med 2001;164(5):858–65.
24. Corren J, Adinoff AD, Buchmeier AD, et al. Nasal beclomethasone prevents the seasonal increase in bronchial responsiveness in patients with allergic rhinitis and asthma. J Allergy Clin Immunol 1992;90(2):250–6.
25. Watson WT, Becker AB, Simons FE. Treatment of allergic rhinitis with intranasal corticosteroids in patients with mild asthma: effect on lower airway responsiveness. J Allergy Clin Immunol 1993;91(1 Pt 1):97–101.
26. Foresi A, Pelucchi A, Gherson G, et al. Once daily intranasal fluticasone propionate (200 micrograms) reduces nasal symptoms and inflammation but also attenuates the increase in bronchial responsiveness during the pollen season in allergic rhinitis. J Allergy Clin Immunol 1996;98(2):274–82.
27. Polosa R, Li Gotti F, Mangano G, et al. Effect of immunotherapy on asthma progression, BHR and sputum eosinophils in allergic rhinitis. Allergy 2004; 59(11):1224–8.
28. Niggemann B, Jacobsen L, Dreborg S, et al. Five-year follow-up on the PAT study: specific immunotherapy and long-term prevention of asthma in children. Allergy 2006;61(7):855–9.
29. Crystal-Peters J, Neslusan C, Crown WH, et al. Treating allergic rhinitis in patients with comorbid asthma: the risk of asthma-related hospitalizations and emergency department visits. J Allergy Clin Immunol 2002;109(1):57–62.
30. Bjermer L. Montelukast in the treatment of asthma as a systemic disease. Expert Rev Clin Immunol 2005;1(3):325–36.
31. Dykewicz MS, Hamilos DL. Rhinitis and sinusitis. J Allergy Clin Immunol 2010; 125(2 Suppl 2):S103–15.
32. Slavin RG, Spector SL, Bernstein IL, et al. The diagnosis and management of sinusitis: a practice parameter update. J Allergy Clin Immunol 2005;116(6 Suppl): S13–47.

33. Schubert MS, Goetz DW. Evaluation and treatment of allergic fungal sinusitis. II. Treatment and follow-up. J Allergy Clin Immunol 1998;102(3):395–402.

34. Schubert MS, Goetz DW. Evaluation and treatment of allergic fungal sinusitis. I. Demographics and diagnosis. J Allergy Clin Immunol 1998;102(3):387–94.

35. Berrettini S, Carabelli A, Sellari-Franceschini S, et al. Perennial allergic rhinitis and chronic sinusitis: correlation with rhinologic risk factors. Allergy 1999;54(3):242–8.

36. Hamilos DL, Leung DY, Wood R, et al. Evidence for distinct cytokine expression in allergic versus nonallergic chronic sinusitis. J Allergy Clin Immunol 1995;96(4): 537–44.

37. al Ghamdi K, Ghaffar O, Small P, et al. IL-4 and IL-13 expression in chronic sinusitis: relationship with cellular infiltrate and effect of topical corticosteroid treatment. J Otolaryngol 1997;26(3):160–6.

38. Pant H, Ferguson BJ, Macardle PJ. The role of allergy in rhinosinusitis. Curr Opin Otolaryngol Head Neck Surg 2009;17(3):232–8.

39. Farabollini B, Braschi MC, Bonifazi F. Allergic rhinitis and associated pathologies: the rationale for steroid options. Eur Ann Allergy Clin Immunol 2009;41(3):67–79.

40. Venekamp RP, Sachs AP, Bonten MJ, et al. Intranasal corticosteroid monotherapy in acute rhinosinusitis: an evidence-based case report. Otolaryngol Head Neck Surg 2010;142(6):783–8.

41. Mori F, Barni S, Pucci N, et al. Upper airways disease: role of corticosteroids. Int J Immunopathol Pharmacol 2010;23(1 Suppl):61–6.

42. Kalish LH, Arendts G, Sacks R, et al. Topical steroids in chronic rhinosinusitis without polyps: a systematic review and meta-analysis. Otolaryngol Head Neck Surg 2009;141(6):674–83.

43. Leung DY, Boguniewicz M, Howell MD, et al. New insights into atopic dermatitis. J Clin Invest 2004;113(5):651–7.

44. Spergel JM. From atopic dermatitis to asthma: the atopic march. Ann Allergy Asthma Immunol 2010;105(2):99–106 [quiz: 107–9, 117].

45. van der Hulst AE, Klip H, Brand PL. Risk of developing asthma in young children with atopic eczema: a systematic review. J Allergy Clin Immunol 2007;120(3): 565–9.

46. Kulig M, Bergmann R, Klettke U, et al. Natural course of sensitization to food and inhalant allergens during the first 6 years of life. J Allergy Clin Immunol 1999; 103(6):1173–9.

47. Kapoor R, Menon C, Hoffstad O, et al. The prevalence of atopic triad in children with physician-confirmed atopic dermatitis. J Am Acad Dermatol 2008;58(1):68–73.

48. Gustafsson D, Sjoberg O, Foucard T. Development of allergies and asthma in infants and young children with atopic dermatitis–a prospective follow-up to 7 years of age. Allergy 2000;55(3):240–5.

49. Cork MJ, Robinson DA, Vasilopoulos Y, et al. New perspectives on epidermal barrier dysfunction in atopic dermatitis: gene-environment interactions. J Allergy Clin Immunol 2006;118(1):3–21 [quiz: 22–3].

50. Baurecht H, Irvine AD, Novak N, et al. Toward a major risk factor for atopic eczema: meta-analysis of filaggrin polymorphism data. J Allergy Clin Immunol 2007;120(6):1406–12.

51. Smith FJ, Irvine AD, Terron-Kwiatkowski A, et al. Loss-of-function mutations in the gene encoding filaggrin cause ichthyosis vulgaris. Nat Genet 2006;38(3):337–42.

52. Hanifin JM. Evolving concepts of pathogenesis in atopic dermatitis and other eczemas. J Invest Dermatol 2009;129(2):320–2.

53. Weidinger S, O'Sullivan M, Illig T, et al. Filaggrin mutations, atopic eczema, hay fever, and asthma in children. J Allergy Clin Immunol 2008;121(5):1203. e1–9. e1.

54. Akei HS, Brandt EB, Mishra A, et al. Epicutaneous aeroallergen exposure induces systemic TH2 immunity that predisposes to allergic nasal responses. J Allergy Clin Immunol 2006;118(1):62–9.
55. Spergel JM, Mizoguchi E, Brewer JP, et al. Epicutaneous sensitization with protein antigen induces localized allergic dermatitis and hyperresponsiveness to methacholine after single exposure to aerosolized antigen in mice. J Clin Invest 1998;101(8):1614–22.
56. He R, Oyoshi MK, Jin H, et al. Epicutaneous antigen exposure induces a Th17 response that drives airway inflammation after inhalation challenge. Proc Natl Acad Sci U S A 2007;104(40):15817–22.
57. Demehri S, Morimoto M, Holtzman MJ, et al. Skin-derived TSLP triggers progression from epidermal-barrier defects to asthma. PLoS Biol 2009;7(5):e1000067.
58. Barberio G, Pajno GB, Vita D, et al. Does a 'reverse' atopic march exist? Allergy 2008;63(12):1630–2.
59. Warner JO. A double-blinded, randomized, placebo-controlled trial of cetirizine in preventing the onset of asthma in children with atopic dermatitis: 18 months' treatment and 18 months' posttreatment follow-up. J Allergy Clin Immunol 2001;108(6):929–37.
60. Simons FE. Safety of levocetirizine treatment in young atopic children: an 18-month study. Pediatr Allergy Immunol 2007;18(6):535–42.
61. del Giudice MM, Rocco A, Capristo C. Probiotics in the atopic march: highlights and new insights. Dig Liver Dis 2006;38(Suppl 2):S288–90.
62. Lee J, Seto D, Bielory L. Meta-analysis of clinical trials of probiotics for prevention and treatment of pediatric atopic dermatitis. J Allergy Clin Immunol 2008;121(1):116.e11–21.e11.
63. Cingi C, Demirbas D, Songu M. Allergic rhinitis caused by food allergies. Eur Arch Otorhinolaryngol 2010;267(9):1327–35.
64. Branum AM, Lukacs SL. Food allergy among children in the United States. Pediatrics 2009;124(6):1549–55.
65. Eigenmann PA, Sicherer SH, Borkowski TA, et al. Prevalence of IgE-mediated food allergy among children with atopic dermatitis. Pediatrics 1998;101(3):E8.
66. Novembre E, de Martino M, Vierucci A. Foods and respiratory allergy. J Allergy Clin Immunol 1988;81(5 Pt 2):1059–65.
67. Penard-Morand C, Raherison C, Kopferschmitt C, et al. Prevalence of food allergy and its relationship to asthma and allergic rhinitis in schoolchildren. Allergy 2005;60(9):1165–71.
68. Sahin-Yilmaz A, Nocon CC, Corey JP. Immunoglobulin E-mediated food allergies among adults with allergic rhinitis. Otolaryngol Head Neck Surg 2010;143(3):379–85.
69. Kusunoki T, Morimoto T, Nishikomori R, et al. Allergic status of schoolchildren with food allergy to eggs, milk or wheat in infancy. Pediatr Allergy Immunol 2009;20(7):642–7.
70. Wallace DV, Dykewicz MS, Bernstein DI, et al. The diagnosis and management of rhinitis: an updated practice parameter. J Allergy Clin Immunol 2008;122(2 Suppl):S1–84.
71. Blumchen K, Ulbricht H, Staden U, et al. Oral peanut immunotherapy in children with peanut anaphylaxis. J Allergy Clin Immunol 2010;126(1):83.e1–91.e1.

Does Allergen Avoidance Work?

Robert K. Bush, MD

KEYWORDS

• Allergic rhinitis • Allergen avoidance • Indoor allergens
• Polysensitization

Ten percent to 25% of individuals globally are sensitized to allergens.[1] In the United States, it is estimated that 30 to 60 million persons are affected by allergic rhinitis.[2] The National Health and Nutrition Examination Survey (NHANES) III study from the United States indicated that 25.7% of individuals in this large cohort were sensitive to house dust mite, 26% to cockroach, and 17% to cat allergen.[3] Because individuals are exposed to indoor allergens throughout the year, allergic rhinitis owing to sensitization to these allergens tends to be perennial.

Exposure to indoor allergens is widespread. Surveys conducted in the United States showed that more than 80% of homes and 85% of day care facilities have detectable dust mite allergen levels.[4] In addition, pet allergens from dogs and cats are detected in most US homes, even where there has never been an animal.[5] Similarly, pet allergens have been detected in schools as well. Recent studies have indicated that in US housing, dust mites, cockroaches, cats, dogs, and mice are important contributors to indoor allergen levels.[6] Water leaks, visible mold growth, poor housekeeping, and homes constructed before 1951 contribute to these increased allergen concentrations in the indoor environment.[6] Thus, allergic rhinitis is a common condition, it is often a result of sensitization to indoor allergens, and exposure in indoor environments is frequent.

Genetics also play an important role in the development of sensitization to allergens and to allergic respiratory disease. It is well known that strong family history increases the likelihood that a child born of an atopic parent is likely to become sensitized and eventually develop allergic respiratory disease. Interestingly, gender differences may have an effect on allergen exposure and disease expression. Bertelsen and colleagues[7] found that girls had higher exposure levels to cat and dog allergens than boys, whereas no differences were found in dust mite allergen exposure between boys and girls. However, increased levels of exposure to house dust mite allergen significantly increased the risk of a diagnosis of current allergic rhinitis in girls, whereas there was no significant association found in boys.[7] In addition to the affects of

Department of Medicine, University of Wisconsin–Madison, K4/910 CSC #9988, 600 Highland Avenue, Madison, WI 53792, USA
E-mail address: rkb@medicine.wisc.edu

Immunol Allergy Clin N Am 31 (2011) 493–507
doi:10.1016/j.iac.2011.05.005   immunology.theclinics.com
0889-8561/11/$ – see front matter © 2011 Elsevier Inc. All rights reserved.

genetics on the risk of immunoglobulin (Ig) E antibody productions to allergen, the environment can also interplay with genetic processes known as epigenetics. Indoor exposures to tobacco smoke, microbial allergens, airborne particulate matter, diesel exhaust particles, nutritional factors, and other exposures may affect DNA methylation, alter histone modifications, affect specific micro RNA expression, and other alternations that orchestrate the immune responses, which may lead to allergic diseases.[8] Although specific allergen sensitization is generally thought not to be directly inherited, recent data suggest that sensitization to specific allergens in the parents increases the likelihood of sensitization to same allergen in their offspring.[9] This may not indicate the specific sensitization is genetically determined, but the risk factors for the development of sensitization and similar exposures between parent and the early life of the child are likely, and this may account for this observation.

It is well known that sensitization (ie, development of specific IgE antigens to a specific allergen) occurs early in life. At most time points, boys are significantly more likely to be sensitized and sensitization increases from childhood and into adolescence. Among the first sensitivities to develop is to house dust mites, because exposure to these allergens are ubiquitous in bedding and in most homes. Although controversial, early exposure to animal allergens from cats and dogs may actually provide some protective effect on the development of sensitization (to these allergens).[10]

The affects of allergen exposure can influence epigenetics, as mentioned previously. Moreover, various exposures can act as adjuvants to the generation of IgE responses. Chitin particles, which arise from fungi, insects, and other allergens, can act as T helper cell 2 (Th2) adjuvants to increase specific allergen sensitization.[11] Ingress into the indoor environment of various pollutants, such as diesel exhaust particles, may also enhance IgE production.[12] In addition, it is well known that endotoxin may influence Th2 expression and can, in and of itself, act as a respiratory irritant.[13] Proteases from sources such as fungi, dust mites, and other sources, have also been shown to affect eosinophilic inflammation and other factors can influence the innate immune system that bias Th2 responses.[14]

In conclusion, allergen exposure, as well as other exposures in the indoor environment, contribute to the pathophysiology and generation of allergic sensitization and allergic inflammation. Therefore, indoor allergen exposure plays a central role in the development of allergic rhinitis and must be addressed in any comprehensive management plan.

BIOLOGY AND CHARACTERIZATION OF INDOOR ALLERGENS
House Dust Mite

In most humid areas of the world, house dust mites are the major source of allergens in house dust.[15] Dust mites are microscopic arthropods that feed on human skin scales. They depend on water from the ambient air. Typically, house dust mites are found in abundance where indoor relative humidity is higher than 50%. High altitude and cold dry air inhibit dust mite proliferation. There may be some seasonal fluctuation in indoor house dust mite allergen levels because indoor humidity is typically higher in summer months than in winter months in the United States. In the home, mites are found in fabrics, such as mattresses, pillows, stuffed animals, upholstered furniture, and carpeted floors and rugs. Higher concentrations are found in older homes where there is high humidity and heating other then forced air systems are used. Mite bodies and fecal pellets are the major sources of allergens, which become airborne when disturbed.[16] Because of the aerodynamic features of the particles, which are 10 μm or larger in diameter, they remain suspended in the air for a relatively short period of time, which prevents air filtration from being an effective measure to reduce airborne levels. The most commonly encountered house dust mites are *Dermatophagoides pteronyssinus* and *Dermatophagoides farinae*. In tropical areas, *Blomia tropicalis* predominates. Storage mites may also be important indoor allergens in areas such as farms, where grain and other sources of food for these arthropods are available. To date, approximately 22 to 23 different house dust mite allergens have been identified.[17] IgE responses to house dust mite allergen occur early in life.[18] Sensitization may rarely remit. Approximately 3% of children followed over 18 years show a decrease in IgE response to dust mite.[19] The IgE response to dust mites typically contributes significantly to the total IgE level and there is little evidence that tolerance or IgG_4 responses occur.[20]

Cats

Pets are a major cause of indoor sensitization and contribute to allergic rhinitis. However, in contrast to house dust mite allergens, cat allergens are distributed on both large aerodynamic and smaller particles, which tend to remain airborne for longer periods of time and thus are amenable to air filtration. The cat allergens are produced in sebaceous glands of the cat and are present on the skin and fur. The major allergen is found in the salivary gland, and additional allergens are added to the hair when the animals groom themselves.[21] Because of electrostatic charges, cat allergens can stick to surfaces such as walls.[22] The major cat allergen (*Fel d 1*) is under androgenic hormonal control and is, therefore, produced in higher concentrations by male cats than female cats. In contrast to dust mite allergens, exposure to cat allergens, especially at high levels, may induce IgG_4 immune responses, which may reduce the risk of the development of allergic disease.[23] However, this phenomenon is dependent on high exposure levels.[24] Because cat allergen is distributed outside the home, allergen avoidance in the home alone may not be of particular value in diminishing sensitization,[25] because cat allergens are found in 90% of all homes and in most public indoor areas (even those without pets).[26]

Dogs

Exposure to cat and dog allergens is common, as 56% to 63% of US households have indoor pets.[26]

The major dog allergens have been shown to have physical properties similar to cat allergens, and there may be a synergistic effect between exposure to cats and dogs in the home that results in a lowered risk for the development of atopy in childhood and young adulthood.[27]

Mouse Allergens

Sampling in residential homes in the United States indicates that 82% have detectable levels of mouse allergen.[28] Some geographic areas, such as inner-city dwellings, have high levels of mouse allergen, and subsequently it has been shown that 25% of inner-city children have evidence of IgE sensitivity to mouse.[29] Socioeconomic conditions may not be of potential importance in women sensitized to mouse allergen, as shown in a recent report.[30]

Cockroaches

Cockroach allergens are an important factor in allergic sensitization, particularly in children in inner-city environments.[31] The major species of cockroaches are *Blattella germanica* (German cockroach) and *Periplaneta americana* (American cockroach). At least 9 to 10 cockroach allergens have been described.[17] Seasonal variations in exposure may occur, with higher levels of exposure occurring during the summer and fall months.[32]

Other Insect Allergens

In addition to cockroaches, seasonal indoor allergen symptoms may be attributable to a newly identified insect allergen, the Asian lady beetle (*Harmonia axyridis*).[33] Cross-reactivity between German cockroach and Asian lady beetle allergens has recently been reported.[34]

Fungi

Fungi, or molds, are widely distributed throughout the world. These organisms are found in most temperate climates globally. The optimal conditions for growth vary among species but all require oxygen, a carbon source, and water. Typically, fungi are found where water leaks or standing water is found in the indoor environment. These organisms are often detected by visible mold growth or by a "musty" or "mildew" odor. Sensitization to fungi, such as *Alternaria*, is strongly associated with allergic rhinitis in children.[35] Many homes have high levels of fungal allergens detectable in the indoor environment. However, in contrast, others have found that outdoor fungal exposure may be more important in causing allergic symptoms than indoor exposures.[36] Fungal exposure in the indoor environment may result from 1 of 2 routes: intrusion from the outdoor environment or growth within the indoor environment. These can be ascertained by conducting studies on both the indoor and the outdoor environment simultaneously, and if the indoor environment shows a higher level of fungal propagals by culture (spore counts) it can be assumed that the exposure is the result of indoor contamination.

Pollen Intrusion

Last, pollens can intrude from the exterior into the interior environment from open windows, cracks, and so forth. Thus, during seasonal pollination of plants, indoor exposures can occur, although outdoor exposure is the primary route. Further, in addition to intrusion through outdoor sources, pollens may also enter through clothing[37] and are occasionally carried in on the fur of pets, but the overall contribution of this exposure appears to be relatively small, and its overall role is unknown.

Effects of Climate Change

The indoor environment is an important source of allergen exposure. Concerns have arisen regarding the effect of climate change on allergic disease.[38] The effect of global climate change may have dramatic effects on the indoor as well as the outdoor environment, where it has been studied more carefully. Future research is needed in this regard.

Molecular Biology of Indoor Allergens

Molecular biology developments over the past 2 decades have led to a better understanding of allergic sensitization and disease processes. The molecular cloning of a number of allergenic proteins has shed light on their structure and biologic functions. There are more than 23 known dust mite allergens identified to date,[17] several of which have enzymatic activity, that can either act as adjuvants to enhance IgE production or increase penetration of allergens through epithelial barriers. Reviews of the characteristics of allergens can be found in Chapman and colleagues[39] and Radauer and colleagues.[40]

At least 7 allergens have been identified in cats and dogs.[17] *Fel d 1* is the major cat allergen, and Canis familiaris allergen 1 (*Can f 1*) and *Can f 2* are important dog allergens. Recently, a carbohydrate, galactose-alpha-1,3-galactose has been shown to be the major IgE-binding epitope on cat IgA, which is a minor allergen.[41] This allergen has been shown to be cross-reactive in patients with food allergy to nonprimate mammalian species. In addition, serum albumins of furred animals may also play a role in some cases of allergy to furred animals.[42]

Of the cockroach allergens, 9 to 10 different allergens have been identified.[17] The major cockroach allergen, *Bla g 2*, has been the most extensively studied. Although characterized as an enzyme, based on its protein structure, it is not known to possess any active enzymatic activity.

A number of fungal allergens have been identified in the indoor environment. Several species are considered to be more likely to be indoor than outdoor allergens. The main species involved are *Penicillium* and *Aspergillis*; however, a number of fungal species can be found in the indoor environment based on substrate and humidity factors. *Alternaria* antigens have been detected in many US homes.[43] At least 9 *Alternaria* allergens have been characterized.[17] The most important of these is *Alt a 1*, which is the major allergen. *Penicillium* and *Aspergillus* species often have cross-reactive allergens, some 34 to 35 allergens from both *Penicillium* species and *Aspergillus fumigatus* have been identified.[17] Many of these have proteolitic activity and, therefore, may act as adjuvants in Th2-driven mechanisms.

DIAGNOSIS OF INDOOR ALLERGEN SENSITIZATION

It is clear that self-reported histories of allergic rhinitis symptoms alone are only modest predictors of true sensitization.[44] Testing for the presence of IgE sensitization by either skin test or in vitro assay is necessary to establish the correct diagnosis.

The assessment of allergic status and true diagnosis cannot be based on history alone but requires additional supporting data, such as a positive skin-prick test.[45] Because symptoms of dust mite and cockroach sensitivity, for example, are perennial, the diagnosis can be achieved only by appropriate testing. The molecular biology of allergens has improved diagnostic capabilities. Microarray techniques,[46] in which specific molecules produced recombinantly are displayed on a microarray and subsequently probed with serum from a patient with suspected sensitization, can improve clinical diagnosis and are very helpful in epidemiologic studies of allergic disease.

The Importance of Polysensitization

Polysensitization to indoor as well as outdoor allergens in the development of allergic rhinitis has been demonstrated in several studies.[47,48] Although sensitization appears to decrease with age, 40% or more of individuals older than 60 years have been shown to have sensitization to one or more indoor allergens.[49] It would, therefore, seem appropriate to conduct skin testing or in vitro assays for specific IgE sensitization in patients presenting for evaluation of chronic rhinitis symptoms so that allergen avoidance measures can be tailored to the patient's specific sensitivities.

ASSESSMENT OF INDOOR ENVIRONMENTAL EXPOSURE

Attempts have been made to establish a threshold of allergen exposure levels that are associated with sensitization and subsequent allergic disease. Such attempts have proven challenging because exposures in the indoor environment are complex and the relationships between exposure and sensitization and/or symptoms in particular are nonlinear.[50,51] Nonetheless, techniques for environmental sampling have been developed to measure specific allergens via the use of monoclonal antibody–based immunoassays. The major source of house dust mite exposure is in bedding and carpeting, as mentioned previously. Settled dust samples are collected by vacuuming bedding or floors using specific protocols, and the concentration of a major dust mite allergen can be measured through the use of immunoassays, which are commercially available (for example, Indoor Biotechnologies, Charlottesville, VA, USA). Such sampling techniques have been useful in ascertaining the concentration of the major allergen, as well as evidence for exposure reduction in outcome studies.

Similarly, for the major cat allergen, settled dust samples can be assayed; however, airborne samples using air-sampling technology can also be adapted to detect the major cat allergen, Fel d 1. Fewer studies have been conducted with major dog allergen. There are several reports of the use of immunoassays for assaying mouse allergens in the indoor environment.

Assessing exposure to fungal allergens has proven more problematic. Although one study used polyclonal antibodies to detect Alternaria allergens in indoor environments,[43] few studies have used monoclonal antibody–based immunoassays. Most often, fungal allergen presence is performed by quantitative culturing techniques of air samples or by spore counts,[52] as exposure can originate from outdoor intrusion of fungal spores or from an indoor source. Simultaneous tests need to be conducted on both indoor and outdoor samples to determine whether an indoor source is present. A guide to interpretation of indoor fungal spore assessments has been published.[53]

As with in vitro diagnostic tests for IgE sensitization, molecular biology has advanced the technology for assessing exposure to indoor allergens. Using a microarray assay system, a number of indoor allergens (Der p 1, p 2, f 1, f 2, Fel d 1, and Can f 1) can be analyzed in a single settled dust sample.[54] Further investigations that will expand the capabilities of these multiplex assay systems are ongoing.

ALLERGEN AVOIDANCE MEASURES

Although it seems intuitive that avoidance of allergen exposure should lead to improvement in allergic rhinitis symptoms, this has been difficult to achieve, particularly in home environments. It is well known that when seasonal pollen allergen exposures cease, symptoms abate shortly thereafter. Likewise, in occupational asthma, removal from exposures tends to improve symptoms as well. Evidence that allergen avoidance is beneficial has been verified in several studies. It should be pointed out that many of the studies involved in allergen avoidance are aimed at asthma, as opposed to rhinitis. The key to success is that exposure levels have to be reduced to near negligible amounts to achieve a positive effect. Use of settled dust or airborne samples for concentrations of major indoor allergens, as discussed previously, can be used as a marker for effective allergen exposure reduction. However, indoor environments contain complex mixtures of allergens and other factors that can affect symptoms of allergic rhinitis. The complexity and nonlinearity of dose response relationships also makes such evaluations of the effectiveness of allergen avoidance difficult.

In one of the earliest allergen avoidance studies, Platts-Mills and colleagues[55] demonstrated that putting patients who are allergic to dust mites in a hospital room for 2 months or more (where the exposure to house dust mite was negligible) resulted in improvement in symptoms and medication use. Further investigations have been conducted at high altitude, where house dust mite concentrations tend to be low as a result of the low humidity and colder temperatures.[56,57] These studies showed beneficial effects on airway inflammation symptoms and other markers of allergic disease.

Using a multifaceted approach in children with asthma with multiple indoor allergen exposures, including such interventions as using impermeable encasements for the mattress and pillows, vacuuming with a HEPA-filtered vacuum, and using a HEPA air purifier, had modest benefits on their symptoms.[58] However, interventions for control of house dust mite avoidance in subjects with asthma, when examined by meta-analyses, demonstrated that chemical and physical methods aimed at reducing exposure to house dust mite allergens cannot be recommended.[59] These and other meta-analyses have come under some criticism because of inclusion and exclusion criteria used in the evaluation.[60]

Because there is some evidence to support strict allergen avoidance, strategies that optimize the reduction of allergen exposure in homes have not been fully determined. There are complex issues regarding the efficacy of measures that target a variety of allergens in the home. One approach that may be particularly useful is educating patients or their caregivers so that they may intervene and perhaps lead to more successful outcomes.[61]

Nonetheless, allergen control measures, although difficult, should be an integral part of the overall management of sensitized patients. Which interventions are the most cost effective remains to be determined, and further trials are warranted.[62]

House Dust Mites

Specific recommendations for reducing house dust mite exposure are shown in **Box 1**. These include fitting of allergen-proof mattress, pillow, and box spring encasements, washing bedding regularly in hot water, and possibly by reducing indoor humidity. Acaricides designed to kill dust mites in carpets have, in and of themselves, proved largely ineffective because the mite populations return shortly after their application, and they may also cause skin and respiratory irritation. Pillow, mattress, and box spring encasements are often used as a single approach to house dust mite allergen avoidance. Randomized controlled trials of such encasements did not seem to provide any benefit in mite-sensitized adults.[63] However, encasements as part of a comprehensive approach can be effective.[64] If such encasements are to be used,

---

Box 1
House dust mite allergen avoidance measures[a]

Primary focus: Bedroom

- Use dust mite impermeable pillow and encasements (woven preferable to nonwoven material). Encase box springs.
- Wash bedclothes in hot water (130°F) weekly. Dry on hot cycle.

Long-term:

- Maintain indoor relative humidity ≤50% (dehumidifiers, air conditioning)
- Minimize wall-to-wall carpets
- Minimize draperies
- Minimize upholstered furniture
- Avoid carpets on cement slabs (eg, basement floors). Condensation under carpet provides moisture conducive to mite proliferation.
- Vacuum with double-layer vacuum bag

[a] To be effective, measures must reduce HDM allergen levels to <0.5 μg/g of settled dust.

a woven mattress encasement is preferred because nonwoven materials can actually accumulate mite and cat allergens.[65] Washing bed clothing in hot water has been shown to kill dust mites and washing is necessary to remove allergens from the bedclothes. Alternatively, freezing conditions also will kill dust mites; therefore, stuffed animals may be placed in a plastic bag in a freezer and then, if possible, washed to remove any remaining allergen. Likewise, hanging rugs outside in freezing conditions may also kill dust mites, but a thorough cleaning is then necessary. Reduction in humidity with improved ventilation control may have little effect on house dust mite allergen levels; however, some minor improvement in respiratory outcomes can be demonstrated.[66] The use of impermeable casings, which can cost up to several hundred dollars, is one of the limiting factors in their use in patients with symptomatic allergic disease. In a recent study, it was shown that in patients receiving immunotherapy, few if any were practicing dust mite avoidance measures.[67] Nonetheless, the studies on dust mite allergen avoidance as a preventive and therapeutic strategy indicate that such stringent measures may reduce potential sensitization[68] but there is little evidence to support the use of single approaches, such as mite-proof encasements, as an intervention in adults for symptomatic control. In children, however, single or multiple-faceted interventions may have some benefit.[68]

Pets

For individuals sensitized to pet allergens (**Box 2**), removal of the pet from the home is the most useful technique, although this has not been studied in any systematic way. Many pet owners, however, are unlikely to relinquish the pet. It should be borne in mind that cat allergen levels can persist for longer than 6 weeks once the pet has been removed. Washing walls and other washable surfaces may be helpful in reducing allergen exposure once the pet has been removed.[22] Efforts have been made to reduce allergen exposure with the animal in situ. Such measures include the use of HEPA filters,[69] and although HEPA filters can reduce the airborne cat allergen concentration, their use does not improve allergen-related symptoms. Other measures include use of HEPA-filtered vacuum cleaners and washing the cat. Although these also have been shown to reduce allergen levels, improvement in symptoms has not been addressed. Likewise, a combination of mattress encasements and cat exclusion from the bedroom reduced airborne cat allergen levels, but no effect on disease activity was detected.[70] A Cochrane analysis of the available data suggests that the

---

Box 2
Animal dander allergen avoidance measures

Focus: Remove pet(s) from environment

- Find suitable alternative home for pet
- Thorough cleaning after pet removed[a]

Measures to reduce exposure with pet in situ are NOT effective.

- Washing pet
- Confining pet to certain areas in home
- Vacuuming with HEPA filter vacuum
- HEPA air filtration

[a] May require 6 months for allergen levels to decline.

studies are too small to provide evidence for or against the use of air-filtration units in the management of pet allergy.[71]

Cockroaches and Other Pests

Particularly in inner-city environments, cockroach allergen (**Box 3**) is a major sensitizer and cause of allergic symptoms. Approaches include pesticides; sanitation, such as making sure that there is no food available to the cockroaches; control of water leaks; and control of entrances. An integrated pest-management program that involves sanitation building management and limited use of pesticides has been helpful in reducing allergen exposure.[72] Once cockroaches have been eliminated from the environment, a thorough cleaning is necessary, not only immediately after pesticide treatment, but continued for long periods of time (up to several months) to remove the allergen.

Likewise, mouse exposure, particularly in bedrooms, is prevalent, especially in inner-city dwellings. Methods for effective rodent control have been shown to reduce allergen exposure and improvement in patient activities.[73]

Fungi

The role of fungal allergen avoidance (**Box 4**) in respiratory disease has had limited investigation.[74] Most instances of fungal growth in the indoor environment are caused by moisture issues (leaks, condensation, and other causes for water accumulation). Repair of any water leaks and humidity control are key factors that can be used. Control of the indoor environmental humidity with reductions to below 50% relative humidity has been recommended.[52] Contaminated materials that can be discarded should be removed. Surfaces that can be washed should be treated with dilute 5% bleach solution with a detergent.[52] A study of the use of hypochlorite bleach solutions to reduce exposure demonstrated that there was a reduction in sensitization to cat and overall sensitization[75]; however, fungal allergen sensitization was not studied.

Box 3
Cockroach allergen avoidance measures

Focus: Integrated pest management program (professional pest control)

- Thorough cleaning of infested areas
  - Mopping floors
  - Washing counter tops and appliances with detergent, water-dilute bleach
  - Vacuuming
- Seal portals of entry
  - Wall cracks, and so forth
- Remove food sources
  - Clean up spills
  - Keep sinks clear of dirty dishes
- Remove water sources
  - Repair leaks, and so forth
- Wash bedclothes
- ? Mattress, pillow encasements
- ? HEPA air filters

Box 4
Indoor fungal allergen avoidance measures[a]

Focus: Remove moisture sources

- Repair leaks
- Remove standing water, eg, humidifiers
- Maintain indoor relative humidity ≤50% with dehumidifiers, air conditioning
- Remove contaminated materials—clothing, books, carpets, and so forth
- Wash washable surfaces with 5% chlorine bleach–water solution containing a detergent
- Proper HVAC (heating, air conditioning) system maintenance
- ? Use of HEPA air filtration

[a] All recommendations are empiric.

Such remediation efforts can reduce spore counts; however, the effectiveness of this in the overall management of allergic disease attributable to fungal sensitization is not clear. Air filtration and air cleaners may also reduce concentrations of fungal spores and indoor pollen in theory. A recent review has been conducted regarding the use of these systems.[76]

Most allergen avoidance approaches are directed at reducing symptoms in patients with established sensitivities. Any approach to allergen avoidance needs to be targeted at the allergen to which the patient is sensitized; therefore, appropriate skin testing or in vitro testing for specific sensitivities is necessary before recommending any environmental control measures that have some costs associated with them.

Alternatively, environmental controls can be directed toward the prevention of allergic sensitization. Studies are under way[77] in which pregnant women at risk for having children who will develop allergic disease are instructed in specific avoidance measures. These studies are designed to determine if control measures are effective in preventing allergic sensitization in the infants. Substantial reductions in levels of major house dust mite, as well as pet allergen concentrations, have been demonstrated in these environments, but the long-term outcomes are not known. Among the difficulties with this type of approach is that not only are allergens reduced, but other environmental factors that influence the outcome are also affected. Consequently, studies that look at genetics as well as the environment and their interactions are important in future investigations.

Education plays an important role in allergen avoidance strategies. One study[78] demonstrated that intensive education of patients at risk for developing allergic disease were able to reduce exposures, but this also occurred in a control group as well. There was a slight reduction in incidence of respiratory symptoms in the group that achieved some measure of environmental control. Environmental control practices were more likely to be instituted by the caregivers of children with allergic rhinitis symptoms than those who had asthma.[79] Applying allergen avoidance measures in the treatment of children who live in poverty is difficult because of the multiple sensitivities and problems with applying protocols, often because of cost concerns. However, home visiting by professionals demonstrates positive influences on management of such patients. In addition to the study by Morgan and colleagues,[58] a tailored, multifaceted environmental program designed to reduce airborne indoor allergen levels as well as airborne particulates in inner-city homes had some modest effects on symptoms.[80] For patients who have poorly controlled respiratory disease, home intervention by nurses or other professionals could improve outcomes.[81,82] Such visits can identify ways of improving the home environment. A more recent study indicates that home environmental assessment and case management through environmental education and assessments may improve outcomes for allergic rhinitis and reduce emergency room visits for asthma.[82]

Because of the complexities of the indoor environment, single interventions in comparison with combined strategies may not be effective.[83] Further research is necessary to establish the cost-effectiveness of approaches that have been recommended to date.[84]

SUMMARY

Exposure and sensitization to indoor allergens play a critical role in allergic rhinitis. The principal allergens are derived from house dust mites, pets, cockroaches and other insects, and fungi. A complex interplay of genetics, allergen, and other environmental exposures is present. Interventions that have been successful in reducing allergen exposure are multifaceted and may be relatively expensive. Nonetheless, reducing allergen exposure to negligible levels has been shown to improve clinical outcomes. Studies that allow better insights into the complex interplay between the environment and genetics are necessary. Strategies to prevent allergic sensitization in at-risk populations are under ongoing investigation to provide improved allergen avoidance recommendations. Any avoidance measure should be targeted at the specific sensitivity demonstrated by the patient.

REFERENCES

1. Cingi C, Kayabasoglu G, Nacar A. Update on the medical treatment of allergic rhinitis. Inflamm Allergy Drug Targets 2009;8(2):96–103.
2. Dykeqicz MS, Hamilos DL. Rhinitis and sinusitis. J Allergy Clin Immunol 2010; 125(2 Suppl 2):S103–15.
3. Arbes SL Jr, Gergen PJ, Elliott L, et al. Prevalence of positive skin test responses to 10 common aeroallegens in the US population: results from the Third National Health and Nutrition Examination Survey. J Allergy Clin Immunol 2005;116: 377–83.
4. Arbes SL Jr, Cohn RD, Uin M, et al. House dust mite allergen in US homes: results from the First National Survey of Lead and Allergens in Housing. J Allergy Clin Immunol 2003;111:408–14.
5. Arbes SL Jr, Cohn RD, Yin M, et al. Dog allergen (Can f 1) and cat allergen (Fel d1) in US homes: results from The National Survey of Lead and Allergens in Housing. J Allergy Clin Immunol 2004;114:111–7.
6. Wilson J, Dixon SL, Breysse P, et al. Housing and allergens: a pooled analysis of nine US studies. Environ Res 2010;110(2):189–98.
7. Bertelsen RJ, Instanes C, Granum B, et al. Gender differences in indoor allergen exposure and association with current rhinitis. Clin Exp Allergy 2010;40:1388–97.
8. Ho SM. Environmental epigenetics of asthma: an update. J Allergy Clin Immunol 2010;126:453–65.
9. Misiak RT, Wegienka G, Havstad S, et al. Specific allergic sensitization in parents and their 18-year-old offspring in the suburban Detroit childhood allergy study. J Allergy Clin Immunol 2009;123(6):1401.e2–6e2.
10. Perzanowski MS, Ronmark E, Platts-Mills TA, et al. Effect of cat and dog ownership on sensitization and development of asthma among preteenage children. Am J Respir Crit Care Med 2002;166(5):696–702.

11. Da Silva CA, Pochard P, Lee CG, et al. Chitin particles are multifaceted immune adjuvants. Am J Respir Crit Care Med 2010;182:1482–91.

12. Eggleston PA. Complex interactions of pollutant and allergen exposures and their impact on people with asthma. Pediatrics 2009;123(Suppl 3):S160–7.

13. Bertelsen RJ, Carlsen KC, Carlsen KH, et al. Childhood asthma and early life exposure to indoor allergens, endotoxin and beta(1,3)-glucans. Clin Exp Allergy 2010;40(2):307–16.

14. Horner AA. Regulation of aeroallergen immunity by the innate immune system: laboratory evidence for a new paradigm. J Innate Immun 2010;2(2):107–13.

15. Arlian LG, Platts-Mills TA. The biology of dust mites and the remediation of mite allergens in allergic disease. J Allergy Clin Immunol 2001;107(Suppl 3):S406–13.

16. Tovey ER, Chapman MD, Platts-Mills TA. Mite feces are a major source of house durt allergens. Nature 1981;289:592–3.

17. Available at: http://www.allergome.org. Accessed September 18, 2010.

18. Matricardi PM, Sockelbrink A, Keil T, et al. Dynamic evolution of serum immuno-globulin E to airborne allergens throughout childhood: results from the Multi-Centre Allergy Study birth cohort. Clin Exp Allergy 2009;39(10):1551–7.

19. Jacobs KD, Brand PL. Can sensitization to aeroallergens disappear over time in children with allergic disease? Acta Paediatr 2010;99:1361–4.

20. Erwin EA, Ronmark E, Wickens K, et al. Contribution of dust mite and cat specific IgE to total IgE: relevance to asthma prevalence. J Allergy Clin Immunol 2007; 119(2):359–65.

21. DeBlay F, Chapman MD, Platts-Mills TA. Airborne cut allergen (Feld 1). Environ-mental control with the cat in situ. Am Rev Respir Dis 1991;143:1334–9.

22. Wood RA, Mudd KE, Eggleston PA. The distribution of cat and dust mite allergens on wall surfaces. J Allergy Clin Immunol 1992;89:126–30.

23. Erwin EA, Wickens K, Custis NJ, et al. Cat and dust mite sensitivity and tolerance in relation to wheezing among children raised with high exposure to both allergens. J Allergy Clin Immunol 2005;115(1):74–9.

24. Lau S, Illi S, Platts-Mills TA, et al, Multicentre Allergy Study Group. Longitudinal study on the relationship between cat allergen and endotoxin exposure, sensiti-zation, cat-specific IgG and development of asthma in childhood: report of the German Multicentre Allergy Study (MAS 90). Allergy 2005;60(6):766–73.

25. Erwin EA, Custis N, Ronmark E, et al. Asthma and indoor air: contrasts in the dose response to cat and dust-mite. Indoor Air 2005;15(Suppl 10):33–9.

26. Wallace DV. Pet dander and perennial allergic rhinitis: therapeutic options. Allergy Asthma Proc 2009;30(6):573–83.

27. Mandhane PJ, Sears MR, Poulton R, et al. Cats and dogs and the risk of atopy in childhood and adulthood. J Allergy Clin Immunol 2009;124(4):745–50.

28. Salo PM, Jaramillo R, Cohn RD, et al. Exposure to mouse allergen in US homes associated with asthma symptoms. Environ Health Perspect 2009;117(3):387–91.

29. Matsui EC. Role of mouse allergens in allergic disease. Curr Allergy Asthma Rep 2009;9(5):370–5.

30. Phipatanakul W, Litonjua A, Platts-Mills TA, et al. Sensitization to mouse allergen and asthma and asthma morbidity among women in Boston. J Allergy Clin Immu-nol 2007;120(4):954–6.

31. Perzanowski MS, Platts-Mills TA. Further confirmation of the relevance of cock-roach and dust mite sensitization to inner-city asthma morbidity. Clin Exp Allergy 2009;39(9):1291–3.

32. Han YY, Lee YL, Guo YL. Indoor environmental risk factors and seasonal variation of childhood asthma. Pediatr Allergy Immunol 2009;20(8):748–86.

33. Nakazawa T, Satinover SM, Naccara L, et al. Asian ladybugs (*Harmonia axyridis*): a new seasonal indoor allergen. J Allergy Clin Immunol 2007;119(2):421–7.
34. Clark MT, Levin T, Dolen W. Cross-reactivity between cockroach and ladybug using the radioallergosorbent test. Ann Allergy Asthma Immunol 2009;103(5):432–5.
35. Stark PC, Celedon JC, Chew GL, et al. Fungal levels in the home and allergic rhinitis by 5 years of age. Environ Health Perspect 2005;113(10):1405–9.
36. Pongracic JA, O'Connor GT, Muilenberg ML, et al. Differential effects of outdoor versus indoor fungal spores on asthma morbidity in inner-city children. J Allergy Clin Immunol 2010;125(3):593–9.
37. Takahaski Y, Tahano K, Suzuki M, et al. Two routes for pollen entering indoors: ventilation and clothes. J Investig Allergol Clin Immunol 2008;18(5):382–8.
38. Shea KM, Truckner RT, Weber RW, et al. Climate change and allergic disease. J Allergy Clin Immunol 2008;122:443–53.
39. Chapman MD, Pomes A, Breiteneder H, et al. Nomenclature and structural biology of allergens. J Allergy Clin Immunol 2007;119:414–20.
40. Radauer C, Bublin M, Wagner S, et al. Allergens are distributed into few protein families and possess a restricted number of biochemical functions. J Allergy Clin Immunol 2008;121:847–52.
41. Ueta M, Uematsu S, Akira S, et al. The carbohydrate galactose-a-1,3-galactose is a major IgE-bilding epitope on cat IgA. J Allergy Clin Immunol 2009;123(5):1189–91.
42. Liccardi G, Dente B, Restani P, et al. Respiratory allergy induced by exclusive polysensitization to serum albumins of furry animals. Eur Ann Allergy Clin Immunol 2010;42(3):127–30.
43. Salo PM, Arbes SJ Jr, Sever M, et al. Exposure to *Alternaria* in US homes is associated with asthma symptoms. J Allergy Clin Immunol 2006;118:892–8.
44. Abrahma CM, Ownby DR, Peterson EL, et al. The relationship between seroatopy and symptoms of either allergic rhinitis or asthma. J Allergy Clin Immunol 2007;119(5):1099–104.
45. Smith HE, Hogger C, Lallemant C, et al. Is structured allergy history sufficient when assessing patients with asthma and rhinitis in general practice? J Allergy Clin Immunol 2009;124(2):388–9.
46. Lin J, Bardina L, Shreffler WG. Microarrayed allergen molecules for diagnostics of allergy. Methods Mol Biol 2009;524:259–72.
47. Ciprandi G, Alesina R, Ariano R, et al. Characteristics of patients with allergic polysensitization: the POLISMAIL study. Eur Ann Allergy Clin Immunol 2008;40(3):77–83.
48. Brockow I, Zutavern A, Hoffmann U, et al. Early allergic sensitizations and their relevance to atopic diseases in children aged 6 years: results of the GINI study. J Investig Allergol Clin Immunol 2009;19(3):180–7.
49. Busse PJ, Lushslurchachai L, Sampson HA, et al. Perennial allergen-specific immunoglobulin E levels among inner-city elderly asthmatics. J Asthma 2010;47:781–5.
50. Platts-Mills TA, Wrwin EA, Heymann PW, et al. Pro: the evidence for a causal role of dust mites in asthma. Am J Respir Crit Care Med 2009;180:109–13.
51. Hertzen L, Haahtela T. Con: house dust mites in atopic diseases. Am J Respir Crit Care Med 2009;108:113–9.
52. Bush RK, Portnoy JM. The role and abatement of fungal allergens in allergic diseases. J Allergy Clin Immunol 2001;107:S430–40.
53. Horner WE, Barnes C, Codina R, et al. Guide for interpreting reports from inspections/investigations of indoor mold. J Allergy Clin Immunol 2008;121:592–7.

54. Earle CD, King EM, Tsay A, et al. High-throughput fluorescent multiplex array for indoor allergen exposure assessment. J Allergy Clin Immunol 2007;119(2): 428–33.
55. Platts-Mills TA, Tovey EF, Mitchell EB, et al. Reduction of bronchial hyperreactivity during prolonged allergen avoidance. Lancet 1982;2(8300):675–8.
56. Van Velzen E, van den Bos JW, Benckhuijsen JA, et al. Effect of allergen avoidance at high altitude on direct and indirect bronchial hyperresponsiveness and markers of inflammation in children with allergic asthma. Thorax 1996;51(6):582–4.
57. Grootendorst DC, Dahlen SE, Van Den Bos JW, et al. Benefits of high altitude allergen avoidance in atopic adolescents with moderate to severe asthma, over and above treatment with high dose inhaled steroids. Clin Exp Allergy 2001; 31(3):400–8.
58. Morgan WJ, Crain EF, Gruchalla RS, et al. Results of a home-based environmental intervention among urban children with asthma. N Engl J Med 2004; 351(11):1068–80.
59. Gotzsche PC, Johansen HK. House dust mite control measures for asthma: systematic review. Allergy 2008;63(6):646–59.
60. Platts-Mills TA. Allergen avoidance in the treatment of asthma: problems with the meta-analyses. J Allergy Clin Immunol 2008;122(4):694–6.
61. Platts-Mills TA, Vaughan JW, Carter MC, et al. The role of intervention in established allergy: avoidance of indoor allergens in the treatment of chronic allergic disease. J Allergy Clin Immunol 2000;106(5):787–804.
62. Custovic A, Murray CS, Gore RB, et al. Controlling indoor allergens. Ann Allergy Asthma Immunol 2002;88(5):432–41.
63. Simpson A, Simpson B, Custovic A, et al. Stringent environmental control in pregnancy and early life: the long-term effects on mite, cat, and dog allergen. Clin Exp Allergy 2003;33(9):1183–9.
64. Luczynska C, Tredwell E, Smeeton N, et al. A randomized controlled trial of mite allergen-impermeable bed covers in adult mite-sensitized asthmatics. Clin Exp Allergy 2003;33(12):1613–7.
65. Miller JD, Naccara L, Satinover S, et al. Nonwoven in contrast to woven encasings accumulate mite and cat allergen. J Allergy Clin Immunol 2007;120(4):977–9.
66. Wright GR, Howieson S, McSharry C, et al. Effect of improved home ventilation on asthma control and house dust mite allergen levels. Allergy 2009;64(11): 1671–80.
67. White KM, Nugent JS, Rathkopf MM. Dust-mite avoidance measures in patients on immunotherapy. Allergy Asthma Proc 2008;29(1):40–4.
68. Semic Jusufagic S, Simpson A, Woodcock A. Dust mite allergen avoidance as a preventive and therapeutic strategy. Curr Allergy Asthma Rep 2006;6(6):521–6.
69. Wood RA, Johnson EF, Van Natta ML, et al. A placebo-controlled trial of a HEPA air cleaner in the treatment of cat allergy. Am J Respir Crit Care Med 1998;158(1): 115–20.
70. Sheehan WJ, Rangsithienchai PA, Wood RA, et al. Pest and allergen exposure and abatement in inner-city asthma: a work group report of the American Academy of Allergy, Asthma & Immunology Indoor Allergy/Air Pollution Committee. J Allergy Clin Immunol 2010;125(3):575–81.
71. Kilburn S, Lasserson TJ, McKean M. Pet allergen control measures for allergic asthma in children and adults. Cochrane Database Syst Rev 2003;1:CD002989.
72. Kass D, McKelvey W, Carlton E, et al. Effectiveness of an integrated pest management intervention in controlling cockroaches, mice, and allergens in New York City public housing. Environ Health Perspect 2009;117(8):1219–25.

73. Pongracic JA, Visness CM, Gruchalla RS, et al. Effect of mouse allergen and rodent environmental intervention on asthma in inner-city children. Ann Allergy Asthma Immunol 2008;101(1):35–41.
74. Barnes CS, Dowling P, Van Osdol T, et al. Comparison of indoor fungal spore levels before and after professional home remediation. Ann Allergy Asthma Immunol 2007;98(3):262–8.
75. Zock JP, Plana E, Anto J, et al. Domestic use of hypochlorite bleach, atopic sensitization, and respiratory symptoms in adults. J Allergy Clin Immunol 2009;124: 731–8.
76. Sublett JL, Seltzer J, Burkhead R, et al. Air filters and air cleaners: rostrum by the American Academy of Allergy, Asthma & Immunology Indoor Allergen Committee. J Allergy Clin Immunol 2010;1285(1):32–8.
77. Simpson A, Custovic A. Prevention of allergic sensitization by environmental control. Curr Allergy Asthma Rep 2009;9(5):363–9.
78. Persky V, Piorkowski J, Hernandez E, et al. The effect of low-cost modification of the home environment on the development of respiratory symptoms in the first year of life. Ann Allergy Asthma Immunol 2009;103(6):480–7.
79. Hansel NN, Eggleston PA, Krishnan JA, et al. Asthma-related health status determinants of environmental control practices for inner-city preschool children. Ann Allergy Asthma Immunol 2006;97(3):409–17.
80. Carter MC, Perzanowski MS, Raymond A, et al. Home intervention in the treatment of asthma among inner-city children. J Allergy Clin Immunol 2001;108(5): 732–7.
81. Eggleston PA, Butz A, Rand C, et al. Home environmental intervention in inner-city asthma: a randomized controlled clinical trial. Ann Allergy Asthma Immunol 2005; 95(6):496–7.
82. Bracken M, Fleming L, Hall P, et al. The importance of nurse-led home visits in the assessment of children with problematic asthma. Arch Dis Child 2009;94(1): 780–4.
83. Liccardi G, Cazzola M, Walter Canonica G, et al. New insights in allergen avoidance measures for mite and pet sensitized patients. A critical appraisal. Respir Med 2005;99(11):1363–76.
84. Bush RK. Indoor allergens, environmental avoidance, and allergic respiratory disease. Allergy Asthma Proc 2008;29(6):575–9.

Antihistamine Therapy in Allergic Rhinitis

Flavia C.L. Hoyte, MD, Rohit K. Katial, MD*

KEYWORDS

- Antihistamine • Rhinitis • Allergy • Allergic • Therapy
- Histamine

Histamine, one of the key mediators of allergic disease, has been a target of allergic rhinitis therapy for some time. More than 40 oral antihistamines are currently available and can be classified as first-generation and second-generation drugs, depending on their pharmacokinetic and pharmacodynamic properties and their side-effect profiles. Intranasal antihistamines were introduced more recently and have shown promise in their efficacy, rapid onset of action, and minimal side effects. The choice of antihistamine for a given individual should be based on patient characteristics that could affect drug metabolism, the specific symptoms experienced, cost concerns, and patient preference. This article discusses the history and classification of antihistamines as well as their role in the treatment of allergic rhinitis and the evidence supporting this use.

HISTORY OF HISTAMINE DISCOVERY AND ANTIHISTAMINE DEVELOPMENT

The mast cell, which is the main source of histamine, was first identified by Paul Ehrlich in 1870. It was not until 1910, however, that histamine itself was discovered by British physiologist Sir Henry Dale as a bacterial product contaminating Ergot. Experiments by Dale and his colleagues demonstrated that this substance could produce smooth muscle contraction in isolated guinea pig ileum and respiratory tissue, stimulate cardiac contractility, and lead to vasodepression and a shock-like state when injected into animals.[1,2] Histamine was initially termed *H substance* by Lewis, whose 1924 article described the "triple response" of vasodilation, wheal, and flare that occurred after intradermal injection of this substance into human skin. Lewis' subsequent experiments demonstrated that other stimuli could produce a similar response,

Flavia C.L. Hoyte has nothing to disclose. Disclosures for Rohit K. Katial: GSK, TEVA, MEDA, Alcon, MedImmune.
Division of Allergy, Asthma, and Immunology, National Jewish Health, 1400 Jackson Street, Room K624, Denver, CO 80206, USA
* Corresponding author.
E-mail address: katialr@njhealth.org

Immunol Allergy Clin N Am 31 (2011) 509–543
doi:10.1016/j.iac.2011.05.003   immunology.theclinics.com
0889-8561/11/$ – see front matter © 2011 Elsevier Inc. All rights reserved.

suggesting an intrinsic molecule similar to H substance produced by the body in response to these stimuli. H substance was later characterized further as β-aminoethyl-imidazole, also known as 2-(4-imidazolyl)-ethylamine, which is the molecule currently known as histamine. The understanding of histamine's clinical impact grew with the identification of histamine in human liver and lung tissue in 1927[3] and with the identification of histamine as the main mediator of anaphylaxis in 1932.[4]

The first antihistamine was identified in 1937 with the discovery of 933F, also known as adrenolytic benzodioxan or piperoxan, a substance that blocked the effect of histamine on guinea pig ileum. In that same year, Bovet and Staub identified 929F, thymol ether, as a substance that protected guinea pig from histamine-induced anaphylaxis. Having been deemed too toxic, 929F was altered by replacing one of the oxygen groups with an amino group to develop aniline ethylene diamine derivatives. Five years later, in 1942, phenbenzamine/pyribenzamine was developed as the first clinically useful antihistamine,[1] followed by the discovery of diphenhydramine, tripelennamine, chlorpheniramine, and promethazine. By 1943, central nervous system (CNS) toxicity had been observed and was unfortunately a feature of all of these first-generation antihistamines. It was not until 1985 that terfenadine, the first nonsedating antihistamine approved for use in the United States, was introduced for clinical use, thus expanding the potential benefit of this family of medications.[5] More recently, the introduction of ocular antihistamines and intranasal antihistamines as therapeutic options has furthered the impact of antihistamines by providing an option for local administration of these medications for the treatment of chronic conjunctivitis and rhinitis.

HISTAMINE BIOLOGY AND HISTAMINE RECEPTORS

Histamine is produced from L-histidine through the action of histidine decarboxylase, an enzyme produced by inflammatory cells, neurons of the CNS, and parietal cells in the gastric mucosa.[6–10] Although most of these cells produce histamine without storing it, mast cells and basophils are capable of storing histamine within their granules and releasing it when these cells degranulate due to various stimuli.[10] Specific to allergic rhinitis, mast cells and basophils in the nasal mucosa release large quantities of histamine after the binding and cross-linking of surface IgE molecules on allergen exposure. Compared with other mediators that are released in picogram quantities when these cells degranulate, histamine is released in microgram quantities with 3 μg to 5 μg per million mast cells and 1 μg per million basophils.[8] Histamine exerts its effect through its interaction with 4 different 7-transmembrane G protein–coupled receptors—H_1, H_2, H_3, and H_4—which are described in **Table 1**. Because each of these receptors predominates on different cell types throughout the body, they exert different biologic effects. Although the H_1 receptor is the most important regarding rhinitis, all 4 histamine receptors contribute to the pathophysiology of this condition.

H_1 receptors are located on endothelial cells and vascular smooth muscle cells, allowing for histamine-mediated vasodilatation and vasopermeability, which are central hallmarks of the pathophysiology of allergic rhinitis, specifically the symptoms of rhinorrhea and congestion.[9] The histamine-mediated parasympathetic reflex stimulation of glandular secretions also contributes to rhinorrhea.[8,9] In addition, H_1 receptors are present on sensory nerves of the upper airway, contributing to the sneezing and itching of the nose, palate, and throat that are prominent symptoms in rhinitis. Furthermore, the presence of these receptors on inflammatory cells, such as neutrophils, eosinophils, lymphocytes, monocytes/macrophages, and dendritic cells, increases trafficking of these cells to areas of inflammation, thus exerting a delayed proinflammatory effect contributing to the late phase allergic response.[8,9]

The H_2 receptor was the next to be discovered and is now most recognized for its role as a receptor for gastric acid secretion. These receptors are also found on the systemic vasculature, hence their role in the cardiovascular instability sometimes seen during anaphylaxis. H_2 receptors are also found on the submucosal glands and epithelial cells of the nasal mucosa, thereby contributing to rhinitis through increased glandular secretions and vascular permeability.[8,9]

The H_3 receptor is found mainly in the presynaptic nerves of the peripheral sympathetic system, leading to suppression of norepinephrine release. Through this mechanism, activation of the H_3 receptor can lead to increased nasal congestion, which is further enhanced by activation of these receptors on the nasal submucosal glands.[11]

Most recently, in 2000, the H_4 receptor was identified and was found present in multiple areas of the body, including the nerves of the nasal turbinates and on multiple inflammatory cells, including eosinophils and mast cells. As such, the H_4 receptor is thought to play a role in the inflammatory aspect of rhinitis, although further work is needed to fully understand the role of this receptor in rhinitis. Data regarding the localization of the H_4 receptor in the CNS are conflicting, although one recent report demonstrates its presence in both human and rodent CNS while postulating its role in pain and itch.[12]

All 4 histamine receptors alternate between an active and inactive form and have a low level of constitutive activity even in the absence of histamine.[13,14] Histamine acts as an agonist of these receptors, preferentially binding to the active conformation and stabilizing the receptor in this form. Antihistamines act as inverse agonists, preferentially binding to and stabilizing the histamine receptors in their inactive form, thereby inhibiting signal transduction.[13] This inhibition has been tested for many of the H_1 antihistamines available for clinical use using gene reporter assays. In these studies, antihistamines inhibit nuclear factor κB activation resulting from upstream signaling initiated by the activated H_1 receptor.[15] The antihistamine molecules on binding to the histamine receptor cause a shift from the active to the inactive form. This holds true for all antihistamines, even those lacking an ethylamine side chain that resembles that of histamine, thereby disproving previous theories that antihistamines inhibit the histamine receptor through competitive inhibition of the groove where this side chain of histamine binds. As shown in **Table 2**, there are more than 40 antihistamines available for clinical use, most of which target the H_1 receptor. A handful of antihistamines that target the H_2 receptor are also currently in clinical use, but there are no commercially available antihistamines that target the H_3 and H_4 receptors.

ORAL ANTIHISTAMINES IN RHINITIS THERAPY
First-Generation and Second-Generation Oral Antihistamines

The antihistamines used in the therapy for rhinitis are those that target the H_1 receptor. There are 2 classes of H_1 antihistamines: first-generation antihistamines and the newer second-generation antihistamines, first developed in the early 1980s. Unlike second-generation antihistamines, first-generation antihistamines readily cross the blood-brain barrier due to their lipophilicity, have a low molecular weight and a positive electrostatic charge, and are often not recognized by the P-glycoprotein efflux pump. These properties of first-generation antihistamines lead to adverse CNS effects, especially sedation, which can impair performance during work, school, or even activities of daily living. The use of these medications is, therefore, often limited to the evening hours, but even bedtime administration sometimes results in sedation and impaired performance the morning after ingestion.[25] Sedation has decreased the use of first-generation antihistamines in favor of second-generation antihistamines,

Table 1
Histamine receptors: expression, function, and available inverse agonists

Receptor	Receptor Expression	General Function	Function in Allergic Inflammation and Immune Modulation	Inverse Agonists Available Clinically
H_1 Receptor	• Nerve cells • Airway and vascular smooth muscle cells • Endothelial cells • Epithelial cells • Neutrophils, eosinophils, monocytes/macrophages, DCs, T and B cells • Hepatocytes • Chondrocytes	• Pruritis, pain • Vasodilation, vascular permeability, hypotension • Flushing, headache, tachycardia • Bronchoconstriction, cough receptor stimulation, airway vagal afferent nerve stimulation • ↓ AV node conduction time	• ↑ Release of histamine and other mediators • ↑ Cellular adhesion molecule expression • ↑ Eosinophil and neutrophil chemotaxis • ↑ APC capacity and costimulatory activity on B cells	More than 40 available for allergic disease and urticaria (see **Table 2**)
H_2 Receptor	• Nerve cells • Airway and vascular smooth muscle cells • Endothelial cells • Epithelial cells • PMNs, eosinophils, monocytes, DC, T and B cells • Hepatocytes • Chondrocytes	• Gastric acid secretion • Vascular permeability, hypotension • Flushing, headache • Tachycardia, chronotropic and inotropic activity • Bronchodilation, airway mucus production	• Suppresses T_h2 cells and cytokines • ↑ Humoral immunity • ↓ Cellular immunity • ↓ IL-12 by DCs • ↓ Eosinophil and neutrophil chemotaxis, • Role in graft rejection, autoimmunity, malignancy • ↑ IL-10 and induced development of T_h2 or tolerance-inducing DCs	Cimetidine, famotidine, nizatidine, ranitidine for PUD, GERD, and related disorders

Receptor			
H₃ Receptor	• High expression in histaminergic neurons • High expression in eosinophils, monocytes, DC • Low expression in peripheral tissues	• Pruritis independent of mast cells • Nasal congestion • Controls degree of bronchoconstriction	• Likely plays a role in neurogenic inflammation through local neuron-mast cell feedback loops • ↑ APC capacity and proinflammatory activity	Currently being developed for narcolepsy, dementia, schizophrenia, and other CNS disorders
H₄ Receptor	• Bone marrow and peripheral hematopoietic cells • PMNs, eosinophils, DC, T cells, mast cells, basophils • Hepatocytes • Chondrocytes	• Pruritus independent of mast cells • Nasal congestion • Differentiation of myeloblasts and promyelocytes	• ↑ Calcium flux in eosinophils • ↑ Eosinophil chemotaxis • ↑ IL-16 production with help of H₂ receptor	Currently being developed for allergic rhinitis

Abbreviations: APC, antigen presenting cell; AV, atrioventricular; DC, dendric cell; GERD, gastroesophageal reflux disease; IL, interleukin; PUD, peptic ulcer disease; Tₕ2, helper T cells type 2; ↑, increase; ↓, decrease.
Data from Refs.[7–9]

Table 2
Pharmacokinetics and pharmacodynamics of Oral H1 Antihistamines[a]

H1 Antihistamines	Onset of Action (h)[b]	Duration of Action (h)[c]	T_{max} After a Single Dose (h)[c]	$T_{1/2}$ (h); Name and $T_{1/2}$ (h) of Metabolite, if Active[16]	Skin Test Suppression Mean (max) in Days[16]	Usual Adult Dose	Dose Adjustment in Renal/Hepatic Impairment[9]
First-Generation							
Chlorpheniramine	3	24	2.8 ± 0.8	–; 27.9 ± 8.7 for Mono- and didesmethyl chlorpheniramine	3[17] (6[18])	4 mg TID or QID; 12 mg (sustained-release formulation) TID	Neither
Diphenhydramine	2	12	1.7 ± 1.0	–; 9.2 ± 2.5 for Nordophenhydramine	2[17] (5)[17]	25–50 mg TID or QHS	Hepatic
Doxepin[19]	—	—	2	13; 31 for N-desmethyldoxepin	6[20]	25–50 mg TID or QHS	Hepatic
Hydroxyzine	2	24	2.1 ± 0.4	20 ± 4.1[21]	5[17] (8)[17]	25–50 mg TID or QHS	Hepatic
Second-Generation							
Acrivastine	1	8	1.4 ± 0.4	1.4–3.1[21]	~3, $T_{1/2}$ = 1.7 h	8 mg TID	Renal/hepatic
Cetirizine	1	24	1.0 ± 0.5	7–11[21]	3[22]	5–10 mg QDay	Renal/hepatic
Desloratadine	2	24	1–3	27; 7/8 ± 4.2 for 3-OH-desloratadine	~7 ($T_{1/2}$ = 31 h)[23]	5 mg QDay	Renal/hepatic

Ebastine[d]	2	24	2.6–5.7	–; 10.3–19.3 for Carebastine	—	10–20 mg QDay	Renal/hepatic
Fexofenadine	2	24	2.6	14.4–14.6	2[22]	60 mg TID; 180 mg QDay	Renal
Levocetirizine	1	24	0.8 ± 0.5	7 ± 1.5	3–4[8]	5 mg QDay	Renal/hepatic
Loratadine	2	24	1.2 ± 0.3	7.8 ± 4.2; 24 ± 9.8 for Descarboethoxyloratadine	7[22]	10 mg QDay	Hepatic
Mizolastine[d]	1	24	1.5	12.9	—	10 mg QDay	Neither
Intranasal							
Azelastine hydrochloride	15 min	12	2–4	22–25; 52–57 for Desmethylazelastine	2[22,24]	1–2 Sprays per nostril BID	Neither
Olapatadine hydrochloride	30 min	12	0.25–2	8–12	Unknown	2 Sprays per nostril BID	Neither

Abbreviations: BID, twice a day; max, maximum; QDay, daily; TID, 3 times daily; $T_{1/2}$, half-life; T_{max}, time to peak plasma concentration, measured from the time of oral intake; QID, 4 times daily.

[a] Unless otherwise indicated, results expressed as means ±SD or as a range of values.

[b] In general, onset of action is based on wheal-and-flare studies.

[c] In general, duration of action is based on wheal-and-flare studies.

[d] Second-generation H1 antihistamines were not available in the United States at the time of publication.

Data from Refs.[8,9,16–22,24]

which are able to distribute widely throughout the body, usually with little CNS penetration. Fexofenadine, in particular, is readily recognized by the P-glycoprotein efflux pump in both the gastrointestinal tract and CNS, keeping it out of these regions and thereby theoretically eliminating CNS side effects completely.[26] One of the main benefits of second-generation antihistamines is their increased selectivity for the H_1 receptor compared with first-generation antihistamines that also bind to and inhibit muscarinic cholinergic, α-adrenergic, and serotonin receptors. The increased selectivity of second-generation antihistamines decreases the anticholinergic side effects of dry mouth, urinary retention, constipation, and tachycardia that can be seen with many first-generation antihistamines.[23,26–29]

Since the discovery of the first clinically useful H_1 antihistamine in 1942, there have been more than 40 such antihistamines discovered, and they have become one of the mainstays of treatment in allergic diseases.[9] All H_1 antihistamines have an ethylamine group, making them structurally similar to each other and to histamine (**Fig. 1**). Many of the newer antihistamines are metabolites or enantiomers of older antihistamines. For example, levocetirizine is an enantiomer of cetirizine, which is a metabolite of the first-generation antihistamine hydroxyzine. Similarly, desloratadine is a metabolite of loratadine, and fexofenadine is a metabolite of terfenadine, although the latter is no longer used in most countries due to cardiotoxicity.[9] Based on their side group, most of the H_1 antihistamines fall into 1 of the following 6 categories: alkylamines, piperazines, piperidines, ethanolamines, ethylenediamines, and phenothiazines. Among the first-generation antihistamines, foxepin is unique in that it has potent H_1 antihistamine activity that is approximately 800 times stronger than diphenhydramine as measured by receptor antagonism as well as significant H_2 antihistamine activity that is approximately 5 times weaker than cimetidine, in addition to its tricyclic antidepressant properties.[30,31]

The pharmacokinetics and pharmacodynamics of oral H_1 antihistamines vary from one drug to the next, as shown in **Table 2**. In general, second-generation antihistamines tend to have more favorable pharmacokinetics than first-generation drugs with rapid and near-complete absorption as well as a relatively long half-life that allows for daily dosing, features that further enhance their use in clinical practice.[27] The following drug-drug interactions are particularly important: fexofenadine binds to aluminum-containing or magnesium-containing antacids taken within 15 minutes of ingestion, decreasing fexofenadine plasma concentrations in a clinically relevant manner; grapefruit juice inhibits the P-glycoprotein pump in vitro and can decrease the plasma concentration of fexofenadine up to 40%[27]; inhibitors of the cytochrome P450 system, such as macrolide antibiotics or imidazole antifungals, increase concentrations of all first-generation H_1 antihistamines and some second-generation antihistamines, such as loratadine, desloratadine, and rupatadine, that use this system for their metabolism.[9,28,32]

The allergic response consists of 2 phases, the early phase and the late phase. The early phase, triggered by the binding of allergen to IgE on mast cells with subsequent IgE cross-linking and mast cell degranulation, is characterized by the release of preformed mediators, such as histamine, and the synthesis of newly formed mediators, such as prostaglandin D_2, cysteinyl leukotrienes, and platelet activating factor. The late phase response, which generally occurs with a several-hour delay, consists of tissue infiltration with eosinophils, basophils, T cells, neutrophils, and macrophages and subsequent cytokine release perpetuating the inflammatory response.[27] In vivo and in vitro studies have demonstrated that second-generation antihistamines decrease both phases of the allergic response, possessing both antiallergic and anti-inflammatory properties. They do so in part by directly inhibiting the calcium ion

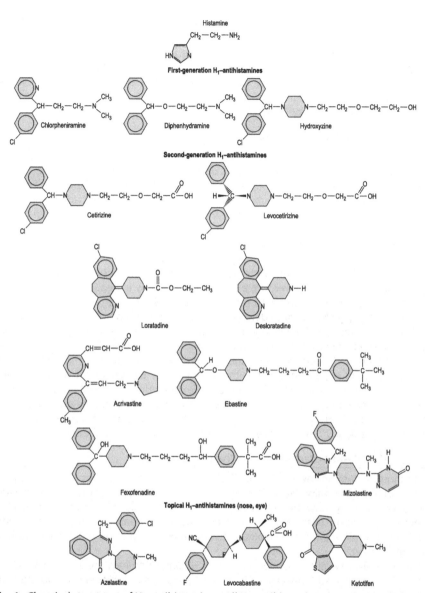

Fig. 1. Chemical structures of H₁ antihistamines. All H₁ antihistamines contain an ethylamine group and thus have some resemblance to histamine. In part because of this, many H₁ antihistamines are structurally similar to each other. As shown in the figure, cetirizine and levocetirizine are enantiomers and are thus structurally similar. Metabolites also tend to resemble their parent drug, which is shown here for cetirizine and hydroxyzine as well as desloratadine and loratadine. (*From* Simons FE, Akdis CA. Histamine and H1-antihistamines. In: Adkinson NF Jr, Bochner BS, Busse WW, et al, editors. Middleton's allergy: principles and practice. 7th edition. St Louis (MO): Mosby; 2009; with permission.)

channels of mast cell and basophils[13] as well as by decreasing eosinophil chemotaxis,[3] inhibiting intercellular adhesion molecule 1 expression on nasal epithelium,[33] and curbing inflammation mediated by various other cell types, such as epithelial cells and lymphocytes.[34,35] In clinical trials, H_1 antihistamine administration before allergen challenge has been shown to decrease the levels of cytokines, proinflammatory cell adhesion molecules, and other mediators, such as leukotrienes and prostaglandins, in addition to histamine.[36–38]

Dosing of Oral Antihistamines for Rhinitis Therapy

Dosing for most of the first-generation antihistamines has been determined based on clinical experience rather than studies as opposed to the second-generation antihistamines where dose-ranging studies have been performed. As shown in **Table 3**, dosing recommendations for each of the oral antihistamines varies according to the population treated, with special consideration given to the elderly, children, and those with renal or hepatic impairment.[27] Dose-ranging studies performed with cetirizine have shown that higher doses provide greater suppression of the wheal and flare reaction and have greater impact on allergic rhinitis symptoms and quality-of-life (QOL) scores, particularly in patients with higher nasal symptom scores at baseline.[39–42] Such dose increases, however, are also accompanied by increased sedation, hence the current recommendation for 10-mg daily dosing. Similarly, the dosing recommendation of 10 mg daily for loratadine comes from a study comparing this dose with a 40-mg daily dose, which showed an increase in sedation at the higher dose with no added effectiveness.[43,44] Dose-ranging studies for fexofenadine have led to the current United States dosing regimens (60 mg twice daily or 180 mg daily), which were each found significantly better than placebo for the treatment of both rhinitis and conjunctivitis symptoms.[45,46] In Europe, fexofenadine is dosed at 120 mg daily based on these same studies. No benefit was found to increasing the dose of fexofenadine in the twice-daily dosing studies,[45,46] and there was no statistically significant difference in efficacy or QOL between the 120-mg and 180-mg dosages.[47]

Efficacy of Oral Antihistamines in the Treatment of Rhinitis

Regarding efficacy in the treatment of allergic rhinitis, few studies have been performed of first-generation H_1 antihistamines.[8,9,48–52] Second-generation H_1 antihistamines, alternatively, have been studied in many rigorous clinical trials (summarized in **Table 3**) that demonstrate the efficacy of these agents in treating both intermittent and persistent allergic rhinitis with minimal adverse effects and good patient acceptance and satisfaction.[8,9]

The currently available second-generation H_1 antihistamines are listed in **Table 2**. Those commonly used in the United States include cetirizine, levocetirizine, loratadine, desloratadine, and fexofenadine. Of these agents, cetirizine and levocetirizine are considered sedating and are, therefore, prohibited for people in certain occupations that demand high psychomotor skills, such as flying airplanes or operating heavy machinery.[53–55] Loratadine, desloratadine, and fexofenadine, alternatively, are considered nonsedating antihistamines if prescribed at their recommended doses.[56,57]

Cetirizine and its enantiomer levocetirizine are zwitterions, molecules with an overall neutral charge despite portions of the molecule having a positive or negative charge, a property that allows for lower serum concentrations, reduced volume of distribution, and less cardiotoxicity due to decreased affinity for the myocardium without compromising efficacy.[53,54,58] As shown in **Table 3**, cetirizine and levocetirizine have proved more efficacious than placebo for the treatment of intermittent and persistent allergic rhinitis in several trials studying symptom relief and QOL. To a lesser degree, both

Table 3
Recommended daily[a] dosage of second-generation oral antihistamines and intranasal antihistamines in various populations

Drug	Adults (≥12 y)	Children	Elderly	Adjustment for Renal Impairment	Adjustment for Hepatic Impairment
Cetirizine	5–10 mg	6–12 mo[b]: 2.5 mg; 12 mo–2 y[b]: 2.5 mg; May increase to 2.5 mg BID; 2–5 y: 2.5 mg; May increase to 2.5 mg BID or 5 mg; 6–11 y: 5–10 mg	Same	<6 y: Not recommended; 6–11 y: <2.5 mg; ≥12 y: Depends on creatinine clearance[c]	<6 y: Not recommended; 6–11 y: <2.5 mg; ≥12 y: 5 mg
Levocetirizine	5 mg[d]	6 mo–5 y[b]: 1.25 mg; 6–11 y: 2.5 mg	2.5–5 mg	6 mo–11 y: Contraindicated; ≥12 y: Depends on creatinine clearance[e]	None
Loratadine	10 mg	2–5 y[f]: 5 mg; 6–11 y[f]: 10 mg	Same	2–5 y: 5 mg QOD; ≥6 y: 10 mg QOD	2–5 y: 5 mg QOD; ≥6 y: 10 mg QOD
Desloratadine	5 mg	6–11 mo: 1 mg; 12 mo–5 y: 1.25 mg; 6–11 y: 2.5 mg	Same	Children: not established; ≥12 y: 5 mg QOD	5 mg QOD
Fexofenadine	180 mg or 60 mg BID	2–11 y: 30 mg BID	Start at 60 mg	2–11 y: 30 mg; ≥12 y: 60 mg	None
Azelastine (intranasal)	SAR: 1–2 sprays per nostril BID; VMR: 2 sprays per nostril BID	5–11 y: 1 spray per nostril BID	Same	None	None
Olopatadine (intranasal)	SAR: 2 sprays per nostril BID	Not approved for <12 y	Same	None	None

Abbreviations: BID, twice daily; QDay, daily; QOD, every 48 hours; PAR, perennial allergic rhinitis; SAR, seasonal allergic rhinitis; VMR, vasomotor rhinitis.
a Unless specified.
b Approved down to 6 mo for PAR but only down to 2 y for SAR.
c Some adults may respond to 2.5 mg daily.
d Creatinine clearance <11 mL/min, not on dialysis: not recommended; 11–31 mL/min or hemodialysis: 5 mg daily.
e Creatinine clearance <10: contraindicated; 10–30 mL/min: 2.5 mg every 3 or 4 days; 30–50 mL/min: 2.5 mg every other day; 50–80 mL/min: 2.5 mg daily.
f Approved only for SAR in children.
Data from Golightly LK, Greos LS. Second-generation antihistamines: actions and efficacy in the management of allergic disorders. Drugs 2005;65(3):341–84; and LexiComp Online drug reference.

cetirizine and levocetirizine have demonstrated efficacy in allergic conjunctivitis symptoms and on nasal congestion, which has traditionally not been a feature of oral antihistamines unless combined with a decongestant.[59,60] QOL can be improved with regular use of either drug,[59,61] and an added benefit has been observed from daily rather than on demand use.[59,62] Higher doses of cetirizine (20 mg daily) improved not only rhinitis symptoms and nasal obstruction but also lower airway symptoms, peak flow measurements, and the need for rescue inhalers in patients with concurrent asthma.[63] In one study of patient preference, the majority of patients who had previously used cetirizine, loratadine, or desloratadine preferred levocetirizine over these other antihistamines.[61]

Loratadine and its metabolite desloratadine are also effective therapies for intermittent and persistent allergic rhinitis, as demonstrated by the studies summarized in **Table 3**. For intermittent allergic rhinitis, loratadine (10 mg daily) helps decrease rhinitis symptoms, with less benefit on nasal obstruction compared with other nasal symptoms.[41] Similar symptomatic relief has been reported for persistent allergic rhinitis, for which one study of loratadine (10 mg daily) demonstrated a gradual increase in symptom improvement over the course of a 28-day treatment period. An additional benefit loratadine is the decrease in both early and late phases of the conjunctival allergic reaction,[37,43] a finding also true for desloratadine.[64]

Fexofenadine, another second-generation antihistamine, has been shown efficacious in various placebo-controlled trials, as depicted in **Table 3**. Like other antihistamines (discussed previously), fexofenadine has an impact on nasal itching, rhinorrhea, and sneezing as well as conjunctival symptoms, with only a small effect on nasal obstruction.[34] Several studies have demonstrated an improvement in QOL for subjects treated with fexofenadine compared with placebo or other antihistamines.[34,47,65] As discussed previously, fexofenadine is unique in that it does not penetrate the CNS due to the effect of the P-glycoprotein efflux pump, translating clinically into less sedation, which was found in comparison trials between fexofenadine and other antihistamines.[66] Unlike its parent drug, terfenadine, fexofenadine does not have cardiotoxic effects.

As shown in **Table 4**, although several studies have compared the second-generation antihistamines, no single drug is considered the best. As such, the decision about which antihistamine to prescribe remains a personalized decision depending on cost and insurance concerns, side-effect profile, and a patient's symptom complex and preference. One placebo-controlled, double-blind study of 688 patients with intermittent allergic rhinitis compared fexofenadine (120 mg daily) with loratadine (10 mg daily) over a 2-week period and demonstrated similar decreases in sneezing, nasal itching, and rhinorrhea but more benefit in nasal congestion and conjunctivitis symptoms in the fexofenadine group.[34] In addition to symptomatic benefit, fexofenadine had a significantly greater improvement in QOL, as measured by the Rhinoconjunctivitis Quality of Life Questionnaire (RQLQ), when compared with placebo or loratadine.[34] Another study by Lee and colleagues[105] compared a single dose of levocetirizine, desloratadine, and fexofenadine in a crossover study assessing the ability of each drug to improve nasal peak inspiratory flow in 16 persistent allergic rhinitis patients challenged with adenosine monophosphate. All 3 antihistamines improved nasal peak inspiratory flow to a similar degree, which was higher than for placebo. As shown in **Table 4**, several studies have compared the efficacy of cetirizine and fexofenadine, demonstrating significant benefit of both drugs over placebo but similar efficacy between them.[59,66,94] One finding when comparing the 2 drugs, however, is decreased sedation with fexofenadine compared with cetirizine.[94] A similar conclusion can be drawn from 2 studies that compare standard dosing of desloratadine and fexofenadine in the treatment of intermittent allergic rhinitis.[100,101] Comparison studies between cetirizine and loratadine, alternatively, demonstrate a fairly consistent benefit in the efficacy of cetirizine over loratadine.[97–99,106] The 2 studies comparing loratadine and fexofenadine showed that either antihistamine is superior to placebo, with 1 study demonstrating equal efficacy between the 2 drugs and the other showing superior efficacy for fexofenadine over loratadine therapy.[34,102,103] In the 2 studies comparing levocetirizine and desloratadine, both drugs demonstrated superior efficacy compared with placebo in decreasing the symptoms of allergic rhinitis, doing so to a similar degree, except for nasal congestion where levocetirizine was overall superior.[60,107]

Oral Antihistamines as Add-on Therapy to Intranasal Corticosteroids in the Treatment of Rhinitis

Although oral antihistamines are beneficial in the treatment of rhinitis, as discussed previously, several studies have demonstrated that combining an oral antihistamine with intranasal steroid does not provide added benefit to the use of intranasal steroid spray alone.[108–111]

The first of these studies was performed in 1989 and compared intranasal beclomethasone (400 μg daily), astemizole (10 mg daily), and combination therapy. In this 6-week study of 90 adult subjects evaluating nasal symptom scores, intranasal beclomethasone was superior to that of astemizole alone with no added benefit from combination therapy in rhinitis symptoms compared with intranasal beclomethasone alone.[108] A similar study in 1998 compared fluticasone (200 μg once daily), loratadine (10 mg daily), and combination therapy of these 2 agents. This 2-week study of 600 patients showed a similar improvement in RQLQ for the fluticasone only and combination therapy groups.[109] A 2004 study of 100 patients examining intranasal steroid, oral antihistamine, and leukotriene antagonist therapy in various combinations over the course of 6 weeks demonstrated similar results. All groups treated with intranasal steroid (monotherapy with fluticasone [200 μg once daily], fluticasone plus cetirizine [10 mg each morning], and fluticasone plus montelukast [10 mg each evening]) demonstrated similar improvements in nasal congestion, both on awakening and during the day. Again, there was no benefit to adding oral antihistamine to intranasal steroids regarind congestion, and this study demonstrated an advantage in decreasing nasal itching for the fluticasone-only group over combination therapy ($P = .003$).[110] In 2006, 27 patients were treated with fluticasone (200 μg daily) and either levocetirizine (5 mg) or placebo for 2 weeks during allergy season with no benefit to combination therapy over fluticasone therapy alone in any of the following categories: RQLQ; domiciliary peak nasal inspiratory flow; total nasal symptom score (TNSS), which assesses itchy nose, runny nose, stuffy nose, and sneezing; and nasal nitric oxide concentrations.[111] Ocular symptoms were not evaluated in any of these studies and may represent an area of potential benefit for the addition of oral antihistamines to intranasal steroid therapy.

INTRANASAL ANTIHISTAMINES IN RHINITIS THERAPY

A major advance in the treatment of rhinitis has been the development of intranasal antihistamines as a way of delivering antihistamine therapy directly to the nasal mucosa. The advantages of such therapy include attaining higher concentrations of active drug directly to the target tissue with the added benefit of reduced systemic side effects.[112] Since the development of the first intranasal antihistamine, several studies have been performed to determine their proper role in the treatment of rhinitis, and their use has increased considerably. In the most recent practice parameters

Table 4
Studies evaluating efficacy of second-generation antihistamines

Medication	Dose	Type of AR	# of Patients	Age Range	Duration (weeks)	Symptom Decrease (%)	Comparative Efficacy	References
Cetirizine	CTZ 10 mg	SAR	20	19–48	4	50	CTZ > PLA	62
	CTZ 10 mg	SAR	375	>15	4	49	CTZ > PLA	67
	CTZ 10 mg	SAR	865	18–65	2	29	CTZ > PLA	68
	CTZ 10 mg	SAR	403	18–65	2	28	CTZ > PLA	69
	CTZ 20 mg	PAR	28	13–59	26	36	CTZ > PLA	63
	CTZ 10–20 mg	PAR	220	18–70	4	43	CTZ > PLA	70
	CTZ 5 mg	PAR	24	18–32	n/a	39	CTZ > PLA	71
	CTZ 10 mg	PAR	274	18–60	6	35	CTZ > PLA	59
	CTZ 10 mg	PAR	143	17–67	52	33	NS	72
Levocetirizine	LEVO 5 mg	SAR	577	NS	2	NS	LEVO > PLA	73
	LEVO 5 mg	SAR	596	18–65	2	NS	LEVO = PLA	74
	LEVO 5 mg	SAR	1290	NS	4	NS	LEVO > previous AH	61
	LEVO 5 mg	PAR	294	≥12	6	86	LEVO > PLA	75
	LEVO 5 mg	PAR	551	>18	4	NS	LEVO > PLA	76
	LEVO 5 mg	PAR	551	>18	24	NS	LEVO > PLA	77
Fexofenadine	FEX 120 mg	SAR	99	14–62	n/a	85	FEX > PLA	78
	FEX 60 mg	SAR	651	12–65	2	74	FEX > PLA	79
	FEX 180 mg	SAR	861	12–65	2	59	FEX > PLA	80
	FEX 120 mg	SAR	545	12–65	2	21	FEX > PLA	45
	FEX 180 mg	SAR	845	12–65	2	63	FEX > PLA	47
	FEX 240 mg	SAR	570	12–66	2	28	FEX > PLA	46
	FEX 120–180 mg	PAR	31	Adult	4	66	FEX > PLA	81
Loratadine	LOR	SAR	338	12–82	1	38	LOR > PLA	82

LOR 10 mg	PAR	14	Adult	2	36	NS	83
LOR 10 mg	SAR	835	12–60	1	NS	LOR > PLA	84
Desloratadine							
DES 5 mg	SAR	346	12–65	2	44	DES > PLA	85
DES 5 mg	SAR	46	19–34	2	43	DES > PLA	86
DES 5 mg, 7.5 mg	SAR	677	12–72	2	NS	DES > PLA	87
DES	SAR	407	NS	2	NS	DES > PLA	88
DES 5 mg	SAR	331	15–75	4	36	DES > PLA	89
DES 2.5–20 mg	SAR	1026	12–75	n/a	29–38	DES > PLA	90
DES 5 mg	PAR	634	≥12	4	38	DES > PLA	91
DES 5 mg	SAR	547	≥12	2	NS	DES > PLA	92
DES 5 mg	PAR	716	≥12	12	NS	DES > PLA	93
Comparative Studies							
CTZ 10 mg / FEX 120 mg	SAR	39	20–36	n/a	48 / 47	CTZ = FEX > PLA	94
CTZ 10 mg / FEX 180 mg	SAR	722	12–66	2	45 / 45	CTZ = FEX > PLA	95
CTZ 10 mg / FEX 180 mg	SAR	495	12–70	2	22 / 19	CTZ = FEX	66
CTZ 10 mg / LOR 10 mg	SAR	278	13–62	n/a	57 / 35	CTZ > LOR > PLA	96
CTZ 10 mg / LOR 10 mg	SAR	111	14–70	n/a	70 / 50	CTZ > LOR > PLA	97
CTZ 10 mg / LOR 10 mg	SAR	360	16–65	n/a	25 / 11	CTZ > LOR > PLA	98
CTZ 10 mg / LOR 10 mg	SAR	194	16–80	n/a	37 / 15	CTZ > LOR > PLA	99
DES 5 mg / FEX 180 mg	SAR	49	NS	2	24 / 22	DES = FEX > PLA	100

(continued on next page)

Table 4
(continued)

Medication	Dose	Type of AR	# of Patients	Age Range	Duration (weeks)	Symptom Decrease (%)	Comparative Efficacy	References
	DES 5 mg FEX 180 mg	SAR	722	NS	2	NS	DES = FEX > PLA	101
	LOR 10 mg FEX 120 mg	SAR	680	12–75	2	32 44	FEX > LOR > PLA	34,102
	LOR 10 mg FEX 120 mg	SAR	569	≥12	2	~79 ~79	FEX = LOR > PLA	103
	DES 5 mg previous AH	SAR/CIU	77	≥12	5.5	NS	DES > previous AH	104
	LOR 10 mg EBAS 10 mg EBAS 20 mg	PAR	317	12–68	1	32 44 47	EBAS > LOR	64

Abbreviations: AH, antihistamine; AR, allergic rhinitis; CTZ, cetirizine; DES, desloratadine; EBAS, ebastine; FEX, fexofenadine; LEVO, levocetirizine; LOR, loratadine n/a, not applicable; NS, not stated; PAR, perennial allergic rhinitis; PLA, placebo; SAR, seasonal allergic rhinitis.
Data from Refs. 9,34,41,45–47,59,61,63,64,66–94,96–104

released by the American Academy of Asthma Allergy and Immunology in 2008 to help guide rhinitis therapy, nasal antihistamines are considered "efficacious and equal to or superior to oral second-generation antihistamines for treatment of intermittent allergic rhinitis" with a similar role in the treatment of episodic allergic rhinitis given their rapid onset of action.[16] Although the parameters cite evidence that "intranasal antihistamines are generally less effective than intranasal corticosteroids for treatment of allergic rhinitis," the literature is sparse and at times conflicting on this issue.[113] As such, the parameters conclude that intranasal antihistamines should be considered "first-line treatment for allergic and nonallergic rhinitis" and an "appropriate choice for mixed rhinitis" given the approved indication of azelastine for vasomotor rhinitis. Two unique features of intranasal antihistamines highlighted in these parameters are the "clinically significant effect on nasal congestion" and a potential benefit for ocular allergic symptoms.[16]

Intranasal Antihistamines Available for Clinical Use

Azelastine hydrochloride and olopatadine hydrochloride are the 2 antihistamines currently commercially available in intranasal form in the United States (see **Table 2**). Three formulations of azelastine hydrochloride nasal spray have been developed, the original 0.1% aqueous solution and a reformulated solution using sorbitol and sucralose to mask the bitter taste of the original formulation. Two head-to-head comparisons of the original formulation with the sucralose-based 0.1% formulation demonstrated a comparable safety profile and similar pharmacokinetics.[114] Although the reformulated solution originally came in the same 0.1% strength as the original formulation, this strength was recently discontinued and replaced by the same formulation in a new 0.15% strength. A 2009 study by Shah and colleagues[115] comparing the 0.1% and 0.15% strengths of azelastine found that both decreased TNSS scores compared with placebo, but the higher dose did so to a greater degree ($P<.05$) with only a slight increase in somnolence. The other intranasal antihistamine currently available in the United States is olopatadine, which comes only as a 0.6% aqueous solution. The main side effects of intranasal antihistamines are bitter taste and somnolence,[16] both of which are less for olopatadine compared with azelastine. Although somnolence was greater with azelastine nasal spray than placebo in earlier studies, more recent trials of azelastine in the treatment of nonallergic rhinitis have not shown a statistical difference in somnolence between azelastine and placebo groups (3.2% vs 1.0%).[16,116,117]

Efficacy of Intranasal Antihistamines in the Treatment of Rhinitis

The efficacy of azelastine and olopatadine nasal sprays has been assessed in various randomized, double-blind, placebo-controlled trials. Azelastine was first evaluated in 1994 through 2 day-in-the-park studies where more than 500 patients were exposed to aeroallergens for 8 hours on 2 consecutive days and then randomized to varying doses of azelastine nasal spray, oral chlorpheniramine, or placebo. In both studies, patients receiving azelastine demonstrated an improvement in rhinitis symptoms compared with the placebo group, as measured by symptom diaries in the first study and by major symptom complex (MSC), assessing nose blows, sneezes, runny nose/sniffles, itchy nose, and watery eyes, and total symptom complex (TSC), assessing those symptoms incorporated in the MSC as well as cough, postnasal drip, and itchy eyes, ears, throat, and palate scores in the second study. Both studies demonstrated duration of action ranging from 12 to 24 hours after a single dose of azelastine, thus supporting a once-daily to twice-daily dosing regimen.[118,119] These studies were followed by two 2-week trials and one 4-week trial of azelastine for the treatment of intermittent allergic rhinitis. The 2-week trials randomized 498 patients to once-daily or twice-daily azelastine, daily chlorpheniramine, or placebo during pollen season. Azelastine administered twice daily again demonstrated a significant decrease in TSC and MSC compared with placebo ($P<.01$), and once-daily dosing trended toward a similar benefit for azelastine over placebo.[120,121] The 4-week trial evaluated 264 patients randomized to these same treatment arms for 2 extra weeks and demonstrated a statistically significant difference in overall mean percentage of MSC improvement ($P = .04$) with a nonstatistically significant trend in overall mean percentage of TSC improvement for those patients receiving azelastine compared with placebo.[122] Although the standard dosing for azelastine is 2 sprays per nostril twice daily, 2 recent placebo-controlled trials evaluated the efficacy of lowering this dose to 1 spray per nostril twice daily in 554 patients over a 2-week period during the spring pollen season and found a significant reduction in TNSS as well as individual symptom scores compared with placebo, with fewer reports of somnolence or bitter taste than the incidences published for the dose of 2 sprays per nostril twice daily.[123]

The data supporting the use of olopatadine nasal spray in the treatment of intermittent allergic rhinitis come mainly from two 3-week multicenter trials that evaluated 1233 patients randomized to receive olopatadine 0.4%, olopatadine 0.6%, or placebo. The 0.6% strength of olopatadine demonstrated a statistically significant decrease in both reflective TNSS and instantaneous TNSS as well as a decrease in ocular symptoms and nasal congestion, although the latter only reached statistical significance in 1 of the 2 studies.[124,125] When data from these 2 studies were pooled, reduction in TNSS correlated with a beneficial impact on QOL as measured by the overall RQLQ score and correlated with decreased impact on work and daily activities as measured by the Work Productivity and Activity Impairment Questionnaire-Allergy Specific ($r = 0.45$ to 0.61, $P<.001$).[125] An improvement in RQLQ with olopatadine treatment was also reported in a trial of 677 patients randomized to treatment with olopatadine 0.4%, olopatadine 0.6%, or placebo. Based on allergen chamber studies, the 0.6% formulation was superior in efficacy and is thus the marketed concentration.[126]

In previous comparisons of olopatadine and azelastine nasal sprays, the 2 medications seem to have similar efficacy. A 2009 study of 544 patients compared olopatadine 0.6%, azelastine 0.1%, and placebo (2 sprays per nostril administered twice daily for 16 days). There was a greater reduction in TNSS for both the olopatadine and azelastine groups compared with placebo, with no difference between the different antihistamine sprays. Although adverse effects were rare for both antihistamine nasal sprays, there were more complaints of bitter taste in the azelastine group ($P = .05$).[127] Comparable efficacy between these 2 medications was also shown in a smaller 2008 study of 20 patients comparing symptom relief from olopatadine 0.1%, olopatadine 0.2%, and azelastine 0.1% (2 sprays per nostril administered before an allergen challenge), with similar benefit from all 3 sprays.[128]

Comparison of Intranasal Antihistamines and Intranasal Corticosteroids

The contention that intranasal corticosteroids are superior to intranasal antihistamines, as stated in the 2008 practice parameters, is based largely on the results of a meta-analysis published in 2002 and required further consideration. Of the 9 studies incorporated in the 2002 meta-analysis, 3 evaluated intranasal levocabastine, which is currently unavailable in the United States, and the other 6 compared varying doses of azelastine with several intranasal corticosteroids, including beclomethasone, budesonide, and fluticasone. These studies suggested that intranasal corticosteroids were overall more effective than intranasal antihistamines in reducing TNSS and in reducing the symptoms of rhinorrhea and nasal itching, although to a more variable degree than with overall TNSS. The conclusions drawn from this meta-analysis must be taken with caution because several of the studies of azelastine used subtherapeutic doses of the drug. In addition, intranasal steroids did not prove beneficial for ocular symptoms and nasal congestion when these symptoms were taken alone, whereas intranasal antihistamines have been shown to benefit both.[129]

Since the publication of this meta-analysis, a recent trial has brought the superiority of intranasal corticosteroids into question. In 2009, Kaliner and colleagues[130] published a double-blind, randomized, parallel-group, 2-week noninferiority trial demonstrating no statistically significant difference between olopatadine 0.6% (2 sprays per nostril twice daily) and fluticasone propionate (50 µg, 2 sprays per nostril daily) when analyzing TNSS reduction or individual symptoms of congestion, runny nose, sneezing, itchy nose, and ocular symptoms in 130 symptomatic patients with intermittent allergic rhinitis. The only statistically significant difference between the 2 groups was a faster onset of action of olopatadine compared with fluticasone propionate.

A recent trial by Ratner and colleagues[131] suggests that combination therapy with intranasal corticosteroid and intranasal antihistamine may be the best approach. In this 2-week multicenter trial, the following therapies were compared for their ability to decrease TNSS: azelastine (2 sprays per nostril twice daily), fluticasone (2 sprays per nostril once daily), and combination of the 2. Combination therapy was found superior to each of the monotherapy regimens, with a reduction in TNSS scores of 37.9% in the combined therapy group compared with 27.1% and 24.8% in the azelastine and fluticasone monotherapy groups, respectively.

Onset of Action of Intranasal Antihistamines

As concluded by Kaliner and colleagues[130] in their 2009 study (referenced previously), one benefit of intranasal antihistamines over intranasal corticosteroids is the more rapid onset of action of the former. This benefit was first demonstrated in the 2007 study by Patel and colleagues[132] that compared olopatadine and mometasone nasal sprays in an allergen exposure chamber, yielding an onset of action of 30 and 150 minutes, respectively, based on TNSS recorded by 425 patients every 30 minutes after spray administration. The 30-minute onset of action was confirmed by another 2007 study demonstrating symptom improvement 30 minutes after administration of olopatadine 0.2%, olopatadine 0.4%, or olopatadine 0.6% with a similar study design.[133] Symptoms were not assessed before 30 minutes in the 2007 or 2009 studies of olopatadine versus intranasal steroids; hence, the possibility exists that the onset of action is more rapid than 30 minutes for olopatadine. Original studies of azelastine, alternatively, began symptom assessments at the 15-minute mark; when compared with mometasone nasal spray, the onset of action of azelastine was 15 minutes compared with mometasone's onset of action of 8 hours, respectively.[134] Azelastine had a faster onset of action than oral desloratadine when both were administered 2 hours after an allergen challenge, with 1 spray of azelastine 0.1% decreasing both MSC and TNSS at 15 minutes compared with 150 minutes for desloratadine.[135] As shown in **Table 2**, the onset of action is faster for intranasal antihistamine compared with all available oral antihistamines, a statement that holds true for all intranasal corticosteroids.[136]

COMPARISON STUDIES BETWEEN INTRANASAL AND ORAL ANTIHISTAMINES

Although intranasal and oral antihistamines are both viable therapeutic options for the treatment of rhinitis in most patients, several studies have demonstrated superior efficacy of intranasal antihistamines over therapy with oral antihistamines. In 2003 and

2004, 2 studies were performed to evaluate the efficacy of azelastine nasal spray in patients inadequately controlled on oral antihistamine therapy. The first study compared twice-daily azelastine to therapy with desloratadine, placebo, or a combination of azelastine and loratadine.[137] The second study compared azelastine monotherapy, fexofenadine monotherapy, and therapy with a combination of these 2 agents.[138] Both studies demonstrated a statistically significant decrease in TNSS for all subjects receiving azelastine spray compared with those receiving placebo therapy or monotherapy with either desloratadine or fexofenadine alone.[137,138] Furthermore, in this subset of patients with inadequate benefit from oral antihistamine monotherapy, there was no added benefit to administering an oral antihistamine concurrent with azelastine nasal spray compared with azelastine monotherapy in either study. Two subsequent trials compared azelastine and cetirizine as a way of directly comparing the efficacy of intranasal and oral antihistamines. The first Azelastine Cetirizine Trial was in 2005 and studied 299 patients,[139] followed shortly by the second Azelastine Cetirizine Trial of 360 patients in 2006.[140] Both studied treatment with azelastine (2 sprays per nostril twice daily) plus a placebo capsule versus a placebo nasal spray plus cetirizine (10 mg capsule daily) over a 2-week period. The azelastine group was superior to the cetirizine group with respect to TNSS in the 2005 Azelastine Cetirizine Trial and regarding RQLQ scores for both trials.[139,140]

USE OF ANTIHISTAMINES IN SPECIAL POPULATIONS

When using antihistamines in clinical practice, special consideration must be given to children, pregnant women, the elderly, and patients with hepatic or renal dysfunction. Dosing for several of these special populations is shown in **Table 4**. Although caution should be used when choosing an agent during pregnancy and lactation, dose adjustment is generally not necessary unless the mother also has hepatic or renal dysfunction.

Antihistamine Use for Rhinitis Therapy in Children

In children, antihistamines are considered first-line agents for the treatment of allergic rhinoconjunctivitis, urticaria, and atopic dermatitis. First-generation antihistamines approved for use in children as young as 2 years of age include diphenhydramine, hydroxyzine, chlorpheniramine, brompheniramine, and clemastine. The anticholinergic and CNS effects of sedation and impairment that limit the use of first-generation antihistamines in adults can also be seen in children. As such, their use is generally limited to cases of pruritus so severe that sedation is a desired side effect or to cases of anaphylaxis where intravenous antihistamines serve as an adjunct to epinephrine therapy. For the treatment of chronic rhinitis, however, second-generation antihistamines are an attractive choice given their efficacy and favorable side-effect profile. The current pediatric dosing recommendations for the most common second-generation antihistamines are shown in **Table 4**. In general, these recommendations are determined by the Food and Drug Administration (FDA) using the pediatric rule, which allows for extrapolation of efficacy from adults to children as long as the pathophysiology, disease course, and drug effects are similar enough between adults and children, as is the case for allergic rhinitis. Once efficacy is extrapolated, pharmacokinetic and pharmacodynamic data are collected to ensure that it is similar for children and adults, followed by a safety study in younger children.[141]

Pharmacokinetic and pharmacodynamic data have been obtained in small children for most of the second-generation antihistamines in small children.[142–147] Of these agents, cetirizine, levocetirizine, and desloratadine have been approved for children as young as 6 months of age, and loratadine and fexofenadine have been approved for children as young as 2 years of age. Trials assessing the efficacy and safety of second-generation oral antihistamines are summarized in **Table 5**. In addition to the oral antihistamines, azelastine nasal spray has been shown to provide symptomatic benefit by reducing scores for total rhinitis symptoms, total nasal symptoms, and ocular symptoms in children with allergic rhinitis and is currently approved for use in children 5 years of age and older.[156,157]

One concern particularly relevant to children is the effect that antihistamines may have on academic performance. Allergic rhinitis itself has been shown to affect learning and school performance; therefore, the possible adverse effect of antihistamine therapy on academic performance must be weighed against the potential benefit of these drugs in enhancing academic performance by decreasing rhinitis symptoms. This balance was addressed in a 1999 study by Tanner and colleagues[65] of more than 500 children with allergic rhinitis, 93% of whom reported an effect on classroom productivity, and 23% reporting missed classroom time due to their rhinitis. After treatment with either placebo or fexofenadine (60 mg twice daily for 2 weeks), there was a significant decrease in missed classroom time and in classroom impairment for those children treated with fexofenadine. Taken together, overall impairment decreased by 41% in the fexofenadine group and only 27% in the placebo group after the 2 weeks of treatment. In a 1993 study by Vuurman and colleagues,[158] academic performance was assessed using didactic stimulation, a validated tool that involves acquiring knowledge and subsequently using that knowledge to demonstrate its retention. In this study, atopic patients were pretreated with diphenhydramine, loratadine, or placebo and trained for 1 day, whereas normal controls received no medications but the same training. After 2 weeks of loratadine treatment in the atopic group, both the atopic children and the normal controls were tested about the knowledge taught to them during the training session. In general, the atopic children did worse on this testing compared with the normal controls. Among the atopic children, those treated with diphenhydramine before training had impairment of retention, whereas pretreatment with loratadine seemed to impart a small benefit on learning. In 1996, Vuurman and colleagues[159] performed a similar study on young adults randomized to pretreatment with acrivastine plus pseudoephedrine, diphenhydramine, or placebo and trained for 3 consecutive days instead of just 1 day. The atopic patients were then treated for 2 weeks with the acrivastine/pseudoephedrine combination and compared with a normal control group that received the same training but no medications. Both groups were tested immediately after the 3-day training session as well as at the end of the 2-week treatment period. For each group, test scores improved with each day of training but the amount of improvement differed between groups. Both immediately after training and at the end of 2 weeks, the best results came from the normal control group and the allergic group pretreated with the combination of acrivastine and pseudoephedrine. The allergic patients pretreated with placebo learned less well than these 2 groups, suggesting an inherent impairment in learning from allergic rhinitis itself, and the group receiving diphenhydramine again did significantly worse than all other groups at the end of the training period.

Antihistamine Use for Rhinitis Therapy During Pregnancy

Allergic rhinitis has been estimated to complicate 20% to 30% of pregnancies, with 10% to 30% of women who have underlying allergic rhinitis describing an increase in symptoms during pregnancy.[160,161] Although prospective studies in pregnancy are few and there are no randomized controlled trials, antihistamines are often used to treat rhinitis symptoms given their extensive clinical experience in pregnant females.[160] First-generation antihistamines have been deemed safe during the first trimester and throughout pregnancy based mostly on epidemiogic data and a

Table 5
Studies of antihistamine efficacy and safety in the pediatric population

Medication	Dose	Patient Population	Age Range	Duration	Primary Endpoint	Study Design	Result	References
Cetirizine	5 mg or 10 mg Daily	209 Children with SAR	6–11 y	4 wk	Efficacy (symptoms)	R, DB, PC	Compared with placebo, cetirizine 10 mg daily but not 5 mg daily significantly improves SAR symptoms	148
	10 mg Daily	544 Children with SAR	6–11 y	4 wk	Efficacy (QOL)	OL, NC	Cetirizine 10 mg daily led to a significant improvement in QOL	149
	0.25 mg/kg BID	817 Children with SAR/CIU	12–24 mo	18 mo	Safety	R, DB, PG, P	Cetirizine is considered safe in pediatric patients aged 12–24 months	150
	0.25 mg/kg BID	85 Infants with previous AH use	6–11 mo	1 wk	Safety	R, DB, PC	Compared with placebo, cetirizine 0.25 mg/kg BID did not cause an increase in adverse events or QTc prolongation	151

Fexofenadine	30 mg BID	932 Children with SAR	6–11 y	2 wk	Efficacy (symptoms)	R, DB, PC	Compared with placebo, fexofenadine 30 mg BID significantly reduced symptom scores	[152]
	All 3 studies: 30 mg BID; 2 studies also assessed: 15 mg and 60 mg BID	1810 Children with SAR	6–11 y	2 wk	Efficacy and Safety	Pooled data from 3 studies: R, DB, PC, PG	Fexofenadine is safe, nonsedative, and effective in children ages 6–11 years	[153]
Desloratadine	1.25 mg daily (2–5 y); 2.25 mg daily (6–11 y)	111 (2–5 y) and 120 (6–11 y) children with SAR/CIU	2–5 y; 6–11 y	2 wk	Safety	DB, PC, PG	Desloratadine is considered safe for 2–11 year-old children	[154]
Levocetirizine	0.125 mg/kg BID	510 Atopic children	12–24 mo	18 mo	Safety	R, DB, PC	Levocetirizine is considered safe in pediatric patients aged 12–24 months	[155]

Abbreviations: AH, antihistamine; BID, twice daily; CIU, chronic idiopathic urticaria; DB, double blind; NC, noncomparative; OL, open label; PC, placebo-controlled; PG, parallel group; QTc, QT interval corrected for rate; R, randomized; SAR, seasonal allergic rhinitis.
Data from Refs.[141,148–155]

meta-analysis of more than 200,000 participants, where there was no increase seen in any type of congenital malformation.[162,163]

Several retrospective and prospective studies have been performed to evaluate the safety of cetirizine and loratadine in pregnancy, and both medications are deemed safe as a result of these studies. Loratadine was analyzed in a Swedish registry study of 292 women taking this medication during pregnancy with no increase in the rate of major malformations.[164] A prospective comparative study was subsequently performed on 161 women taking loratadine during pregnancy and 161 pregnant controls, demonstrating similar infant outcomes.[165] In another comparative study, 210 loratadine-exposed pregnant women, 267 women taking other antihistamines during pregnancy, and 929 pregnant women not taking antihistamines had no adverse effects from loratadine ingestion during pregnancy.[166] Although further analysis of the Swedish registry data suggested increased hypospadias risk in male infants exposed to loratadine, a subsequent case-control study using telephone interviews to collect data from the mothers of approximately 2000 male infants demonstrated no significant correlation between first-trimester loratadine exposure and hypospadias.[167] A subsequent meta-analysis of 2694 loratadine-exposed infants and more than 450,000 unexposed controls also refuted this association.[161]

The safety of cetirizine in pregnancy has also been examined through several prospective and retrospective studies. The first of these was a comparative telephone study of 120 women receiving hydroxyzine during pregnancy and 39 women receiving cetirizine (10 mg per day), 37 of whom took the medication during their first trimester. This prospective study showed no difference in pregnancy outcomes for either group.[168] Data from these 39 patients were supplemented with data from 60 other women who also took standard-dose cetirizine early during pregnancy, again with no increase in adverse effects on exposed infants. There was an incidental finding of significantly less pregnancy-induced nausea and vomiting for those women taking cetirizine.[169] The largest study of cetirizine was an analysis of more than 17,000 pregnant females in the Swedish Medical Birth Register from 1995 to 1999, 917 of whom took cetirizine during pregnancy with no increase in malformations or delivery complications when compared with the general population.[164] After this analysis, 144 infants exposed to cetirizine during the first trimester and 196 infants exposed during any trimester were evaluated in a 2004 study by the North Atlantic Treaty Organization[170] and a 2008 analysis of the Berlin teratogen information service, respectively.[161] Neither analysis demonstrated adverse effects on those infants exposed to cetirizine compared with unexposed infants.

Animal studies of cetirizine, levocetirizine, and loratadine have demonstrated safety during pregnancy, yielding an FDA pregnancy category B based on lack of demonstrable risk in animal reproduction studies without well-controlled studies on pregnant women.[53,54] Fexofenadine and desloratadine, alternatively, have been designated pregnancy category C based on adverse effects reported in animal studies without well-controlled studies on pregnant women.[56,171] In animal studies of fexofenadine, animal studies have shown a decrease in pup weight and survival. Limited human data for fexofenadine's parent drug, terfenadine, during pregnancy have not shown an increase in any major malformations for exposed fetuses.[56] Animal studies on desloratadine have been variable, with some showing increased preimplantation loss and a decrease in pup weight and slow righting reflex at doses equivalent to 50 or more times the recommended human dose.[171] Because there have not been any controlled studies examining the safety of antihistamines during human pregnancy, there are no antihistamines that carry an FDA category A rating. Both azelastine and olopatadine intranasal antihistamines are FDA category C for pregnancy due to minor adverse effects on the fetus at high doses in animal studies only.

Antihistamine Use for Rhinitis Therapy During Lactation

Antihistamines considered safe during lactation include fexofenadine, loratadine, and desloratadine based on studies measuring the actual amount excreted into the breast milk of women taking loratadine or fexofenadine during lactation. A pharmacokinetic study performed on the breast milk of 6 lactating women taking loratadine (40 mg) concluded that the breastfeeding baby would ingest approximately 1% of the weight-adjusted recommended dose for adults when combining breast milk excretion of loratadine and its metabolite, desloratadine.[172] A similar study performed on 4 lactating women taking terfenadine showed that the weight-adjusted fexofenadine dose ingested by the baby was approximately 0.45% of the adult-recommended dose.[173] Because the amount of drug to which breastfeeding infants are exposed is minimal, these 3 antihistamines are currently options available to lactating women. Although similar studies have not been performed on cetirizine, its use is not generally recommended during lactation based on dog studies suggesting higher concentrations of drug excreted in breast milk.[52]

SUMMARY

Histamine, one of the key mediators of allergic disease, functions by binding to 1 of 4 histamine receptors. Antihistamines act as inverse agonists of these receptors to prevent the downstream actions of histamine. More than 40 oral antihistamines are currently available and can be classified as first-generation and second-generation drugs, depending on their pharmacokinetic and pharmacodynamic properties and their side-effect profiles. Intranasal antihistamines, which were introduced more recently, have shown promise as efficacious agents with a rapid onset of action and minimal side effects. Although data are conflicting on how intranasal antihistamines compare with intranasal steroids, several studies comparing intranasal and oral antihistamines point to the intranasal formulation as superior. The role of antihistamines in the treatment of allergic rhinitis is variable from one patient to another depending on an individual's symptom complex, cost concerns, and patient preference. Certain patient populations, such as children, pregnant or lactating women, and those taking medications that could interfere with antihistamine metabolism, require special consideration regarding antihistamine choice and dosing as part of rhinitis therapy.

ACKNOWLEDGMENTS

We would like to thank Diedre Versluis for her assistance in the preparation of this manuscript.

REFERENCES

1. Parsons M, Ganellin C. Histamine and its receptors. Br J Pharmacol 2006;147: S127–35.
2. Dale HD, Laidlaw PD. The physiological action of beta-iminazolylethylamine. J Physiol 1910;41:318–44.
3. Best CH, Dale HH, Dudley HW, et al. The nature of the vaso-dilator constituents of certain tissue extracts. J Physiol 1927;62:397–417.
4. Steinhoff M, Griffiths C, Church M, et al. Histamine. In: Burns T, Breathnach S, Cox N, et al, editors. Rok's textbook of dermatology, vol. 9. Oxford (UK): Blackwell Science; 2004. p. 50–2.
5. Masheter HC. Terfenadine: the first nonsedating antihistamine. Clin Rev Allergy 1993;11:5–34.

6. Jutel M, Blaser K, Akdis CA. Histamine receptors in immune regulation and allergen-specific immunotherapy. Immunol Allergy Clin North Am 2006;26: 249–59.

7. Akdis CA, Simons FER. Histamine receptors are hot in immunopharmacology. Eur J Pharmacol 2006;533:69–76.

8. Simons FE, Adkis CA. Antihistamines. In: Adkinson NF Jr, Bochner BS, Busse WW, et al, editors. Middleton's allergy: principles and practice. 7th edition. St Louis (MO): Mosby; 2009. p. 1517–47.

9. Simons FE. Advances in H1-antihistamines. N Engl J Med 2004;351:2203–17.

10. Godot V, Arock M, Garcia G, et al. H4 histamine receptor mediates optimal migration of mast cell precursors to CXCL12. J Allergy Clin Immunol 2007; 120:827–34.

11. Suzuki S, Takeuchi K, Majima Y. Localization and function of histamine H3 receptor in the nasal mucosa. Clin Exp Allergy 2008;38:1476–82.

12. Strakhova MI, Nikkela AL, Manellia AM, et al. Localization of histamine H4 receptors in the central nervous system of human and rat. Brain Res 2009; 1250:41–8.

13. Leurs R, Church MK, Taglialatela M. H1-antihistamines: inverse agonism, anti-inflammatory actions and cardiac effects. Clin Exp Allergy 2002;32:489–98.

14. Milligan G, Bond R, Lee M. Inverse agonism: pharmacological curiosity or potential therapeutic strategy? Trends Pharmacol Sci 1995;16:10–3.

15. Ash AS, Schild HO. Receptors mediating some actions of histamine. 1966. Br J Pharmacol 1997;120:302–14 [discussion: 300–1].

16. Wallace DV, Dykewicz MS, Bernstein DI, et al. The diagnosis and management of rhinitis: an updated practice parameter. J Allergy Clin Immunol 2008;122:S1–84.

17. Cook TJ, MacQueen DM, Wittig HJ, et al. Degree and duration of skin test suppression and side effects with antihistamines: a double blind controlled study with five antihistamines. J Allergy Clin Immunol 1973;51:71–7.

18. Long WF, Taylor RJ, Wagner CJ, et al. Skin test suppression by antihistamines and the development of subsensitivity. J Allergy Clin Immunol 1985;76:113–7.

19. LexiComp Online drug reference [online].

20. Rao KS, Menon PK, Hilman BC, et al. Duration of the suppressive effect of tricyclic antidepressants on histamine-induced wheal-and-flare reactions in human skin. J Allergy Clin Immunol 1988;82(5 Pt 1):752–7.

21. del Cuvillo A, Mullol J, Bartra J, et al. Comparative pharmacology of the H1 antihistamines. J Investig Allergol Clin Immunol 2006;16(Suppl 1):3–12.

22. Simons FE, Simons KJ. Clinical pharmacology of new histamine H1 receptor antagonists. Clin Pharmacokinet 1999;36:329–52.

23. Molimard M, Diquet B, Benedetti MS. Comparison of pharmacokintetics and metabolism of desloratadine, fexofenadine, levocetirizine and mizolastine in humans. Fundam Clin Pharmacol 2004;18:399–411.

24. Pearlman DS, Grossman J, Meltzer EO. Histamine skin test reactivity following single and multiple doses of azelastine nasal spray in patients with seasonal allergic rhinitis. Ann Allergy Asthma Immunol 2003;91:258–62.

25. Kay GG. The effects of antihistamines on cognition and performance. J Allergy Clin Immunol 2000;105(6):S622–7.

26. Hansten PD, Levy RH. Role of P-glycoprotein and organic anion transporting polypeptides in drug absorption and distribution. Clin Drug Investig 2001;21: 587–96.

27. Lehman JM. Selecting the optimal oral antihistamine for patients with allergic rhinitis. Drugs 2006;66(18):2309.

28. Golightly LK, Greos LS. Second-generation antihistamines: actions and efficacy in the management of allergic disorders. Drugs 2005;65(3):341–84.
29. Simons FE, Simons KJ. Clinical pharmacology of H1 antihistamines. In: Simons FE, editor. Histamine and H1-antihistamines in allergic disease. New York: Marcel Dekker; 2002. p. 141–78.
30. Figueiredo A, Ribeiro CA, Goncalo M, et al. Mechanism of action of doxepin in the treatment of chronic urticaria. Fundam Clin Pharmacol 1990;4(2): 147–58.
31. Greene SL, Reed CE, Schroeter AL. Double-blind crossover study comparing doxepin with diphenhydramine for the treatment of chronic urticaria. J Am Acad Dermatol 1985;12:669–75.
32. Passalacqua G, Canonica GW. A review of evidence from comparative studies of levocetirizne and desloratadine for symptoms of allergic rhinitis. Clin Ther 2005;27(7):979–92.
33. Ciprandi G, Tosca MA, Cosentino C, et al. Effects of fexofenadine and other anti-histamines on components of the allergic response: adhesion molecules. J Allergy Clin Immunol 2003;112(Suppl 4):S78–82.
34. van Cauwenberge P, Juniper EF, Meltzer EO, et al. Comparison of the efficacy, safety and quality of life provided by fexofenadine hydrochloride 120mg, loratadine 10mg and placebo administered once daily for the treatment of seasonal allergic rhinitis. Clin Exp Allergy 2000;30:891–9.
35. Paolieri F, Battifora M, Riccio A, et al. Terfenadine and fexofenadine reduce in vitro ICAM-1 expression on human continuous cell lines. Ann Allergy Asthma Immunol 1998;81:601–7.
36. Naclerio RM. The effect of antihistamines on the immediate allergic response: a comparative review. Otolaryngol Head Neck Surg 1993;108(6):723–30.
37. Ciprandi G, Passalacqua G, Canonica GW. Effects of H1 antihistamines on adhesion molecules: a possible rationale for long-term treatment. Clin Exp Allergy 1999;29(Suppl 3):49–53.
38. Schroeder JT, Schleimer RP, Lichtenstein LM, et al. Inhibition of cytokine generation and mediator release by human basophils treated with desloratadine. Clin Exp Allergy 2001;31:1369–77.
39. Slater JM, Zechnich AD, Haxby DG. Second-generation anti-histamines: a comparative review. Drugs 1999;57:31–47.
40. Dubuske L. Dose-ranging comparative evaluation of cetirizine in patients with seasonal allergic rhinitis. Ann Allergy Asthma Immunol 1995;74:345–54.
41. Clissold SP, Sorkin EM, Goa KL. Loratadine: a preliminary review of its pharmacodynamic properties and therapeutic efficacy. Drugs 1989;37:42–57.
42. Haria M, Fitton A, Peters DH. Loratadine: a reappraisal of its pharmacological properties and therapeutic use in allergic disorders. Drugs 1994;48:617–37.
43. Bruttmann G, Pedrali P. Loratadine (SCH 29851) 40mg once daily vs terfenadine 60mg twice daily in the treatment of seasonal allergic rhinitis. J Int Med Res 1987;15:63–70.
44. Bradley CM, Nicholson AN. Studies on the central effects of the H1-antagonist, loratadine. Eur J Clin Pharmacol 1987;32:419–21.
45. Bronsky EA, Falliers CJ, Kaiser HB, et al. Effectiveness and safety of fexofenadine, a new nonsedating H1-receptor antagonist, in the treatment of fall allergies. Allergy Asthma Proc 1998;19:135–41.
46. Bernstein DI, Schoenwetter WF, Nathan RA, et al. Efficacy and safety of fexofenadine hydrochloride for treatment of seasonal allergic rhinitis. Ann Allergy Asthma Immunol 1997;79:443–8.

47. Meltzer EO, Casale TB, Nathan RA, et al. Once-daily fexofenadine HCl improves quality of life and reduces work and activity impairment in patients with seasonal allergic rhinitis. Ann Allergy Asthma Immunol 1999;83:311–7.

48. Raphael GD, Angello JT, Wu MM. Efficacy of diphenhydramine vs desloratadine and placebo in patients with moderate-to-severe seasonal allergic rhinitis. Ann Allergy Asthma Immunol 2006;96:606–14.

49. Bousquet J, Van Cauwenberge PB, Khaltaev N, et al. Allergic rhinitis and its impact on asthma. J Allergy Clin Immunol 2001;108:1A–14A, S147–334.

50. Bonini S, Bonini M, Bousquet J, et al. Rhinitis and asthma in athletes: an ARIA document in collaboration with GA2LEN. Allergy 2006;61:681–92.

51. Juniper EF, Stahl E, Doty RL, et al. Clinical outcomes and adverse effect monitoring in allergic rhinitis. J Allergy Clin Immunol 2005;115:S390–413.

52. Zyrtec (cetirizine hydrochloride) tablets and syrup [package insert]. New York: Pfizer Inc; 2002.

53. Mohler SR, Nicholson A, Harvey RP, et al. The use of antihistamines in safety-critical jobs: a meeting report. Curr Med Res Opin 2002;18:332–7.

54. Xyzal (levocetirizine) tablets [package insert]. Brussels: UCB Pharma Ltd; 2003.

55. Kay GG, Berman B, Mockoviak SH, et al. Initial and steady state effects of diphenhydramine and loratadine on sedation, cognition, mood, and psychomotor performance. Arch Intern Med 1997;157:2350–6.

56. Allegra (fexofenadine hydrochloride) capsules and tablets: activity impairment in patients with seasonal allergic rhinitis [package insert]. Kansas City, MO: Aventis Pharmaceuticals Inc; 2003.

57. Pagliara A, Testa B, Carrupt PA, et al. Molecular properties and pharmacokinetic behavior of cetirizine, a zwitterionic H1-receptor antagonist. J Med Chem 1998; 41:853–63.

58. Lai DS, Lue KH, Hsieh JC, et al. The comparison of the efficacy and safety of cetirizine, oxatomide, ketotifen, and a placebo for the treatment of childhood perennial allergic rhinitis. Ann Allergy Asthma Immunol 2002;89:589–98.

59. Bousquet J, Duchateau J, Pignat JC, et al. Improvement of quality of life by treatment with cetirizine in patients with perennial allergic rhinitis as determined by a French version of the SF-36 questionnaire. J Allergy Clin Immunol 1996;98:309–16.

60. Ciebiada M, Gorska-Ciebiada M, DuBuske LM, et al. Montelukast with desloratadine or levocetirizine for the treatment of persistent allergic rhinitis. Ann Allergy Asthma Immunol 2006;97:664–71.

61. Jorissen M, Bertrand B, Stiels B, et al. Levocetirizine as treatment for symptoms of seasonal allergic rhinitis. B-ENT 2006;2(2):55–62.

62. Ciprandi G, Passalacqua G, Mincarini M, et al. Continuous versus on demand treatment with cetirizine for allergic rhinitis. Ann Allergy Asthma Immunol 1997;79:507–11.

63. Aaronson DW. Evaluation of cetirizine in patients with allergic rhinitis and perennial asthma. Ann Allergy Asthma Immunol 1996;76:440–6.

64. Torkildsen GL, Gomes P, Welch D, et al. Evaluation of desloratadine on conjunctival allergen challenge-induced ocular symptoms. Clin Exp Allergy 2009;39(7): 1052–9.

65. Tanner LA, Reilly M, Meltzer EO, et al. Effect of fexofenadine HCl on quality of life and work, classroom and daily activity impairment in patients with seasonal allergic rhinitis. Am J Manag Care 1999;5(Suppl 2):S235–47.

66. Hampel F, Ratner P, Mansfield L, et al. Fexofenadine hydro-chloride, 180 mg, exhibits equivalent efficacy to cetirizine, 10 mg, with less drowsiness in patients

with moderate-to-severe seasonal allergic rhinitis. Ann Allergy Asthma Immunol 2003;91:354–61.

67. Sabbah A, Daele J, Wade AG, et al. Comparison of the efficacy, safety, and onset of action of mizolastine, cetirizine, and placebo in the management of seasonal allergic rhinoconjunctivitis. Ann Allergy Asthma Immunol 1999;83: 319–25.

68. Murray JJ, Nathan RA, Bronsky EA, et al. Comprehensive evaluation of cetirizine in the management of seasonal allergic rhinitis: impact on symptoms, quality of life, productivity, and activity impairment. Allergy Asthma Proc 2002;23: 391–8.

69. Noonan MJ, Raphael GD, Nayak A, et al. The health-related quality of life effects of once-daily cetirizine HCl in patients with seasonal allergic rhinitis: a randomized double-blind, placebo-controlled trial. Clin Exp Allergy 2003;33:351–8.

70. Mansmann HC Jr, Altman RA, Berman BA, et al. Efficacy and safety of cetirizine therapy in perennial allergic rhinitis. Ann Allergy 1992;68:348–53.

71. Horak F, Toth J, Marks B, et al. Efficacy and safety relative to placebo of an oral formulation of cetirizine and sustained-release pseudoephedrine in the management of nasal congestion. Allergy 1998;53:849–56.

72. Rinne J, Simola M, Malmberg H, et al. Early treatment of perennial rhinitis with budesonide or cetirizine and its effect on long-term outcome. J Allergy Clin Immunol 2002;109:426–32.

73. Segall N, Gawchik S, Georges G, et al. Efficacy and safety of levocetirizine in improving symptoms and health-related quality of life in US adults with seasonal allergic rhinitis: a randomized, placebo-controlled study. Ann Allergy Asthma Immunol 2010;104(3):259–67.

74. Mansfield LE, Hampel F, Haeslui JM, et al. Study of levocetirizine in seasonal allergic rhinitis. Curr Med Res Opin 2010;26(6):1269–75.

75. Potter PC, Study Group. Levocetirizine is effective for symptom relief including nasal congestion in adolescent and adult (PAR) sensitized to house dust mites. Allergy 2003;58:893–9.

76. Bachert C, Bousquet J, Canonica GW, et al. Levocetirizine improves quality of life and reduces costs in longterm management of persistent allergic rhinitis. J Allergy Clin Immunol 2004;114:838–44.

77. Canonica GW, Bousquet J, Van Hammee G, et al. Levocetirizine improves health-related quality of life and health status in persistent allergic rhinitis. Respir Med 2006;100:1706–15.

78. Day JH, Briscoe MP, Welsh A, et al. Onset of action, efficacy, and safety of a single dose of fexofenadine hydrochloride for ragweed allergy using an environmental exposure unit. Ann Allergy Asthma Immunol 1997;79:533–40.

79. Sussman GL, Mason J, Compton D, et al. The efficacy and safety of fexofenadine HCl and pseudoephedrine, alone and in combination, in seasonal allergic rhinitis. J Allergy Clin Immunol 1999;104:100–6.

80. Casale TB, Andrade C, Qu R. Safety and efficacy of once-daily fexofenadine HCl in the treatment of autumn seasonal allergy rhinitis. Allergy Asthma Proc 1999;20:193–8.

81. Ciprandi G, Cosentino C, Milanese M, et al. Fexofenadine reduces nasal congestion in perennial allergic rhinitis. Allergy 2001;56:1068–70.

82. Druce HM, Thoden WR, Mure P, et al. Brompheniramine, loratadine, and placebo in allergic rhinitis: a placebo-control led comparative trial. J Clin Pharmacol 1998;38:382–9.

83. Crawford WW, Klaustermeyer WB, Lee PH, et al. Comparative efficacy of terfenadine, loratadine, and astemizole in perennial allergic rhinitis. Otolaryngol Head Neck Surg 1998;118:668–73.

84. Kaiser HB, Gopalan G, Chung W. Loratadine provides early symptom control in seasonal allergic rhinitis. Allergy Asthma Proc 2008;29(6):654–8.

85. Nayak AS, Schenkel E. Desloratadine reduces nasal congestion in patients with intermittent allergic rhinitis. Allergy 2001;56:1077–80.

86. Horak F, Stübner UP, Zieglmayer R, et al. Comparison of the effects of desloratadine 5mg daily and placebo on nasal airflow and seasonal allergy rhinitis symptoms induced by grass pollen exposure. Allergy 2003;58:481–5.

87. Salmun LM, Lorber R, Danzig M, et al. Efficacy and safety of desloratadine in seasonal allergic rhinitis. J Allergy Clin Immunol 2000;104(Suppl 1):384–5 [abstract no: 1123].

88. Heithoff K, Meltzer EO, Mellars L, et al. Desloratadine improves quality of life in patients with seasonal allergic rhinitis. J Allergy Clin Immunol 2000;104(Suppl 1): 383–4 [abstract no: 1121].

89. Berger WE, Schenkel EJ, Mansfield LE, et al. Safety and efficacy of desloratadine 5mg in asthma patients with seasonal allergic rhinitis and nasal congestion. Ann Allergy Asthma Immunol 2002;89:485–91.

90. Salmun LM, Lorber R. 24-Hour efficacy of once-daily desloratadine therapy in patients with seasonal allergic rhinitis. BMC Fam Pract 2002;3:14–20.

91. Simons FE, Prenner BM, Finn A Jr, et al. Efficacy and safety of desloratadine in the treatment of perennial allergic rhinitis. J Allergy Clin Immunol 2003;111: 617–22.

92. Bousquet J, Bachert C, Canonica GW, et al. Efficacy of desloratadine in intermittent allergic rhinitis: a GA(2)LEN study. Allergy 2009;64(1):1516–23.

93. Bousquet J, Bachert C, Canonica GW, et al. Efficacy of desloratadine in persistent allergic rhinitis–a GALEN study. Int Arch Allergy Immunol 2010;153(4): 395–402.

94. Horak F, Stübner UP, Zieglmayer R, et al. Controlled comparison of the efficacy and safety of cetirizine 10mg daily and fexofenadine 120mg daily in reducing symptoms of seasonal allergic rhinitis. Int Arch Allergy Immunol 2001;125: 73–9.

95. Howarth PH, Stern MA, Roi L, et al. Double-blind, placebo controlled study comparing the efficacy and safety of fexofenadine hydrochloride (120 and 180mg once daily) and cetirizine in seasonal allergic rhinitis. J Allergy Clin Immunol 1999;104:927–33.

96. Meltzer EO, Weiler JM, Widlitz MD. Comparative outdoor study of the efficacy, onset and duration of action, and safety of cetirizine, loratadine, and placebo for seasonal allergic rhinitis. J Allergy Clin Immunol 1996;97:617–26.

97. Day JH, Briscoe MP, Clark RH, et al. Onset of action and efficacy of terfenadine, astemizole, cetirizine, and loratadine rhinitis for the relief of symptoms of allergic rhinitis. Ann Allergy Asthma Immunol 1997;79:163–72.

98. Day JH, Briscoe MP, Rafeiro E, et al. Comparative onset and symptom relief with cetirizine, loratadine, or placebo in an environmental exposure unit in subjects with seasonal allergic rhinitis: confirmation of a test system. Ann Allergy Asthma Immunol 2001;87:474–81.

99. Day JH, Briscoe M, Widlitz MD. Cetirizine, loratadine, or placebo in subjects with seasonal allergic rhinitis: effects after controlled ragweed pollen challenge in an environmental exposure unit. J Allergy Clin Immunol 1998;101:638–45.

100. Wilson AM, Haggart K, Sims EJ, et al. Effects of fexofenadine and desloratadine on subjective and objective measures of nasal congestion in seasonal allergic rhinitis. Clin Exp Allergy 2002;32:1504–9.
101. Berger WE, Lumry WR, Meltzer EO, et al. Efficacy of desloratadine, 5mg, compared with fexofenadine, 180mg, in patients with symptomatic seasonal allergic rhinitis. Allergy Asthma Proc 2006;27(3):214–23.
102. Mösges R, van Cauwenberg P, Purello-D'Ambrosio F, et al. Fexofenadine and loratadine exhibit rapid relief, but only fexofenadine maintains efficacy over a 2-week period [abstract no: 1005]. Allergy 2000;55(Suppl 63):281.
103. Ricard N, Kind P, Christian S, et al. Link between preferences and treatment outcomes in seasonal allergic rhinitis: an empiric investigation. Clin Ther 1999; 20:268–77.
104. Bachert C, Maurer M. Safety and efficacy of desloratadine in subjects with seasonal allergic rhinitis or chronic urticaria: results of four postmarketing surveillance studies. Clin Drug Investig 2010;30(2):109–22.
105. Lee DK, Gardiner M, Haggart K, et al. Comparative effects of desloratadine, fexofenadine, and levocetirizine on nasal adenosine monophosphate challenge in patients with perennial allergic rhinitis. Clin Exp Allergy 2004;34:650–3.
106. Meltzer EO, Weiler JM, Widlitz MD. Comparative outdoor study of the efficacy, onset and duration of action, and safety of cetirizine, loratadine, and placebo for seasonal allergic rhinitis. Life Sci 2002;72:409–14.
107. Ciprandi G, Cirillo I, Vizzaccaro A, et al. Desloratadine and levocetirizine improve nasal symptoms, airflow, and allergic inflammation in patients with perennial allergic rhinitis: a pilot study. Int Immunopharmacol 2005;5:1800–8.
108. Juniper EF, Kline PA, Hargreave FE, et al. Comparison of beclomethasone dipropionate aqueous nasal spray, astemizole, and the combination in the prophylactic treatment of ragweed pollen-induced rhinoconjunctivitis. J Allergy Clin Immunol 1989;83:627–33.
109. Ratner P, VanBavel J, Martin B, et al. A comparison of the efficacy of fluticasone propionate aqueous nasal spray and loratadine, alone and in combination, for the treatment of seasonal allergic rhinitis. J Fam Pract 1998;47: 118–25.
110. Di Lorenzo G, Pacor ML, Pellitteri ME, et al. Randomized placebo-controlled trial comparing fluticasone aqueous nasal spray in mono-therapy, fluticasone plus cetirizine, fluticasone plus montelukast and cetirizine plus montelukast for seasonal allergic rhinitis. Clin Exp Allergy 2004;34:259–67.
111. Barnes M, Ward J, Fardon T, et al. Effects of levocetirizine as add-on therapy to fluticasone in seasonal allergic rhinitis. Clin Exp Allergy 2006;36:676–84.
112. Aurora J. Development of nasal delivery systems: a review. Drug Deliv Technol 2002;2:85.
113. Kaliner MA. Azelastine and olopatadine in the treatment of allergic rhinitis. Ann Allergy Asthma Immunol 2009;103:373–80.
114. Berger WE. Pharmacokinetic characteristics and safety and tolerability of a reformulated azelastine hydrochloride nasal spray in patients with chronic rhinitis. Expert Opin Drug Metab Toxicol 2009;5(1):91–102.
115. Shah S, Berger W, Lumry W. Efficacy and safety of azelastine 0.15% nasal spray and azelastine 0.10% nasal spray in patients with seasonal allergic rhinitis. Allergy Asthma Proc 2009;30:628–33.
116. Bernstein JA. Azelastine hydrochloride: a review of pharmacology, pharmacokinetics, clinical efficacy and tolerability. Curr Med Res Opin 2007;23:2441–52.

117. Banov CH, Lieberman P. Efficacy of azelastine nasal spray in the treatment of vasomotor (perennial nonallergic) rhinitis. Ann Allergy Asthma Immunol 2001; 86:28–35.

118. Meltzer E, Weiler J, Dockhorn R, et al. Azelastine nasal spray in the management of seasonal allergic rhinitis. Ann Allergy Asthma Immunol 1994;72:354–9.

119. Weiler J, Meltzer E, Benson P, et al. A dose-ranging study of the efficacy and safety of azelastine nasal spray in the treatment of seasonal allergic rhinitis with an acute model. J Allergy Clin Immunol 1994;94:972–80.

120. Storms W, Pearlman D, Chervinsky P, et al. The effectiveness of azelastine nasal solution in seasonal allergic rhinitis. Ear Nose Throat J 1994;73:382–94.

121. Ratner P, Findlay S, Hampel F Jr, et al. A double-blind, controlled trial to assess the safety and efficacy of azelastine nasal spray in seasonal allergic rhinitis. J Allergy Clin Immunol 1994;94:818–25.

122. LaForce C, Dockhorn R, Prenner B, et al. Safety and efficacy of azelastine nasal spray (Asteline NS) for seasonal allergic rhinitis: a 4-week comparative multicenter trial. Ann Allergy Asthma Immunol 1996;76:181–8.

123. Lumry W, Prenner B, Corren J, et al. Efficacy and safety of azelastine nasal spray at a dosage of one spray per nostril twice daily. Ann Allergy Asthma Immunol 2007;99:267–72.

124. Ratner P, Hampel F, Amar N, et al. Safety and efficacy of olopatadine hydrochloride nasal spray for the treatment of seasonal allergic rhinitis to mountain cedar. Ann Allergy Asthma Immunol 2005;95:474–9.

125. Fairchild C, Meltzer E, Roland P, et al. Comprehensive report of the efficacy, safety, quality of life, and work impact of Olopatadine 0.6% and Olopatadine 0.4% treatment in patients with seasonal allergic rhinitis. Allergy Asthma Proc 2007;28:716–23.

126. Hampel F, Ratner P, Amar N, et al. Improved quality of life among seasonal allergic rhinitis patients treated with olopatadine HCL nasal spray 0.4% and olopatadine HCL nasal spray0.6% compared with vehicle placebo. Allergy Asthma Proc 2006;27:202–7.

127. Shah S, Nayak A, Ratner P, et al. Effects of olopatadine hydrochloride nasal spray 0.6% in the treatment of seasonal allergic rhinitis: a phase III, multicenter, randomized, double-blind, active- and placebo-controlled study in adolescents and adults. Clin Ther 2009;31:99–107.

128. Pipkorn P, Constantini C, Reynolds C, et al. The effects of the nasal antihistamine olopatadine and azelastine in nasal allergen provocation. Ann Allergy Asthma Immunol 2008;101:82–9.

129. Yáñez A, Rodrigo G. Intranasal corticosteroids versus topical H1 receptor antagonists for the treatment of allergic rhinitis: a systematic review with meta-analysis. Ann Allergy Asthma Immunol 2002;89:479–84.

130. Kaliner MA, Storms W, Tilles S, et al. Comparison of olopatadine 0.6% nasal spray versus fluticasone propionate 50 microg in the treatment of seasonal allergic rhinitis. Allergy Asthma Proc 2009;30:255–62.

131. Ratner P, Hampel F, VanBavel J, et al. Combination therapy with azelastine hydrochloride nasal spray and fluticasone propionate nasal spray in the treatment of patients with seasonal allergic rhinitis. Ann Allergy Asthma Immunol 2008;100:74–81.

132. Patel D, Garadi R, Brubaker M, et al. Onset and duration of action of nasal sprays in seasonal allergic rhinitis patients: olopatadine hydrochloride versus mometasone furoate monohydrate. Allergy Asthma Proc 2007;28:592–9.

133. Patel P, Roland P, Marple B, et al. An assessment of the onset and duration of action of olopatadine nasal spray. Otolaryngol Head Neck Surg 2007;137:918–24.

134. Patel D, D'Andrea C, Sacks HJ. Onset of action of azelastine nasal spray compared with mometasone nasal spray and placebo in subjects with seasonal allergic rhinitis evaluated in an environmental exposure chamber. Am J Rhinol 2007;21:499–503.

135. Horak F, Zieglmayer UP, Zieglmayer R, et al. Azelastine nasal spray and desloratadine tablets in pollen-induced seasonal allergic rhinitis: a pharmacodynamic study of onset of action and efficacy. Curr Med Res Opin 2006;22:151–7.

136. Cassell HR, Katial RK. Intranasal antihistamines for allergic rhinitis: examining the clinical impact. Allergy Asthma Proc 2009;30:349–57.

137. Berger W, White M, The Rhinitis Study Group. Efficacy of azelastine nasal spray in patients with an unsatisfactory response to loratadine. Ann Allergy Asthma Immunol 2003;91:205–11.

138. LaForce C, Corren J, Wheeler W, et al. Efficacy of azelastine nasal spray in seasonal allergic rhinitis patients who remain symptomatic after treatment with fexofenadine. Ann Allergy Asthma Immunol 2004;93:154–9.

139. Corren J, Storms W, Burnstein J, et al. Effectiveness of azelastine nasal spray compared with oral cetirizine in patients with seasonal allergic rhinitis. Clin Ther 2005;27:543–53.

140. Berger W, Hampel F Jr, Berstein J, et al. Impact of azelastine nasal spray on symptoms and quality of life compared with oral tablets in patients with seasonal allergic rhinitis. Ann Allergy Asthma Immunol 2006;97:375–81.

141. Schad CA, Skoner DP. Antihistamines in the pediatric population: Achieving optimal outcomes when treating seasonal allergic rhinitis and chronic urticaria. Allergy Asthma Proc 2008;29:7–13.

142. Simons FE. H1-antihistamines in children. In: Simons FE, editor. Histamine and H1-antihistamines in allergic disease. New York: Marcel Dekker; 2002. p. 437–64.

143. Gupta S, Khalilieh S, Kantesaria B, et al. Pharmacokinetics of desloratadine in children between 2 and 11 years of age. Br J Clin Pharmacol 2007;63:534–40.

144. Gupta SK, Kantesaria B, Banfield C, et al. Desloratadine dose selection in children aged 6 months to 2 years: comparison of population pharmacokinetics between children and adults. Br J Clin Pharmacol 2007;64:174–84.

145. Simons FE, Simons KJ. Levocetirizine: pharmacokinetics and pharmacodynamics in children age 6 to 11 years. J Allergy Clin Immunol 2005;116:355–61.

146. Cranswick N, Turzikova J, Fuchs M, et al. Levocetirizine in 1–2 year old children: pharmacokinetic and pharmacodynamic profile. Int J Clin Pharmacol Ther 2005; 43:172–7.

147. Simons FE, ETAC Study Group. Population pharmacokinetics of levocetirizine in very young children: the pediatricians' perspective. Pediatr Allergy Immunol 2005;16:97–103.

148. Pearlman DS, Lumry WR, Winder JA, et al. Once-daily cetirizine effective in the treatment of seasonal allergic rhinitis in children aged 6 to 11 years: a randomized, double-blind, placebo- controlled study. Clin Pediatr (Phila) 1997;36:209–15.

149. Gillman SA, Blatter M, Condemi JJ, et al. The health-related quality of life effects of once-daily cetirizine HCl syrup in children with seasonal allergic rhinitis. Clin Pediatr (Phila) 2002;41:687–96.

150. Simons FE. Prospective, long-term safety evaluation of the H1- receptor antagonist cetirizine in very young children with atopic dermatitis. ETAC Study Group. Early treatment of the atopic child. J Allergy Clin Immunol 1999;104:433–40.

151. Simons FE, Silas P, Portnoy JM, et al. Pharmd. Safety of cetirizine in infants 6 to 11 months of age: a randomized, double-blind, placebo-controlled study. J Allergy Clin Immunol 2003;111:1244–8.
152. Wahn U, Meltzer EO, Finn AF Jr, et al. Fexofenadine is efficacious and safe in children (aged 6–11 years) with seasonal allergic rhinitis [Erratum in J Allergy Clin Immunol 2003;112:1202 J Allergy Clin Immunol 2003;112:71]. J Allergy Clin Immunol 2003;111:763–9.
153. Meltzer EO, Scheinmann P, Rosado Pinto JE, et al. Safety and efficacy of oral fexofenadine in children with seasonal allergic rhinitis—a pooled analysis of three studies. Pediatr Allergy Immunol 2004;15:253–60.
154. Bloom M, Staudinger H, Herron J. Safety of desloratadine syrup in children. Curr Med Res Opin 2004;20:1959–65.
155. Simons FE, Early Prevention of Asthma in Atopic Children (EPAAC) Study Group. Safety of levocetirizine treatment in young atopic children: an 18-month study. Pediatr Allergy Immunol 2007;18(6):535–42.
156. Fineman SM. Clinical experience with azelastine nasal spray in children: physician survey of case reports. Pediatr Asthma Allergy Immunol 2001;15(1):49–54.
157. Herman D, Garay R, Le Gal M. A randomized double-blind placebo controlled study of azelastine nasal spray in children with perennial rhinitis. Int J Pediatr Otorhinolaryngol 1997;39(1):1–8.
158. Vuurman EF, van Veggel LM, Uiterwijk MM, et al. Seasonal allergic rhinitis and antihistamine effects on children's learning. Ann Allergy 1993;71:121–6.
159. Vuurman EF, van Veggel LM, Sanders RL, et al. Effects of semprex-D and diphenhydramine on learning in young adults with seasonal allergic rhinitis. Ann Allergy Asthma Immunol 1996;76:247–52.
160. Mazzotta P, Loebstein R, Koren G. Treating allergic rhinitis in pregnancy: safety considerations. Drug Saf 1999;20:361–75.
161. So M, Inoue PB, Einarson A. Motherisk update: safety of antihistamines during pregnancy and lactation. Can Fam Physician 2010;56:427–9.
162. Gilbert C, Mazzotta P, Loebstein R, et al. Fetal safety of drugs used in the treatment of allergic rhinitis: a critical review. Drug Saf 2005;28(8):707–19.
163. Seto A, Einarson T, Koren G. Pregnancy outcome following first trimester exposure to antihistamines: meta-analysis. Am J Perinatol 1997;14(3):119–24.
164. Källén B. Use of antihistamine drugs in early pregnancy and delivery outcome. J Matern Fetal Neonatal Med 2002;11(3):146–52.
165. Moretti ME, Caprara D, Coutinho CJ, et al. Fetal safety of loratadine use in the first trimester of pregnancy: a multicentre study. J Allergy Clin Immunol 2003;111(3):479–83.
166. Diav-Citrin O, Shechtman S, Aharonovich A, et al. Pregnancy outcome after gestational exposure to loratadine or antihistamines: a prospective controlled study. J Allergy Clin Immunol 2003;111(6):1239–43.
167. Keleş N. Treatment of allergic rhinitis during pregnancy. Am J Rhinol 2004;18: 23–8.
168. Einarson A, Bailey B, Jung G, et al. Prospective controlled study of hydroxyzine and cetirizine in pregnancy. Ann Allergy Asthma Immunol 1997;78(2):183–6.
169. Einarson A, Levichek Z, Einarson TR, et al. The antiemetic effect of cetirizine in pregnancy [letter]. Ann Pharmacother 2000;34:1486–7.
170. NATO Advanced Research Workshop on "Drugs in pregnancy: consensus conference on teratogen information services," Prague, 16–18 April 2004 [abstract]. Reprod Toxicol 2004;19(2):258.

171. Clarinex (desloratadine) tablets [package insert]. Kenilworth (NJ): Schering Corporation; 2003.
172. Hilbert J, Radwanski E, Affrime M, et al. Excretion of loratadine in human breast milk. J Clin Pharmacol 1988;28(3):234–9.
173. Lucas BD Jr, Purdy CY, Scarim SK, et al. Terfenadine pharmacokinetics in breast milk of lactating women. Clin Pharmacol Ther 1995;57:398–402.

The Role of Nasal Corticosteroids in the Treatment of Rhinitis

Eli O. Meltzer, MD

KEYWORDS

• Allergic rhinitis • Vasomotor rhinitis • Nonallergic rhinopathy
• Intranasal corticosteroids • Corticosteroid pharmacology
• Rhinitis treatment

Intranasal corticosteroids (INSs) have been available for the treatment of rhinitis since 1974. They are extremely effective in reducing the nasal symptoms of sneezing, itching, rhinorrhea, and nasal congestion. It is evident that INSs are the appropriate first-line treatment choice for many patients with rhinitis, particularly those with persistent or more severe symptoms.[1] In addition to efficacy and safety considerations, patients may have a preference for one INS agent over another, which can influence their compliance with therapy. This article reviews the rationale for using INSs in rhinitis and examines the criteria that should be considered when selecting an INS treatment.

NASAL CORTICOSTEROID MECHANISMS OF ACTION

The mechanisms of action of INSs are related to their anti-inflammatory activities. It is important to understand these and the magnitude of INS effects to use them most appropriately.

T Lymphocytes

Corticosteroid therapy provides a modest reduction in the number of lymphocytes because of induction of programmed cell death or apoptosis.[2] Topical corticosteroid administration has been shown to inhibit T-lymphocyte activation, prevent increases

Disclosure Statement: Grant/Research Support: Alcon, Alexza, Amgen, Antigen Labs, Apotex, Astellas, AstraZeneca, Boehringer Ingelheim, GlaxoSmithKline, MAP, MEDA, Merck, Novartis, Proctor & Gamble, Schering-Plough, Teva, UCB; Consultant/Speaker: Alcon, Alexza Pharmaceuticals, Amgen, AstraZeneca, Boehringer Ingelheim, Capnia, Dainippon Sumitomo Pharma, Dey, GlaxoSmithKline, ISTA, Johnson & Johnson, Kalypsys, MAP Pharmaceuticals, Meda, Merck, National Jewish Health, Rady Children's Hospital, Sandoz, sanofi-aventis, Schering-Plough, Sepracor, SRxA, Teva, VentiRx, Wockhardt, Wyeth; Major Stock Shareholder: None; Other Financial or Material Support and Gifts: None.
Allergy & Asthma Medical Group & Research Center, 5776 Ruffin Road, San Diego, CA 92123, USA
E-mail address: eomeltzer@aol.com

Immunol Allergy Clin N Am 31 (2011) 545–560
doi:10.1016/j.iac.2011.05.004
immunology.theclinics.com
0889-8561/11/$ – see front matter © 2011 Elsevier Inc. All rights reserved.

in interleukin (IL)-4, IL-5, and local IgE, and inhibit eosinophil recruitment and activation,[3,4] IL-2 production,[5] and IL-2 generation.[6]

Eosinophils

Corticosteroids have well-recognized effects on the eosinophil component of the inflammatory process through direct induction of eosinophil apoptosis[7] and inhibition of eosinophil recruitment and migration into the nasal airways. Cytokine production in the airways may trigger this cellular infiltration, and therefore inhibition of cytokine production is one of the most important effects of corticosteroid therapy.[8] Corticosteroids are effective and potent inhibitors of cytokines such as tumor necrosis factor α (TNF-α) and IL-1, which induce secretion of the nonspecific endothelial activators.[9] They also inhibit the release of IL-4 and IL-13, thereby preventing expression of specific endothelial cell adhesion molecules, which can bind basophils, eosinophils, monocytes, and lymphocytes.[3]

In addition, corticosteroid treatment has been shown to inhibit the expression of the chemokine RANTES in airway epithelial cells.[10] Furthermore, corticosteroids inhibit the production of IL-3, IL-5, and granulocyte-macrophage colony-stimulating factor (GM-CSF)[11] and reduce eosinophil survival time.[12] Thus, corticosteroids have multiple effects on eosinophils: they reduce the number of eosinophils in the circulation, prevent recruitment of eosinophils to local tissue sites,[13] reduce survival of eosinophils, and prevent production of cytokines that are responsible for, or involved in, all of these processes. Glucocorticosteroids inhibit the production of many cytokines.

Mast Cells and Basophils

Topical corticosteroids can reduce inflammation through affecting the infiltration of mast cells and basophils. Treatment can decrease the number of mast cells in the nasal mucosa.[14,15] Corticosteroid treatment has also been shown to markedly reduce the number of basophils in nasal secretions.[16] An associated reduction in the release of mast cell mediators has been shown after corticosteroid treatment, along with an interference of arachidonic acid metabolism associated with a subsequent decrease in mediator production.[17,18] The reduction in the recruitment and activation of lymphocytes, eosinophils, and basophils and the associated decrease in the production of inflammatory mediators contribute to the value of corticosteroids in relieving the symptoms of rhinitis.

Neutrophils

Corticosteroids are able to inhibit the accumulation of neutrophils,[19] possibly through preventing neutrophil adherence to vascular endothelium because of suppression of the release of endothelial-activating cytokines, for example, IL-1, IL-4, and TNF-α, and by preventing the release of factors that influence migration through the endothelial barrier, for example, IL-8, TNF-α, platelet-activating factor (PAF), and LTB4.[20]

Monocytes and Macrophages

Corticosteroids reduce the number of tissue macrophages and inhibit their release of IL-1, interferon gamma, TNF-α, and GM-CSF (**Table 1**).[8,21]

Epithelial Cells

Human epithelial cells metabolize arachidonic acid. Arachidonic acid metabolites, such as leukotrienes, prostaglandins, thromboxane, and PAF, have several activities, including regulation of vascular tone and vascular permeability, stimulation of mucus secretion, chemotaxis, and regulation of cell proliferation. The cytokines produced by

Table 1	
Effects of corticosteroids on inflammatory cells	
Cells Affected	**Corticosteroid Effect**
T lymphocytes	Reduction of circulating cell number, apoptosis Inhibition of: T-lymphocyte activation IL-2 production IL-2 receptor generation IL-4 production Antigen-driven proliferation
Eosinophils	Reduction of circulating cell number, apoptosis Reduction of epithelial and mucosal cell counts Reduction of cell influx in late-phase response Inhibition of IL-4– and IL-5–mediated cell survival
Mast cells/basophils	Reduction of circulating cell counts Reduction of cell influx in late-phase response Reduction of mast cell-derived mediators after challenge Reduction of histamine content and release
Neutrophils	Reduction of cell influx after challenge
Macrophages/monocytes	Reduction of circulating cell counts Inhibition of release of: IL-1 Interferon-γ TNF-α GM-CSF

Data from Meltzer EO. The treatment of vasomotor rhinitis with intranasal corticosteroids. WAO Journal 2009;2:168.

epithelial cells can also mediate recruitment, activation, and survival of inflammatory cells in the airway.[22] Corticosteroids interfere with the inflammatory response through blocking the production of arachidonic acid metabolites in many cells. This interference is accomplished through inducing the production of the anti-inflammatory protein, lipocortin, which inhibits phospholipase A2, an enzyme central to the arachidonic acid cascade, thereby preventing the generation of cyclooxygenase and lipoxygenase products.[22]

Blood Vessels

Topical corticosteroids reduce blood flow and inhibit vascular permeability. The mechanisms for these actions include a reduction in the cyclooxygenase metabolites that maintain vascular beds, inhibition of phospholipase A2, and the subsequent formation of leukotrienes and PAF,[23] inhibition of the release of endothelial-derived relaxing factor, production of vasocortin (which reduces permeability), and enhancement of vasospasm by α-adrenergic stimulation.[24,25]

Nerve Cells

Steroids have been reported to upregulate neutral endopeptidase that degrades neuropeptides[26] and inhibits neurogenic plasma extravasation.[27]

THE GLUCOCORTICOID RECEPTOR

Corticosteroid activity is mediated by intracellular activation of the glucocorticoid receptor (GR).[28,29] In its inactive state, the GR exists as a cytosolic protein bound to two heat shock protein 90 chaperonin molecules. Binding to the corticosteroid ligand results in a conformational change that allows dissociation of the GR from the protein complex, and a quick translocation into the cell nucleus. The ligand-bound GR can modulate gene expression in the nucleus through binding to glucocorticoid response elements in promoter regions of responsive genes. The GR binds to the glucocorticoid response elements as a homodimer and acts as a transcription factor. It has also become evident that the GR can regulate gene expression unfacilitated by glucocorticoid response elements through direct interaction with transcription factors such as nuclear factor NF-kappa B and activating protein.[28,30,31] The inhibition of these two factors leads to downregulation of the production of cytokines and other inflammatory molecules and is believed to be among the primary mechanisms for the anti-inflammatory effects of corticosteroids.[28,29]

NASAL CORTICOSTEROID PHARMACOLOGY
Corticosteroid Molecules

In recent years, increased understanding of glucocorticoid receptor and corticosteroid pharmacology has enabled the development of molecules designed specifically to achieve potent, localized activity with minimal risk of systemic exposure. Currently, eight INS compounds are approved for the management of allergic rhinitis in the United States: beclomethasone dipropionate, budesonide, ciclesonide, flunisolide, fluticasone furoate, fluticasone propionate, mometasone furoate, and triamcinolone acetonide (**Table 2**).[32]

Corticosteroid molecules are derived from the parent molecule, cortisol.[33] The carbon framework of each corticosteroid is made up of three 6-carbon rings (rings A, B, and C) and one 5-carbon ring (ring D).[32] All anti-inflammatory corticosteroids have features in common with cortisol and with each other: a ketone oxygen at position 3; an unsaturated bond between carbons 4 and 5; a hydroxyl group at position 11; and a ketone oxygen group on carbon 20. The variations occurring off ring D at positions 16, 17, and 21 are the greatest differentiating factors between the individual molecules. Structure–activity relationship studies of this region led to the identification of chemical groups that enhance topical activity and reduce systemic adverse events.[34] For example, the furoate group of mometasone furoate was found to enhance molecular affinity for the glucocorticoid receptor binding site.

Other modifications have improved the activity of corticosteroid compounds. The 21-chloro-17 (2' furoate) group on the mometasone furoate structure improves anti-inflammatory activity, whereas the chloride at position 21 provides the additional benefit of inferring resistance to degradation by esterases.[34] Halogen substitutions at positions 6 and 9 are thought to increase potency, as are side-chain substitutions at position 17.[35]

Pharmacodynamic Properties

Glucocorticoid potency can be measured in various ways, but is thought to be closely related to GR binding affinity.[32] **Fig. 1** illustrates the relative GR binding affinities for most intranasal compounds. Relative receptor affinity studies are highly dependent on assay methodology and prone to error.[36] Although specific values vary between studies, most have shown a similar order of potency. An earlier study of INSs that used competition assay methodology reported a similar rank order of relative binding potency: mometasone furoate > fluticasone propionate > budesonide > triamcinolone acetonide > dexamethasone.[29]

Corticosteroid potency also has been evaluated using the McKenzie assay, which compares the relative cutaneous vasoconstrictor and skin blanching responses of

Table 2
Available intranasal corticosteroids

Generic (Proprietary) Name	Recommended Dosage
Beclomethasone dipropionate (Beconase AQ)	*Adults and children >12 years of age:* 1 or 2 sprays (42–84 μg) per nostril bid (total dose 168–336 μg/d) *Children 6–12 years of age:* 1 spray (42 μg) per nostril bid for total of 168 μg/d, or up to 2 sprays per nostril bid for total of 336 μg/d
Budesonide (Rhinocort Aqua)[a]	*Adults and children >6 years of age:* 1 spray (32 μg/spray) per nostril qd up to a maximum of 128 μg/d (6 to <12 years of age) or 256 μg/d (>12 years of age)
Ciclesonide (Omnaris)	*Adults and children >12 years of age:* 2 sprays (50 μg/spray) per nostril qd
Flunisolide (Nasarel)	*Adults:* 2 sprays (58 μg) per nostril bid, not to exceed 8 sprays per nostril per day (464 μg) *Children 6–14 years of age:* 1 spray (29 μg) per nostril tid or 2 sprays (58 μg) per nostril bid, not to exceed 4 sprays per nostril per day (232 μg)
Fluticasone furoate (Veramyst)	*Adults and children >12 years of age:* 2 sprays (55 μg) per nostril qd *Children 2–11 years of age:* 1 spray (27.5 μg) per nostril qd up to 2 sprays (55 μg) per nostril qd
Fluticasone propionate (Flonase)	*Adults:* 2 sprays (100 μg) per nostril qd or 1 spray (50 μg) bid *Adolescents and children >4 years of age:* 1 spray (50 μg) per nostril per day up to, but not in excess of, 2 sprays (100 μg) per nostril per day
Mometasone furoate (Nasonex)	*Adults and children >12 years of age:* 2 sprays (100 μg) per nostril qd *Children 2–11 years of age:* 1 spray (50 μg) per nostril qd
Triamcinolone acetonide (Nasacort AQ)	*Adults and children >12 years of age:* 2 sprays (110 μg) per nostril qd *Children 6–12 years of age:* 1 spray (55 μg) per nostril or 110 μg qd, up to 2 sprays (110 μg each) per nostril or 220 μg qd

[a] Available in two strengths: 32 and 64 μg per spray.
Data from Derendorf H, Meltzer EO. Molecular and clinical pharmacology of intranasal corticosteroids: clinical and therapeutic implications. Allergy 2008;63:1297.

individual compounds.[37] Using this methodology, the rank order of potency was: fluticasone propionate > mometasone furoate > budesonide > flunisolide > triamcinolone acetonide (**Table 3**).[8,38] This vasoconstriction phenomenon, which occurs in all subjects, has been suggested to partly explain the glucocorticosteroid effect on the nasal mucosa. In a randomized double-blind crossover study, using the 133Xe wash-out method as a measure of nasal mucosal blood flow, the effect of topically administered budesonide was compared with placebo. No difference between the groups was found to occur. A more complex activity than vasoconstriction seems likely to be responsible for the clinical effect of INSs.[39]

Results of studies using another marker of corticosteroid potency, transactivation potency, correlate with receptor binding affinity results. One study found mometasone furoate the most potent GR ligand, requiring the lowest concentration to affect 50% of the maximum level of transcription activation of a glucocorticoid response element reporter gene in cells.[29] Overall rank of potency using this methodology

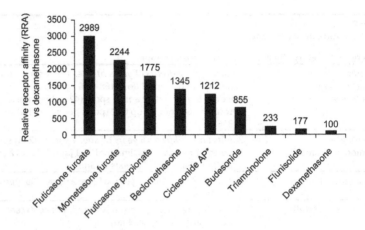

*Ciclesonide active principle (active metabolite)

Fig. 1. Relative glucocorticoid receptor affinity of intranasal corticosteroids. (*From* Derendorf H, Meltzer EO. Molecular and clinical pharmacology of intranasal corticosteroids: clinical and therapeutic implications. Allergy 2008;63:1294; with permission.)

was: mometasone furoate > fluticasone propionate > triamcinolone acetonide > budesonide > dexamethasone.

No evidence is available of a linear association between glucocorticoid potency and clinical response, nor does a known "plateau" exist beyond which greater potency does not add additional benefit. Likewise, no evidence shows that the compound with the highest receptor affinity will have superior clinical efficacy. Although increased potency at intranasal sites would seem desirable, the possibility of greater potency at other sites could theoretically increase the risk of systemic adverse effects, because GRs are similar throughout the body.

Pharmacokinetic Properties

Because the goals of INS therapy are to deposit drug at the site of action, have it remain there as long as possible, and limit the amount that leaves the site and enters the systemic circulation, the pharmacokinetic features of particular interest are lipophilicity and systemic availability.

Table 3
Potency of topical corticosteroids based on receptor binding affinity and the skin-blanching test

Corticosteroid	Receptor Binding Affinity	Skin Blanching Potency
Flunisolide	1.8	330
Triamcinolone acetonide	3.6	330
Beclomethasone dipropionate	0.4	600
Budesonide	9.4	900
Fluticasone propionate	18.0	1200

Data from Meltzer EO. The treatment of vasomotor rhinitis with intranasal corticosteroids. WAO Journal 2009;2:169.

Lipophilicity

The more highly lipophilic compounds are absorbed more quickly and thoroughly by the nasal mucosa and retained longer in nasal tissue, increasing exposure to the GR.[40] Lipophilicity also contributes to increased plasma protein binding. In this sense, lipophilicity is a desired characteristic. In the event of systemic absorption, lipophilicity may contribute to the accumulation of drug in other tissues, possibly contributing to unwanted side effects. Thus, the ideal combination of features would include a high degree of lipophilicity coupled with low systemic absorption and rapid clearance.

The order of lipid solubility for corticosteroids has been reported as: mometasone furoate > fluticasone propionate > beclomethasone dipropionate > budesonide > triamcinolone acetonide > flunisolide.[40] Ciclesonide and des-ciclesonide have greater lipophilicity than fluticasone propionate.[41] The furoate (mometasone) and propionate (fluticasone) ester side chains are pharmacologically similar moieties that contribute greatly to the lipophilicity of their associated compounds.[42] The lipophilicity of fluticasone propionate has been reported as being three times higher than beclomethasone dipropionate, 300 times more than budesonide, and at least 1000-fold greater than flunisolide and triamcinolone acetonide.[38]

Absorption/Bioavailability

After intranasal administration, a drug can enter the systemic circulation through direct local absorption in the nasal mucosa or after gastrointestinal absorption of swallowed material. A large proportion of intranasally administered drug is quickly cleared from the nose into the throat and swallowed, becoming available for absorption in the gastrointestinal tract. A high rate of first-pass metabolism will inactivate the absorbed drug, but direct absorption into the systemic circulation through the nasal tissues bypasses the protective hepatic first-pass mechanism.

Systemic absorption rates are highest among the relatively older compounds, flunisolide, beclomethasone, and budesonide (**Fig. 2**). One-third to one-half of an intranasally administered dose of the older agents may reach the systemic circulation. For budesonide, systemic exposure is primarily through absorption through the nasal

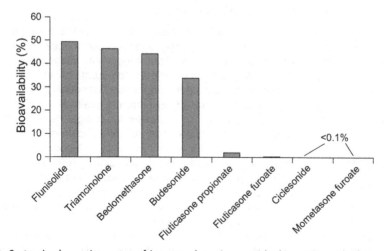

Fig. 2. Systemic absorption rates of intranasal corticosteroids. (*From* Derendorf H, Meltzer EO. Molecular and clinical pharmacology of intranasal corticosteroids: clinical and therapeutic implications. Allergy 2008;63:1294; with permission.)

mucosa.[43,44] The newer compounds, fluticasone propionate, and mometasone furoate, are more lipophilic[34] and undergo rapid and extensive first-pass metabolism after oral administration, contributing to their negligible systemic absorption.[38] A pharmacokinetic study of ciclesonide in both healthy subjects and patients with seasonal allergic rhinitis found that serum levels of ciclesonide and the active metabolite desciclesonide were below the lower limits of quantification (25 and 10 pg/mL, respectively) in most subjects.[45]

CLINICAL CONSIDERATIONS
Onset and Duration of Action

It was traditionally accepted that INSs should be used for days or weeks to achieve significant benefits, and because these agents were used primarily to control chronic symptoms, few studies focused on onset of action.[40] Symptom improvement has been noted within 1 to 2 days after administration of most newer agents.[40] A clinical study of ciclesonide nasal spray in patients with seasonal allergic rhinitis reported a significantly greater effect of treatment on total nasal symptom scores compared with placebo as early as hour 12.[46] In subjects with seasonal allergic rhinitis, mometasone furoate nasal spray significantly improved nasal symptom scores compared with placebo in as little as 7 hours after a single 200-μg dose.[47] It is not uncommon for patients to use intranasal medications intermittently on an "as-needed" basis,[40] and this use may be justified given the potential for a more rapid onset of action than was previously ascribed to these medications.

Lipid conjugation, or fatty acid esterification, is a process through which a corticosteroid molecule forms a reversible chemical bond with fatty acids in the nasal tissues. These drug–lipid complexes serve as a slow-release drug reservoir that holds the corticosteroid within the target area, increasing the local residence time. As the binding process is reversible, the retained corticosteroid remains available for binding to local GRs. This binding process may be partly responsible for the once-daily duration of efficacy of many INSs. Lipid conjugation has been reported for budesonide[48] and des-ciclesonide.[49]

Clinical Efficacy in the Therapy of Allergic Rhinitis

The design of topically active INS formulations has provided a much better therapeutic ratio than oral corticosteroids.[25] The pharmacodynamic and pharmacokinetic properties of these agents play an important role in facilitating local anti-inflammatory activity with a low rate of side effects. However, whether the often-subtle pharmacodynamic and pharmacokinetic differences between the compounds distinguish them in a clinical setting remains to be confirmed. Based on currently available data, no clear evidence shows that any INS is superior to any other for allergic rhinitis symptom relief,[40,50] despite their pharmacologic differences. All have shown efficacy in both seasonal and perennial allergic rhinitis in a large number of well-controlled studies. The possibility exists that the degree of anti-inflammatory activity required for allergic rhinitis symptom relief is low enough that relief is easily achieved with agents of varying potencies, or that GR saturation or near-saturation occurs with all of the preparations.[40,51] These considerations have not been well studied in the treatment of vasomotor rhinitis, also known as nonallergic rhinopathy.

INSs are the single most effective class of medications for allergic rhinitis, and therefore are recommended as first-line therapy by both national and international task forces for those with moderate-to-severe or persistent allergic rhinitis.[52,53] They improve each of the nasal and ocular symptoms of allergic rhinoconjunctivitis. They are superior to oral antihistamines in terms of both total nasal symptom scores and congestion scores.[54,55] They also produce greater symptom relief than oral leuko-triene antagonists[56,57] and, despite limited information, INSs are equivalent[58] or even superior[59,60] to combinations of antihistamines and antileukotrienes. Although intranasal antihistamines have a more rapid onset of benefit compared with INSs, the data are insufficient to conclude that intranasal antihistamines are therapeutically equivalent to INSs, especially after a 14-day treatment period.[61] In addition, INSs show greater effectiveness than intranasal H1 antihistamines in improving nasal blockage.[62] For the most part, the addition of an oral antihistamine to an INS does not seem to confer additional clinical benefits over the use of an INS alone.[63,64] However, adding an intranasal antihistamine to an INS does seem to provide greater efficacy than the monotherapies.[65]

Formulation characteristics may also influence the efficacy and tolerability of INSs. These characteristics can affect patient preference and adherence to allergic rhinitis therapy.[66] All currently available INSs are delivered in aqueous preparations, and beclomethasone and ciclesonide are under development in hydrofluoroalkane nasal aerosol solution formulations. Although INS preparations may vary in the volume emitted per actuated spray and sensory attributes (such as perceived runoff, discom-fort, taste, and smell), and thus patient acceptance and adherence, no clear clinically relevant differences in efficacy have been seen between them.[40]

Clinical Efficacy in the Therapy of Nonallergic Rhinopathy

Beclomethasone dipropionate was first reported to be effective for vasomotor rhinitis in 1976. In Sweden, 39 men and women aged 19 to 66 years (average, 39 years) with perennial nasal obstruction, drip, itching, and sneezing were studied in a randomized, double-blind, placebo-controlled, 4-week treatment period, crossover-designed trial. Intracutaneous specific aeroallergen testing for these subjects was negative. Nasal secretion eosinophilic cells were estimated to be less than 10%. The dosage was one aerosol-delivered puff into each nostril three times daily (300 µg of beclometha-sone dipropionate per day during the active period). No difference was seen in the response of the groups on the first day of treatment. However, a significant reduction in the total symptom score was observed during the second week of the beclometha-sone dipropionate treatment period. This effect remained throughout the remainder of the treatment period. For the individual nasal symptoms, a significantly lower score was registered for sneezing during the first week, for nasal drainage during the second week, for nasal itching during the third week, and for nasal blocking only during the fourth week of beclomethasone dipropionate treatment. After the beclomethasone dipropionate treatment period, 4 patients considered themselves free of trouble, 25 had improved, 10 were unchanged, and none had worsened; 74% considered them-selves free of symptoms or greatly improved. After the placebo period, none was free of trouble, 12 had improved, 20 were unchanged, and 7 patients had worsened; 31% considered themselves free of symptoms or greatly improved. Of the 39 patients who completed the study, 25 preferred the beclomethasone dipropionate period, 5 preferred the placebo period, and 9 found no difference between the periods. The authors concluded that the results were encouraging, because approximately 75% of the patients considered themselves free of trouble or improved when treated with the intranasal corticosteroid.[67] In a small study of nonallergic patients aged 20 to 68 years, budesonide nasal aerosol was found to be significantly more effective than placebo in reducing the symptoms of nasal obstruction, nasal drainage, and sneezing at twice-daily dosing of 50, 200, and 800 µg. Budesonide, in dosages of 200 and

800 μg daily, significantly reduced the methacholine-induced secretions compared with the placebo treatment.[68]

Of the currently available INS preparations in the United States, only fluticasone propionate has an indication approved by the U.S. Food and Drug Administration (FDA) for the treatment of perennial nonallergic rhinitis (PNAR), regardless of the presence of nasal eosinophilia.[69] In a large study of patients with PNAR, administration of fluticasone propionate at 200 μg (two sprays per side, once daily) was as effective as 400 μg once daily, and both doses were statistically better than placebo in achieving symptom reduction over 4 weeks.[70] A separate study in patients with vasomotor rhinitis showed that fluticasone propionate, 200 μg once daily, was significantly superior to placebo in reducing symptoms of nasal obstruction and decreasing inferior turbinate hypertrophy as assessed via CT scan.[71] However, a study of individuals with PNAR showed that treatment with mometasone furoate, 200 μg (2 sprays per side once daily) for 6 weeks, did not show any significant improvement in rhinitis symptoms compared with placebo.[72] Furthermore, another study showed that fluticasone furoate, administered as 110 μg (2 sprays per side once daily) to 699 subjects with vasomotor rhinitis triggered by weather or temperature, was not superior to placebo in reducing congestion, rhinorrhea, or postnasal drip during the 4-week study period.[73]

The evidence for benefit of INSs in nonallergic nasal disease is somewhat inconsistent, probably reflecting the heterogeneous nature of these conditions. Nonetheless, studies to date in the treatment of vasomotor rhinitis, also known as nonallergic rhinopathy, suggest that INS treatment for nonallergic rhinopathy may be of some therapeutic value and should, for now, be considered for first-line therapy.[74]

Safety

Differences in safety between INSs are more theoretical than evidence-based, with the greatest concern being systemic exposure and effects on adrenal function in all patients, and on growth in children. Pharmacokinetic studies confirm that the newer agents, mometasone furoate, fluticasone propionate, fluticasone furoate, and ciclesonide, exhibit negligible systemic absorption and would be expected to pose fewer risks. One could also argue that their greater potency could pose safety risks, even if they were absorbed to only a small degree. To date, these concerns have not been realized. Binding to proteins such as albumin and other biologic material can occur at the local site of action, and also in general circulation if a corticosteroid is systemically absorbed. Most INSs have a high degree of protein binding, ranging from 71% (triamcinolone acetonide) to 99% (ciclesonide, des-ciclesonide). Only free drug is pharmacologically active, and therefore a high degree of serum protein binding for these compounds is desirable to limit potential systemic adverse events.[75]

Special caution is warranted in treating individuals who may be using concomitant corticosteroid therapy for other medical conditions, such as asthma. The safety of overlapping corticosteroid therapy has not been well studied, but combined treatments may be a concern because of the increased total systemic corticosteroid load. Despite potential concerns, the use of INSs at recommended doses does not seem to have a significant effect on the hypothalamic-pituitary-adrenal axis.[76] Osteocalcin, a marker of bone turnover, and eosinophilia were both unaffected by intranasal budesonide, mometasone, and triamcinolone, suggesting that the systemic glucocorticoid burden was clinically insignificant.[77] These results seem to be corroborated by the finding of no increased likelihood of bone fractures among octogenarians using intranasal corticosteroids, regardless of the dose used.[78] The effects of these agents on bone growth and height have also been evaluated in numerous studies, with knemometry considered the most reliable and sensitive indicator.[79] Studies with budesonide, mometasone furoate, and fluticasone propionate using knemometry have not shown significant changes in lower leg growth velocity.[79–81] Among studies based on stadiometry measurements, only one reported a small but significant reduction in height among children treated with intranasal beclomethasone for 1 year compared with placebo.[82] One-year studies involving mometasone furoate, fluticasone propionate, budesonide, triamcinolone, and ciclesonide did not report any significant negative effects on height.[83–87]

Common local side effects of INSs include dryness, stinging, burning, and epistaxis, the frequencies of which are similar in the various compounds. These side effects occur in 5% to 10% of patients, with the exception among the aqueous preparations of flunisolide, which, because of its excipients, causes a higher incidence of discomfort.[88] The administration technique of aiming the spray away from the septum is important because it seems to reduce the incidence of epistaxis.

Nasal mucosal atrophy is a concern with chronic topical steroid use. A long-term study with mometasone furoate found no evidence of atrophy or metaplasia after 12 months of intranasal use.[89] Similar studies with fluticasone propionate did not identify indications of atrophy, and noted only a nonsignificant increase in metaplasia in one patient.[90] Clinically apparent nasal candidiasis, occasionally seen with orally inhaled corticosteroids, is extremely rare with INSs.

SUMMARY

Allergic rhinitis, which has a well-known pathophysiology, and nonallergic rhinopathy, which is less well understood, are common conditions that affect millions of individuals worldwide. INSs diffuse across the respiratory membrane, bind to the intracellular glucocorticoid receptor, and, after transportation to the nucleus, can reduce inflammatory reactions. Their risk/benefit ratio is the best of the pharmacotherapeutic options. Therefore, INSs should be the first-choice treatments for patients with these nasal diseases to improve symptoms and quality of life.

REFERENCES

1. Bousquet J, van Cauwenberge P, Khaltaev N. Allergic rhinitis and its impact on asthma. J Allergy Clin Immunol 2001;108:S147–334.
2. Cohen JJ. Lymphocyte death induced by glucocorticoids. In: Schleimer RP, Claman HN, Oronsky A, editors. Antiinflammatory steroid action: basic and clinical aspects. San Diego (CA): Academic Press; 1989. p. 110–31.
3. Masuyama K, Jacobson MR, Rak S, et al. Topical glucocorticosteroid (fluticasone propionate) inhibits cells expressing cytokine mRNA for interleukin-4 in the nasal mucosa in allergen-induced rhinitis. Immunology 1994;82:192–9.
4. Alvarado C, Reed C, Gleich T, et al. Fluticasone propionate aqueous nasal spray reduces nasal eosinophils and cytokine activity of patients with allergic rhinitis [abstract]. J Allergy Clin Immunol 1995;95:193.
5. Schleimer RP. Glucocorticosteroids: their mechanism of action and use in allergic diseases. In: Middleton E, Reed CE, Ellis EF, editors. Allergy principles and practice. 3rd edition. Washington, DC: Mosby; 1988. p. 739–65.
6. Reed JC, Abidi AH, Alpers JD, et al. Effect of cyclosporin A and dexamethasone on interleukin-2 receptor gene expression. J Immunol 1986;137:150–4.
7. Her E, Frazer J, Austen KF, et al. Eosinophil hematopoietins antagonize the programmed cell death of eosinophils: cytokine and glucocorticoid effects on

eosinophils maintained by endothelial cell conditioned medium. J Clin Invest 1992;88:1982.

8. Meltzer EO. The pharmacological basis for the treatment of perennial allergic rhinitis and non-allergic rhinitis with topical corticosteroids. Allergy 1997;52:33–40.

9. Staruch MJ, Wood DD. Reduction of serum interleukin-1-like activity after treatment with dexamethasone. J Leukoc Biol 1985;37:193–207.

10. Stellato C, Beck LA, Gorgone GA, et al. Expression of the chemokine RANTES by a human bronchial epithelial cell line: modulation by cytokines and glucocorticoids. J Immunol 1995;155:410–8.

11. Kato M, Schleimer RP. Antiinflammatory steroids inhibit GM-CSF production by human lung tissue. Lung 1994;172:113–34.

12. Wallen N, Kita H, Weiler D, et al. Glucocorticoids inhibit cytokine-mediated eosinophil survival. J Immunol 1991;147:3490–5.

13. van As A, Bronsky EA, Dockhorn RJ, et al. Once daily fluticasone propionate is as effective for perennial allergic rhinitis as twice daily beclomethasone dipropionate. J Allergy Clin Immunol 1993;91:1146–54.

14. Schleimer RP. The effects of anti-inflammatory steroids on mast cells. In: Kaliner M, Metcalfe D, editors. The mast cell in health and disease. New York: Marcel Dekker; 1992. p. 483.

15. Gomez E, Claque JE, Gatland D, et al. Effect of topical corticosteroids on seasonally induced increases in nasal mast cells. BMJ 1988;296:1572–3.

16. Bascom R, Wachs M, Naclerio RM, et al. Basophil influx occurs after nasal antigen challenge: effects of topical corticosteroid pretreatment. J Allergy Clin Immunol 1988;81:580.

17. Pipkorn U, Proud D, Lichtenstein LM, et al. Inhibition of mediator release in allergic rhinitis by pretreatment with topical corticosteroids. N Engl J Med 1987;316:1506–10.

18. Meltzer EO, Jalowayski AA, Field EA, et al. Intranasal fluticasone propionate reduces histamine and tryptase in the mucosa of allergic rhinitis patients [abstract]. J Allergy Clin Immunol 1993;91:298.

19. Bascom R, Pipkorn U, Lichtenstein LM, et al. The influx of inflammatory cells into nasal washings during the late response to antigen challenge. Am Rev Respir Dis 1988;138:406–12.

20. Bochner B, Rutledge BK, Schleimer RP. Interleukin-1 production by human lung tissue. II. Inhibition by anti-inflammatory steroids. J Immunol 1987;39:2303.

21. Guyre PM, Munck A. Glucocorticoid action on monocytes and macrophages. In: Schleimer RP, Claman HN, Oronsky A, editors. Antiinflammatory steroid action: basic and clinical aspects. New York: Academic Press; 1991. p. 199–225.

22. Flower RJ, Blackwell GJ. Anti-inflammatory steroids induce biosynthesis of a phospholipase A2 inhibitor which prevents prostaglandin generation. Nature 1979;278:456–9.

23. Flower RJ. Lipocortin and the mechanism of action of the glucocorticoids. Br J Pharmacol 1988;94:987–1015.

24. Williams TJ, Yarwood H. Effect of glucocorticosteroids on microvascular permeability. Am Rev Respir Dis 1990;141:S39.

25. Boschetto P, Rogers DF, Fabbri LM, et al. Corticosteroid inhibition of microvascular leakage. Am Rev Respir Dis 1991;143:605.

26. Borson DB. Roles of neutral endopeptidase in airways. Am J Physiol 1991;260:L212–25.

27. Piedimonte G, McDonald DM, Nadel JA. Glucocorticoids inhibit neurogenic plasma extravasation and prevent virus-potentiated extravasation in the rat trachea. J Clin Invest 1990;86:1409–15.

28. Austin RJ, Maschera B, Walker A, et al. Mometasone furoate is a less specific glucocorticoid than fluticasone propionate. Eur Respir J 2002;20:1386–92.
29. Smith CL, Kreutner W. In vitro glucocorticoid receptor binding and transcriptional activation by topically active glucocorticoids. Arzneimittelforschung 1998;48: 956–60.
30. Ray A, Siegel MD, Prefontaine KE, et al. Anti-inflammation: direct physical association and functional antagonism between transcription factor NF-KB and the glucocorticoid receptor. Chest 1995;107(3 Suppl):139S.
31. Konig H, Ponta H, Rahmsdorf HJ, et al. Interference between pathway-specific transcription factors: glucocorticoids antagonize phorbol ester-induced AP-1 activity without altering AP-1 site occupation in vivo. EMBO J 1992;11:2241–6.
32. Derendorf H, Meltzer EO. Molecular and clinical pharmacology of intranasal corticosteroids: clinical and therapeutic implications. Allergy 2008;63:1292–300.
33. Naclerio RM. Allergic rhinitis. N Engl J Med 1991;325:860–9.
34. Szefler SJ. Pharmacokinetics of intranasal steroids. J Allergy Clin Immunol 2001; 108:S26–31.
35. Bikowski J, Pillai R, Shroot B. The position not the presence of the halogen in corticosteroids influences potency and side effects. J Drugs Dermatol 2006;5: 125–30.
36. Hogger P, Rohdewald P. Binding kinetics of fluticasone propionate to the human glucocorticoid receptor. Steroids 1994;59:597–602.
37. McKenzie AW. Percutaneous absorption of steroids. Arch Dermatol 1962;86: 611–4.
38. Johnson M. Development of fluticasone propionate and comparison with other inhaled corticosteroids. J Allergy Clin Immunol 1998;101:S434–9.
39. Bende M, Lindquist N, Pipkorn U. Effect of a topical glucocorticoid, budesonide, on nasal mucosal blood flow as measured with 133Xe wash-out technique. Allergy 1983;38:461–4.
40. Corren J. Intranasal corticosteroids for allergic rhinitis: how do different agents compare? J Allergy Clin Immunol 1999;104:S144–9.
41. Colice GL, Derendorf H. Shapiro GG. Inhaled corticosteroids: is there an ideal therapy? Medscape Web site. Available at: http://www.medscape.org/viewprogram/2917. Accessed February 22, 2007.
42. Crim C, Pierre LN, Daley-Yates PT. A review of the pharmacology and pharmacokinetics of inhaled fluticasone propionate and mometasone furoate. Clin Ther 2001;23:1339–54.
43. Edsbacker S, Andersson KE, Ryrfeldt A. Nasal bioavailability and systemic effects of the glucocorticoid budesonide in man. Eur J Clin Pharmacol 1985;29:477–81.
44. Rhinocort Aqua [package insert]. Wilmington, DE: AstraZeneca LP; 2004.
45. Nave R, Wingertzahn MA, Brookman S, et al. Safety, tolerability, and exposure of ciclesonide nasal spray in healthy and asymptomatic subjects with seasonal allergic rhinitis. J Clin Pharmacol 2006;46:461–7.
46. Ratner PH, Wingertzahn MA, van Bavel JH, et al. Efficacy and safety of ciclesonide nasal spray for the treatment of seasonal allergic rhinitis. J Allergy Clin Immunol 2006;118:1142–8.
47. Berkowitz RB, Roberson S, Zora J, et al. Mometasone furoate nasal spray is rapidly effective in the treatment of seasonal allergic rhinitis in an outdoor (park), acute exposure setting. Allergy Asthma Proc 1999;20:167–72.
48. Miller-Larsson A, Jansson P, Runstrom A, et al. Prolonged airway activity and improved selectivity of udesonide possibly due to esterification. Am J Respir Crit Care Med 2000;162:1455–61.

49. Nave R, Meyer W, Fuhst R, et al. Formation of fatty acid conjugates of ciclesonide active metabolite in the rat lung after 4-week inhalation of ciclesonide. Pulm Pharmacol Ther 2005;18:390–6.

50. Waddell AN, Patel SK, Toma AG, et al. Intranasal steroid sprays in the treatment of rhinitis: is one better than another? J Laryngol Otol 2003;117:843–5.

51. Stellato C, Atsuta J, Bickel CA, et al. An in vitro comparison of commonly used topical glucocorticoid preparations. J Allergy Clin Immunol 1999;104:623–9.

52. Wallace DV, Dykewicz MS, Bernstein DI, et al. The diagnosis and management of rhinitis: an updated practice parameter. J Allergy Clin Immunol 2008; 122(2 Suppl):S1–84.

53. Bousquet J, Khaltaev N, Cruz AA, et al. Allergic Rhinitis and its Impact on Asthma (ARIA) 2008 update (in collaboration with the World Health Organization, GA(2) LEN and AllerGen). Allergy 2008;63(Suppl 86):8–160.

54. Weiner JM, Abramson MJ, Puy RM. Intranasal corticosteroids versus oral H1 receptor antagonists in allergic rhinitis: systematic review of randomized controlled trials. BMJ 1998;317:1624–9.

55. Rinne J, Simola M, Malmberg H, et al. Early treatment of perennial rhinitis with budesonide or cetirizine and it effects on long-term outcome. J Allergy Clin Immunol 2002;109:426–32.

56. Nathan RA, Yancey SW, Waitkus-Edwards K, et al. Fluticasone propionate nasal spray is superior to montelukast for allergic rhinitis while neither affects overall asthma control. Chest 2005;128:1910–20.

57. Ratner PH, Howland WC 3rd, Arastu R, et al. Fluticasone propionate aqueous nasal spray provided significantly greater improvement in daytime and nighttime nasal symptoms of seasonal allergic rhinitis compared with montelukast. Ann Allergy Asthma Immunol 2003;90:536–42.

58. Wilson AM, Orr LC, Sims EJ, et al. Effects of monotherapy with intra-nasal corticosteroids or combined oral histamine and leukotriene receptor antagonists in seasonal allergic rhinitis. Clin Exp Allergy 2001;31:61–8.

59. Di Lorenzo G, Pacor ML, Pellitteri ME, et al. Randomized placebo-controlled trial comparing fluticasone aqueous nasal spray in mono-therapy, fluticasone plus cetirizine, fluticasone plus montelukast and cetirizine plus montelukast for seasonal allergic rhinitis. Clin Exp Allergy 2004;34:259–67.

60. Pullerits T, Praks L, Ristioja V, et al. Comparison of a nasal glucocorticoid, antileukotriene, and a combination of antileukotriene and antihistamine in the treatment of seasonal allergic rhinitis. J Allergy Clin Immunol 2002;109:949–55.

61. Kaliner MA, Storms W, Tilles S, et al. Comparison of olopatadine 0.6% nasal spray versus fluticasone propionate 50 microg in the treatment of seasonal allergic rhinitis. Allergy Asthma Proc 2009;30:255–62.

62. Yanez A, Rodrigo GJ. Intranasal corticosteroids versus topical H1 receptor antagonists in allergic rhinitis: a systematic review with meta-analysis. Ann Allergy Asthma Immunol 2002;89:479–84.

63. Barnes ML, Ward JH, Fardon TC, et al. Effects of levocetirizine as add-on therapy to fluticasone in seasonal allergic rhinitis. Clin Exp Allergy 2006;36(5):676–84.

64. Ratner PH, van Bavel JH, Martin BG, et al. A comparison of the efficacy of fluticasone propionate aqueous nasal spray and loratadine, alone and in combination, for the treatment of seasonal allergic rhinitis. J Fam Pract 1998;47:118–25.

65. Ratner PH, Hampel F, VanBavel J, et al. Combination therapy with azelastine hydrochloride nasal spray in the treatment of patients with seasonal allergic rhinitis. Ann Allergy Asthma Immunol 2008;100:74–81.

66. Meltzer EO. Formulation considerations of intranasal corticosteroids for the treatment of allergic rhinitis. Ann Allergy Asthma Immunol 2007;98:12–21.
67. Lofkvist T, Svensson G. Treatment of vasomotor rhinitis with intranasal beclomethasone dipropionate. Acta Allergol 1976;31:227–38.
68. Malm L, Wihl JA, Lamm CJ, et al. Reduction of metacholine-induced nasal secretion by treatment with a new topical steroids in perennial non-allergic rhinitis. Allergy 1981;36:209–14.
69. Flonase [prescribing information]. Research Triangle Park, NC: GlaxoSmithKline; 2004. Available at: http://www.flonase.com. Accessed April 2, 2010.
70. Webb DR, Meltzer EO, Finn AF Jr, et al. Intranasal fluticasone propionate is effective for perennial nonallergic rhinitis with or without eosinophilia. Ann Allergy Asthma Immunol 2002;88:385–90.
71. Arikan OK, Koc C, Kendi T, et al. CT assessment of the effect of fluticasone propionate aqueous nasal spray treatment on lower turbinate hypertrophy due to vasomotor rhinitis. Acta Otolaryngol 2006;126:37–42.
72. Lundblad L, Sipila P, Farstad T, et al. Mometasone furoate nasal spray in the treatment of perennial non-allergic rhinitis: a Nordic, multicenter, randomized, double-blind, placebo-controlled study. Acta Otolaryngol 2001;121:505–9.
73. Jacobs R, Lieberman P, Kent E, et al. Weather/temperature-sensitive vasomotor rhinitis may be refractory to intranasal corticosteroid treatment. Allergy Asthma Proc 2009;30:120–7.
74. Meltzer EO. The treatment of vasomotor rhinitis with intranasal corticosteroids. WAO Journal 2009;2:166–79.
75. Derendorf H, Nave R, Drollmann A, et al. Relevance of pharmacokinetics and pharmacodynamics of inhaled corticosteroids to asthma. Eur Respir J 2006;28:1042–50.
76. Boner AL. Effects of intranasal corticosteroids on the hypothalamic–pituitary–adrenal axis in children. J Allergy Clin Immunol 2001;108:S32–9.
77. Wilson AM, Sims EJ, McFarlane LC, et al. Effects of intranasal corticosteroids on adrenal, bone, and blood markers of systemic activity in allergic rhinitis. J Allergy Clin Immunol 1998;102:598–604.
78. Suissa S, Baltzan M, Kremer R, et al. Inhaled and nasal corticosteroid use and the risk of fracture. Am J Respir Crit Care Med 2004;169:83–8.
79. Skoner DP, Gentile D, Angelini B, et al. The effects of intranasal triamcinolone acetonide and intranasal fluticasone propionate on short-term bone growth and HPA axis in children with allergic rhinitis. Ann Allergy Asthma Immunol 2003;90:56–62.
80. Wolthers OD, Pedersen S. Knemometric assessment of systemic activity of once daily intranasal dry-powder budesonide in children. Allergy 1994;49:96–9.
81. Agertoft L, Pedersen S. Short-term lower leg growth rate in children with rhinitis treated with intranasal mometasone furoate and budesonide. J Allergy Clin Immunol 1999;104:948–52.
82. Skoner DP, Rachelefsky GS, Meltzer EO, et al. Detection of growth suppression in children during treatment with intranasal beclomethasone dipropionate. Pediatrics 2000;105:E23.
83. Schenkel EJ, Skoner DP, Bronsky EA, et al. Absence of growth retardation in children with perennial allergic rhinitis after one year of treatment with mometasone furoate aqueous nasal spray. Pediatrics 2000;105:e22.
84. Allen DB, Meltzer EO, Lemanske RF Jr, et al. No growth suppression in children treated with the maximum recommended dose of fluticasone propionate aqueous nasal spray for one year. Allergy Asthma Proc 2002;23:407–13.

85. Moller C, Ahlstrom H, Henricson KA, et al. Safety of nasal budesonide in the long-term treatment of children with perennial rhinitis. Clin Exp Allergy 2003;33: 816–22.
86. Skoner DP, Gentile DA, Doyle WJ. Effect on growth of long-term treatment with intranasal triamcinalone acetonide aqueous in children with allergic rhinitis. Ann Allergy Asthma Immunol 2008;101:431–6.
87. Skoner D, Maspero J, Kundu S, et al. Ciclesonide, administered once daily, has no effect on growth velocity in prepubertal children with mild, persistent asthma [abstract]. J Allergy Clin Immunol 2006;117(Suppl 2):S11 [abstract 44].
88. Welsh PW, Stricker WE, Chu CP, et al. Efficacy of beclomethasone nasal solution, flunisolide, and cromolyn in relieving symptoms of ragweed allergy. Mayo Clin Proc 1987;62:125–34.
89. Minshall E, Ghaffar O, Cameron L, et al. Assessment by nasal biopsy of long-term use of mometasone furoate aqueous nasal spray (Nasonex) in the treatment of perennial rhinitis. Otolaryngol Head Neck Surg 1998;118:648–54.
90. Holm AF, Fokkens WJ, Godthelp T, et al. 1-year placebo-controlled study of intra-nasal fluticasone propionate aqueous nasal spray in patients with perennial allergic rhinitis: a safety and biopsy study. Clin Otolaryngol 1998;23:69–73.

Specific Allergy Immunotherapy for Allergic Rhinitis: Subcutaneous and Sublingual

Linda Cox, MD*, Dana Wallace, MD

KEYWORDS

- Allergen immunotherapy • Sublingual immunotherapy
- Allergic rhinitis • Subcutaneous immunotherapy

Specific allergen immunotherapy (SIT) is a unique therapy for allergic rhinitis because it provides symptomatic relief while modifying the allergic disease by targeting the underlying immunologic mechanisms. Sublingual (SLIT) and subcutaneous (SCIT) immunotherapy are the two most commonly prescribed routes for administering SIT. In Europe, SLIT is prescribed nearly as frequently as SCIT but this varies considerably by region.[1] In southern Europe, SLIT accounts for approximately 80% of immunotherapy prescriptions[1] whereas in the United States, where SCIT is the only route with a Food and Drug Administration (FDA) approved formulation, a relatively small percentage of allergists prescribe SLIT (~6%) (Donald W. Aaronson, MD, JD, MPH, personal communication, 2009).[2] Lack of an FDA-approved SLIT formulation was cited as the most common reason for not prescribing SLIT in two surveys of practicing allergists in the United States (61.7%[2] and 86.3% [Donald W. Aaronson, MD, JD, MPH, personal communication, 2009] of respondents), followed by "effective dose not known" (27.5% and 43.9% [Donald W. Aaronson, MD, JD, MPH, personal communication, 2009] of respondents).

The efficacy of SCIT was demonstrated nearly 100 years ago through the work of two English physicians, Noon and Freeman.[3–5] In a 1911 Lancet article, Leonard Noon reported on his work with immunization of hay fever patients using a distilled aqueous extract of timothy grass pollen.[5] Using conjunctival challenge, he provided objective evidence of immunotherapy efficacy by demonstrating an increase of up to 100-fold of the allergen dose required to produce a conjunctival reaction in an

---

Disclosure: Dr Cox has been a consultant for Stallergenes and Hollister-Steir.
Nova Southeastern University School of Osteopathic Medicine, Davie, FL, USA
* Corresponding author. 5333 North Dixie Highway, Fort Lauderdale, FL 33334.
E-mail address: Lindaswolfcox@msn.com

immunotherapy-treated patient.[3,5] He also used the conjunctival challenge in the first attempts to "standardize" allergen extracts, arbitrarily defining a unit of pollen as the "...quantity of pollen that can be extracted from a thousandth part of a milligrame of Phleum pollen." This became known as the Noon unit.[5] Subsequently, multiple controlled clinical trials have demonstrated that SCIT is effective in the treatment of allergic asthma, rhinitis, and stinging insect hypersensitivity. SCIT may provide lasting benefits after discontinuation,[6] prevent disease progression, including the development of asthma (Table 1),[7,8] as well as prevent the development of new allergen sensitization (Table 2).[9–12] Recognizing the inconvenience of the conventional weekly build-up schedule, which he called "leisurely," Freeman began experimenting with accelerated build-up schedules in 1924.[4] Freeman concluded the advantages of the "rush" method were the saving of time, convenience, and improved patient compliance.

The inconvenience associated with the conventional weekly build-up schedules is probably the reason why, 100 years later, only a small percentage of allergic patients subscribe to this treatment: approximately 2.5 million persons (5%) of the allergic rhinitis and/or asthma population in the United States.[1] Freeman also recognized the potential risks of SCIT, noting that a marked increase in dose may cause "...such unpleasant things as swelling, pain and urticaria at the site of the inoculation, a general malaise and all of the nose and eye symptoms of a thorough attack of hay fever."[3]

In an article summarizing his experience with "rush desensitization," Freeman describes, most likely, one of the earliest cases of SCIT anaphylaxis: a 7-year-old girl with horse-induced asthma who developed urticaria, fluttering of the heart, and felt "funny" during a 4-day rush protocol. Although accelerated SCIT schedules offer greater convenience to patients by reducing the number of visits needed to achieve the therapeutic maintenance dose, concerns about a potentially greater risk of anaphylaxis have limited their use by United States allergists.

Efforts to develop safer and more effective immunotherapy began not long after Freeman's "rush inoculation" publication (Figs. 1 and 2, respectively, show the SCIT and SLIT timelines of historical landmarks). The initial focus was on noninjection routes, with anecdotal reports as early as the1930s on oral immunotherapy. Adverse side effects and limited efficacy are the primary reasons why investigation of this route for inhalant allergies ceased.[13] However, several clinical trials have demonstrated that oral immunotherapy may be effective in increasing tolerance in individuals with food allergies, and investigation of this route has shifted from inhalant to food allergies.[14–16] Randomized controlled trials that included bronchial and nasal routes began in the 1970s and 1980s. Although these trials demonstrated clinical efficacy, there was a fairly high rate of adverse local reactions with the bronchial and nasal routes, and further investigation essentially ceased when SLIT was introduced. The first double-blind, placebo-controlled trial of SLIT was published in 1986. In the following years, more than 60 double-blind placebo-controlled (DBPC) clinical trials of SLIT have been conducted throughout the world primarily in allergic rhinitis patients with or without asthma. In general, these trials have demonstrated an efficacy similar to SCIT with less serious adverse effects. One of the purported advantages of SLIT over SCIT is improved safety, which may allow for administration of this treatment outside of a medical facility (ie, at home). Home administration would decrease the "inconvenience" of SIT and possibly increase the percentage of the allergic population that subscribe to this disease-modifying treatment. This article reviews the benefits, risks, and practical considerations, such as costs and compliance, of these two widely used forms of SIT.

Table 1
Using SIT for treatment of allergic rhinitis and prevention of asthma

Study	SCIT SLIT	Study Design	Year	Age Range of Pts, yr Range (mean)	Pts Active/Control	Duration of SIT (yr)	Follow-Up from Onset of SIT (yr)	New-Onset Asthma SIT, %	New-Onset Asthma Placebo, %	P value	OR During SIT	OR at Follow-Up
Jacobsen et al[33] (subset AR only)	SCIT	Follow-up, open	1997	15–72 (33.2)	17/0	3	6	0	N/A	N/A	N/A	N/A
Moller et al[53] (PAT study part 1) (subset with AR only)	SCIT	DBPC-RCT	2002	6–14 (10.7) 4.6 mean yr with AR	79/72 (1992–1994)	3	3	24	44	<.05	↓2.52	—
PAT Part 2 Niggemann et al[116]	—	Follow-up	2006		75/67 (1996)	N/A	5	20	43	<.01	—	↓3.1
PAT Part 3 Jacobsen et al[7]	—	Follow-up	2007		64/53 (2001)	N/A	10	25	45	.0075	—	↓2.5
Polosa et al[117]	SCIT	DBPC-RCT	2004	20–54 (33)	15/15	3	3	14	47	.056	—	—
Polosa et al[8]	SCIT	Retrospective	2005	18–40	202/130	3	10	42	53	<.05	—	↑OR 7.8 without SIT ↓OR 0.53 with SIT
Novembre et al[68]	SLIT	RCT-open	2004	5–14	54/59	3	3	18	41	.0412	N/A	↑OR 3.8 without SIT
Margona et al[67]	SLIT	RCT-open	2008	5–17	58/27	3	3	<13.1[a]	<45.4	—	—	—

[a] Unable to determine as number of AR developing asthma was not clearly stated.

Table 2
Using SIT for treatment of allergic rhinitis and prevention of new sensitizations

Study	SCIT SLIT	Study Design	Year	Age Range of Pts, yr (mean)	Pts Active/ Placebo	Duration of SIT	Follow-up from Onset of SIT (yr)	New-Onset Allergens in Active, %	New onset Allergens in Placebo, %	P value
Des Roches et al[12]	SCIT House dust mite monosensitized	Case-control prospective	1997	2–6 (median 5 yr A, 4 yr P)	22/22 AR + asthma (73%)	3	3	55	100	<.001
Pajno et al[11]	SCIT Dust mite monosensitized	Case-control prospective	2001	5–8	75/63 (asthma, intermittent ± AR)	3	6	25	67	<.0002
Purello-D'Ambrosio et al[9]	SCIT (polysensitized)	Open retrospective	2001	≥14 (22–23)	7182/1214 (asthma + AR) 2938 AR only	4 (98% ≥2 allergens)	7	All = 27 AR = 24 Asthma + AR = 29	All = 77 AR = 71 Asthma + AR = 81	≤.0001 to .0086
Limb[118]	SCIT (polysensitized)	DBPC-RCT, Follow-up	2006	5–12	61/60 original study (<1995) Asthma moderate to severe Follow-up 41/41 or original group Asthma moderate to severe	≥18 mo (median 27 mo)	10.8 (mean)	30	31	.75
Eng et al[32,119]	SCIT	Prospective RCT, long-term follow-up	2006	5–16 (9.5)	14/14 (1988) 13/10 (1997) 12/10 (2003)	3 (1989–91)	15 (2003)	58	100	<.05
Marogna et al[69]	SLIT	RCT-open	2004	15–65	319/192	3	3	5.9	38	<.001
Marogna et al[67]	SLIT	RCT-open	2008	5–17	58/27	3	3	3	35	—

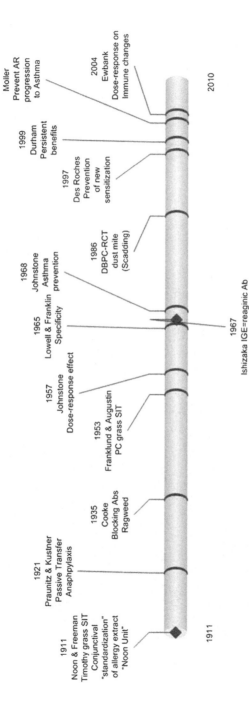

Fig. 1. Subcutaneous immunotherapy (SCIT) timetable. Ab, antibody; AR, allergic rhinitis; DBPC-RCT, double-blind placebo-controlled randomized controlled trial; PC, placebo-controlled.

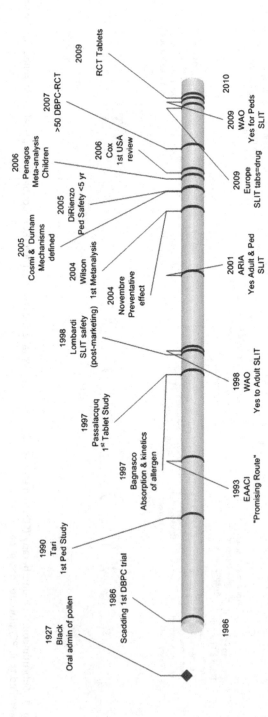

Fig. 2. Sublingual immunotherapy (SLIT) timetable. ARIA, Allergic Rhinitis and its Impact on Asthma; EAACI, European Academy of Allergy and Clinical Immunology; Ped, pediatric patients; WAO, World Allergy Organization.

EFFICACY OF SUBCUTANEOUS AND SUBLINGUAL IMMUNOTHERAPY
Subcutaneous Immunotherapy

The work of Noon and Freeman essentially formed the basis for SCIT as it is practiced today, but the efficacy was not confirmed in a DBPC until 1954 in a study of grass-pollen–allergic patients performed by Frankland and Augustin[17] (see **Fig. 1**). In the following decade, Franklin and Lowell demonstrated that SCIT was specific for the treated allergen[18] and that efficacy was dose dependent.[19] In the same decade, John-stone and Dutton[20] demonstrated a dose-response effect on persistence of asthma in a 14-year study that compared 3 doses of multiallergen SCIT with placebo. Subsequently, numerous studies using different allergens confirmed that SCIT efficacy was dose dependent. For most of the allergens studied, the effective dosing range was between 5 and 20 μg of the major allergen.[21–25] The efficacy of SCIT also appears to be dependent on duration of treatment.[26]

Poor response to SCIT may be due to several reasons, including (1) ongoing significant allergenic exposures (eg, 5 cats in the house), (2) continued exposure to nonallergen triggers (eg, tobacco smoke), (3) missing clinically relevant allergens, or (4) failure to treat with adequate doses of each allergen. The most recent document on allergen immunotherapy from the Joint Task Force of Practice Parameters (JTFPP) recommends "if clinical improvement is not apparent after 1 year of maintenance therapy, possible reasons for lack of efficacy should be evaluated. If none are found, discontinuation of immunotherapy should be considered, and other treatment options should be pursued."[27]

In most studies, the primary outcome of SCIT efficacy was determined by changes in symptoms and medication scores as compared with a placebo group (see **Table 3** on SCIT efficacy). Clinical efficacy often correlated with changes in objective measures, such as titrated skin tests, changes in allergen-specific IgG_4 and IgE, and allergen-provocation organ challenges, which are secondary outcomes that are often monitored in many of in SIT clinical trials. The overall efficacy of SCIT for allergic rhinitis was confirmed in a Cochrane meta-analysis, which analyzed 1111 studies published between 1950 and February of 2006.[28] In the 51 trials that met the review's inclusion criteria, there were 2871 participants (1645 active, 1226 placebo). Overall, a significant overall reduction in the symptoms scores, namely Standardized Mean Difference (SMD) −0.73; 95% confidence interval [CI] −0.97 to −0.50; $P<.00001$) and medication scores (SMD −0.57; 95% CI −0.82 to −0.33; $P<.00001$) was seen in the SCIT-treated groups compared with placebo (**Fig. 3** for comparison of SCIT and SLIT meta-analysis). In terms of secondary outcomes, all studies that provided information demonstrated the following:

- Skin testing: all 21 trials reported reduction in skin test reactivity
- Nasal challenge: most reported reduction in allergen provocation dose
- Conjunctival challenge: 4 of 6 studies showed significant increase in allergen provocation dose
- Allergen-specific IgG_4: 10 of 11 studies demonstrated a significant increase with SCIT
- Allergen-specific IgE: Of 30 studies, 20 showed an increase in specific IgE, 9 showed no change, and 1 showed a decrease in specific IgE.

This meta-analysis validates the efficacy of SCIT in improving both clinical and objective parameters of allergic rhinitis. Clinical improvement can be demonstrated very shortly after the patient reaches a maintenance dose.[23,29–31] One study of cat-allergic patients, who achieved the maintenance dose in 5 weeks with a cluster

Table 3
Efficacy of subcutaneous immunotherapy

Author	Year	Age Range, yr	Active/Placebo	Dropout Active/Placebo	Allergen	Duration	Dose	Symptom ↓, %	Medication ↓, %
Balda et al[120]	1998	18–58	51/60	1/5	Mixed trees (3)	7 wk preseasonal	1–3 µg	28	62
Jutel et al[121]	2005	25 (median)	29/28	0	Mixed grass (5)	21 mo	Cumulative: 490 µg total	36.5	36.5
Corrigan et al[122]	2005	18–60	77/77	11/15	Mixed grass (6) Allergoid absorbed	2 consecutive pre-seasons	30 µg (median max.)	31	69
Frew et al[23]	2006	18–60	203/104	16/15	Single grass	10 wk	2 µg 20 µg depot (8 injections)	22 29	16 32
Colas et al[123]	2006	18–50	41/19	2/1	Russian thistle	4 wk preseasonal	Cluster 45 µg/ml 450 µg/ml Polymerized Cumulative: 597.65 µg	33	11 (NS)
Pauli et al[124]	2008	18–50	98/36	15/6	Birch	2 yr	Recombinant Licensed Natural Maintenance 15 µg	52	65

Studies were selected that fit the following criteria: 25 or more subjects in active group; Past 12 years; DBPC-RCT; Symptom and Medication Scores included.

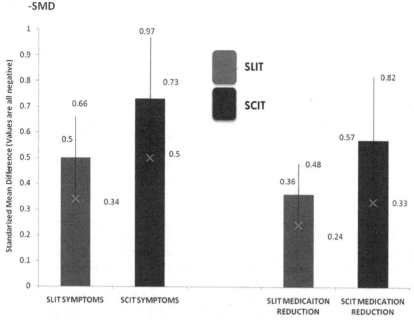

Fig. 3. Comparison of the systematic reviews of sublingual and subcutaneous immunotherapy for seasonal allergic rhinitis symptom and medication score improvement. SMD, standard mean difference. Graph bars have negative value, with higher number representing better results. Superimposed lines represent confidence interval (CI). See associated table for details.

	Studies Published	No. of Studies Included	Participants Active/Placebo	Symptoms/Medications	
				P value	I^2
SLIT[164]	1966–2009	49	2333/2256	<.00001 for both	81%/55%
SCIT[28]	1984–2006	51	1645/1226	<.00001 for both	63.2%/64.0%

schedule, reported that the response to titrated nasal allergen challenge, titrated skin-prick testing, and allergen-specific IgG_4 measurement to cat immunotherapy at 5 weeks was predictive of the response at 1 year.[25] In addition to clinical improvement while receiving treatment, SCIT may provide persistent benefits after discontinuation of treatment.[6,32,33] It may also prevent the development of asthma and new allergen sensitizations in patients with allergic rhinitis.[7,9–12]

Sublingual Immunotherapy

Seventy-five years after Noon first reported on the efficacy of SCIT, the first clinical trials of SLIT for the treatment of allergic rhinitis commenced in Europe (see **Fig. 2** for the SLIT timeline). The first meta-analysis on SLIT for the treatment of allergic rhinitis included 979 patients in 22 trials that were published up to September 2002.[34] Overall, the meta-analysis found a significant reduction in both symptoms (SMD −0.42, 95% CI −0.69 to −0.15; P = .002) and medication use (SMD −0.43, 95% CI −0.63 to −0.23; P = .00003) in the SLIT-treated groups compared with placebo (see **Fig. 3**). A subgroup analysis revealed no significant reduction in symptoms and medication scores in those studies involving only children. However, the total numbers of pediatric patients was too small to make lack of SLIT efficacy a reliable conclusion. The meta-analysis concluded that SLIT was significantly more effective than placebo. Subsequently, several large clinical trials demonstrated that grass-pollen SLIT was as efficacious in the pediatric allergic rhinitis population as in the adult populations (see **Table 4** for summary of SLIT efficacy).[35,36] Another meta-analysis of SLIT for allergic rhinitis in pediatric patients (aged 4–18 years) analyzed 10 studies published between 1990 and 2004 that included 484 patients (245 SLIT and 239 placebo).[37] Overall, a significant reduction in both symptoms (SMD 0.56, 95% CI 1.01–0.10; $P = .02$) and medication use (SMD 0.76, 95% CI 1.46–0.06; $P = .03$) was found in the SLIT group compared with placebo. A subanalysis showed that SLIT for longer than 18 months was more effective than treatment for less than 18 months, and that treatment using pollen extracts was more effective than those employing dust mite extracts.

The early SLIT trials had considerable study design heterogeneity, with small patient populations, variable dosing regimens (once a week to daily administration), and cumulative monthly doses (CMD), ranging from a fraction of (0.017) to more than 500 times the customary subcutaneous maintenance dose (CMD) (see **Table 5** for comparison between SCIT and SLIT dosing range). The relationship between efficacy and allergen dose has not been as clearly established with SLIT as with SCIT. In a comprehensive review of SLIT studies published through October 2006, efficacy was demonstrated over a wide range of doses: from 10 ng of Fel d 1[38] to 314 µg of Amb a 1,[39] with the effective CMD SLIT dose being as high as 300 times the usual monthly SCIT maintenance dose.[40] In this review, only 35% of the DBPC or randomized-controlled studies demonstrated significant improvement in both symptom and medication scores in the first year of treatment, whereas 38% showed no improvement on either measure. However, in subsequent years of treatment, several studies that showed no improvement in the first treatment year did demonstrate significant clinical improvement in symptoms, medication use, or both parameters.

Since 2006, several large clinical trials investigating the efficacy of grass-pollen tablets in allergic rhinitis have demonstrated a clear dose-response relationship in terms of improvement in symptoms, rhinitis quality of life, and medication scores compared with placebo.[41,42] A dose response was also seen in the immunologic markers studied: grass-pollen–specific-IgG_4, grass-pollen–specific IgE, and IgE-blocking antibody.[43] Subsequent studies demonstrated sustained clinical improvement in the second and third year, which was accompanied by these immunologic changes.[43,44] Following a 3-year course of grass-pollen tablets, these benefits were maintained for 1 year after discontinuation of treatment.[44] This result suggests that SLIT, like SCIT, may have a disease-modifying effect and may provide long-term benefits after discontinuation.

The magnitude of effect on clinical parameters in these large clinical grass-tablet trials[41–43] is similar to that of SCIT,[23] with reductions compared with placebo of:

- Symptom score reduction: SLIT 21%–37% versus SCIT 32%
- Medication score reduction: SLIT 29%–46% versus SCIT 41%.

A consistent relationship with treatment duration, dosing frequency, and efficacy has not been clearly established.[40] One study found that significant improvement in both symptom and medication scores during the first season required at least 8 weeks of preseasonal treatment.[41] Whereas another DBPC study using an environmental challenge chamber to assess efficacy found a significant effect on rhinoconjunctivitis symptoms during challenge as early as 1 month after beginning grass-pollen SLIT treatment.[45]

There have been few studies that have compared SLIT dosing frequency regimens. All of the comparative dosing regimen studies included more than one variable, usually dose and dosing frequency, and none have compared the same dose administered at different frequencies. In most of the recent large clinical SLIT trials, treatment is begun about 4 months before season and administered 3 times a week to daily. The rationale for daily administration is that it may improve patient compliance. Further studies are needed to determine the optimal SLIT dosing regimen.

EFFICACY OF MULTIALLERGEN SUBCUTANEOUS AND SUBLINGUAL IMMUNOTHERAPY

One important consideration is that most SCIT and SLIT clinical trials have been performed with single allergens, whereas most of the United States population is polysensitized. In a study designed to assess the prevalence of positive skin test responses to 10 common allergens in the United States population, the median number of positive reactions was 3.[46] In another study, 81% of the 1338 mild to moderate asthmatics had positive reactions to 3 or more of the 14 allergens tested.[47]

The prevalence of polysensitization raises two questions: (1) is monoallergen immunotherapy effective in polysensitized patients, and (2) is multiallergen subcutaneous or sublingual immunotherapy effective?

Many of the SCIT and SLIT monoallergen clinical trials have been performed in polysensitized patients. Several SLIT studies that examined the question of monoallergen efficacy in polysensitized patients found similar efficacy in both patient populations.[48–50] Whereas there have been no SCIT studies specifically designed to address this question, many of the single-allergen trials have included polysensitized patients.[51] Thus it appears that single-allergen SIT is effective in polysensitized individuals.

However, the efficacy of multiallergen immunotherapy has been debated. There have been few studies that have specifically investigated the efficacy of multiallergen subcutaneous or sublingual immunotherapy (**Table 6**). A review on this subject identified 13 SIT studies that used 2 or more unrelated allergen extracts: 11 subcutaneous, 2 sublingual, and 1 using both.[52] These studies have produced conflicting results, and some have provided general results without specific information on response to each of the treated allergens.[53–56] Four of the 7 studies using 2 non–cross-reacting allergens found similar efficacy when compared with single-allergen extract treatment. In the 5 studies that used multiple allergens, 3 demonstrated efficacy[18–20] whereas 2 did not.[57,58] One of the "ineffective" multiallergen studies did not include an important allergen,[57] cockroach, which was shown to correlate with asthma severity in inner-city asthmatic children.[59]

There have been few studies that have evaluated the efficacy of multiallergen SLIT.[60–62] One open-label trial of rhinitis patients allergic to birch and grass pollen, who were treated with either a single allergen, both allergens, or pharmacotherapy, demonstrated significant improvement in symptom and medication scores, nasal eosinophils, and bronchial hyperresponsiveness in both the single-allergen and multiallergen groups.[60] However, a greater improvement in clinical symptoms and inflammation was found in the multiallergen treatment group compared with the single-allergen SLIT groups. One DBPC trial of grass-pollen–allergic rhinitis patients compared the efficacy of multiallergen and single-allergen SLIT on various objective and clinical parameters.[62] In the patients who received timothy extract alone, there were significant changes in multiple objective parameters, whereas improvement was only seen in

Table 4
Efficacy of sublingual immunotherapy

Author	Year	Age Range, yr	Active/ Placebo	Dropout Active/ Placebo	Allergen	Duration	Single Dose (If Mix Total is Given), µg	Cumulative Monthly Dose	Symptom, ↓ %	Medication, ↓ %
Durham et al[41]	2006	18–66	569/286	39/26	Grass Phl p5 3 doses Tablets	6 mo	0.5 5 15	15 µg 150 µg 450 µg	NS NS 16	NS NS 28
Dahl et al[82]	2006	18–65	316/318	42/46	Grass Phl p5 Tablets	6 mo	15	450 µg Cumulative 6-mo dose: 4.5 mg	30	38
Dahl et al[125]	2006	18–64	74/40	13/8	Grass Phl p5 Tablets	5 mo	15	450 µg	37	41
Roder et al[126]	2007	6–18	108/96	26/24	5 Grass (G5) Mix Solution	2 yr	21	168 µg	None	None
Didier et al[42]	2007	25–47	472/156	59/10	5 Grass (G5) Mix Tablet	6 mo	8 25 42	240 µg 750 µg 1.2 mg	4 27 24	23 46 47
De Blay et al[127]	2007	12–41	61/57	8/8	3 Grass Mix (G3) Solution	10 mo	21	250 µg Cumulative 10-mo dose: 2.5 mg	None	22 (P = .02)
Pfaar and Klimek[128]	2008	17–59	94/91	17/9	6 Grass (G6) Mix Solution	2 yr	40	1.2 mg	Combined symptom-medication score benefit for AUC (<.01) and VAS	

Study	Year	Age	N		Allergen	Duration		Dose		
Wahn et al[36]	2009	5–17	139/139	4/8	5 Grass (G5) Mix Tablets	8 mo	20	600 µg	28	24
Ott et al[129]	2009	20–50	142/67	3/1	5 Grass (G5) Mix Solution	5 yr, 4 seasons	21	630 µg Cumulative dose: 1.5 mg major allergen/season	47	None
Bufe et al[130]	2009	5–16	126/127	12/7	Grass Phl p5 Tablets	6 mo	15	450 µg	24	34
Horak et al[45]	2009	18–50	45/44	3/4	5 Grass (G5) Mix Tablets	4 mo	20	600 µg	29	N/A (out-of-season challenge study)
Durham et al[41,44]	2006	18–65	170/138	—	Grass Phl p5 Tablets	3 yr No Tx	15 Off Tx	450 µg	29	40
	2010	—	↓	—		4 yr	—	—	—	—
	2010	—	157/126	13/12					26	29
Skoner et al[131]	2010	18–50	75/40	12/6	Ragweed Amb a 1 Solution	23 wk	4.8 / 48	83 µg low / 823 µg high	15 (NS) / 15 (NS)	37 / 51

Studies were selected that fit the following criteria: 100 subjects; Past 10 years; DBPC-RCT.

G5 = 5-grass mix: orchard (*Dactylis glomerata*), meadow (*Poa pratensis*), perennial rye (*Lolium perenne*), sweet vernal (*Anthoxanthum odoratum*), timothy (*Phleum pratense*); G6 = 6-grass mix: velvetgrass (*Holcus lanatus*), orchard (*Dactylis glomerata*), perennial rye (*Lolium perenne*), timothy (*Phleum pratense*), meadow (*Poa pratensis*), and fescue (*Festuca elatior*); G3 = 3-grass mix: orchard (*Dactylis glomerata*), meadow (*Poa pratensis*), perennial rye (*Lolium perenne*), timothy (*Phleum pratense*).

Abbreviations: AUC, area under the curve; NS, not significant; Tx, therapy; VAS, visual analog score.

Table 5
Major allergen effective dose range for SCIT and SLIT

Allergen Extract	Major Allergen	Single Dose at Maintenance Level Mixtures (Total µg per Treatment)		Monthly Dose at Maintenance Level	
		SCIT	SLIT	SCIT (Usually Same As Single Dose)	SLIT Cumulative Monthly Dose (CMA)
Dust Mite F	Der f 1	10 µg[132]	No studies using only Der F1	10 µg[132]	No studies using only Der F1
Dust Mite P	Der p 1	7–11.9 µg[51,132,133]	.86–3.75 µg[134–136]	7–11.9 µg[51,132,133]	10.4–320 µg; Cumulative: 57 µg to 1.7 mg[134–137]
Dust mite P + F or unlisted	Der P 1 and Der F 1	7–21 µg[51]	7.6–84 µg[137–140]	7–21 µg[51]	60.8–2520 µg; Cumulative: 1.46–25 mg[137–140]
Ragweed, short	Amb a 1	6–12 µg[21,141,142] (6–12 µg 1000–4000 AU)[27]	314 µg tablets,[39,143] 314 µg solution 314 µg[143]	6–12 µg[21,141,142]	3.8 mg[39,143]–9.4 mg[143]; Cumulat: 25.7 mg[39] –375 mg[143]
Grass, timothy	Phl p 5	4–50 µg[23] va[144] (1000–4000 BAU)[27]	15 µg[41,44,82,125]	4–50 µg[23,144] every 2–6 wk	450 µg[41,44,82,125]
Grass, Bermuda	Cyn d 1	4.6–63.3 µg (300–1500 BAU)[27]	None	4.6–63.3 µg	None
3,5,6, Grass mix	G3, G5, G6	4–44 µg[121,122,145–147] (1000–4000 BAU)[27]	20–25 µg[42,45,127,129,148]	4–44 µg[121,122,145–147]	600–750 µg[42,129,148,149]
Birch	Bet v 1	3.28 µg[150], 12 µg[151]; 15 µg[124] (No US standardized product)	49.2 µg[150] Not provided[152,153]	3.28 µg[150], 12 µg[151]; 15 µg[124]	738 µg[150], 62 µg[152], 90 µg[153]
Mixed Trees	Group 1 major allergen[120] T3 = Bet v 1, Cor a 1, Aln g 1[154]	1–12 µg[120] (No US standardized product)	1.8–15 µg[154]	1–12 µg[120]	14.4–120 µg[154]
Dog	Can f 1	15 µg[24,27] (No standardized US product)	None	15 µg[24,27]	None

G5 = 5-grass mix: orchard (*Dactylis glomerata*), meadow (*Poa pratensis*), perennial rye (*Lolium perenne*), sweet vernal (*Anthoxanthum odoratum*), timothy (*Phleum pratense*); G6 = 6-grass mix: velvet grass (*Holcus lanatus*), orchard (*Dactylis glomerata*), perennial rye (*Lolium perenne*), timothy (*Phleum pratense*), meadow (*Poa pratensis*), fescue (*Festuca elatior*); G3 = 3-grass mix: orchard (*Dactylis glomerata*), meadow (*Poa pratensis*), perennial rye (*Lolium perenne*), timothy (*Phleum pratense*); T3 = mixed trees: birch (*Betula verrucosa*), hazel (*Corylus avellana*), alder (*Alnus glutinosa*).

Abbreviations: AU, allergy unit; BAU, bioequivalent allergy unit.

titrated skin-prick testing in the group that received timothy extract mixed with 9 additional pollens. This study suggests that the clinical efficacy of SLIT may be reduced with the addition of multiple allergens, potentially limiting its use in polysensitized individuals.

In considering the conflicting results in these very heterogeneous studies, a firm conclusion about the efficacy—or lack of—mulitallergen SIT cannot be made. Further research is clearly needed for both multiallergen SCIT and SLIT.

PREVENTIVE EFFECT OF SUBCUTANEOUS AND SUBLINGUAL IMMUNOTHERAPY

Allergic rhinitis is an identified risk factor for the development of asthma, with up to 40% of individuals with allergic rhinitis developing asthma later in life.[63–66] Allergen immunotherapy may alter the natural history of allergic disease, sometimes referred to as the "atopic march," by preventing the development of asthma as well as the development of new allergen sensitizations (see **Tables 1** and **2**). One placebo-controlled trial of polysensitized asthmatic children who were randomized to receive 1 of 3 doses of an allergen mixture or placebo found a dose-dependent difference in being "free of asthma" at age 16 years.[20]

One prospective randomized, controlled open study of 147 children, aged 16 to 25 years, evaluated the effect of a 3-year course SCIT with grass and/or birch pollen allergy on the development of asthma compared with pharmacotherapy alone (PAT study).[8] There was a significantly lower incidence of asthma in the SCIT group compared with the pharmacotherapy group 7 years after discontinuation of treatment (odds ratio [OR] 2.5, 95% CI 1.1–5.9). One 11-year retrospective study of 436 nonasthmatic adults found that treatment with SCIT was significantly and inversely related to the development of new-onset asthma (OR 0.53, 95% CI 0.32–0.86).[8]

Two randomized, open controlled studies suggest that SLIT also reduces the risk of asthma onset in children with rhinitis.[67,68] One of these studies prospectively followed 113 children, aged 5 to 14 years, with grass pollen allergic rhinitis, who were randomized to receive either coseasonal grass-pollen SLIT or pharmacotherapy for 3 years. The incidence of asthma after 3 years was 3.8 times more frequent in the pharmacotherapy-alone group compared with the SLIT group (95% CI 1.5–10.0).[68] The rate of prevention of the onset of asthma in children in this SLIT study was similar to the aforementioned SCIT trial (the PAT study).

Several randomized controlled and open studies have demonstrated that SCIT[9–12,32] and SLIT[67,69] may reduce the onset of new allergen sensitizations (see **Table 1**). Three studies demonstrated a significantly lower incidence of new allergen sensitizations in monosensitized patients who received SCIT compared with the untreated matched control groups, with new sensitizations developing in 23%, 24%, and 54% of the SCIT patients versus 68%, 67%, and 100% of the untreated control patients.[9,11,12] Similar results were found in a 3-year open study of 511 patients with allergic rhinitis ± asthma patients randomized to SLIT or pharmacologic treatment.[69] New allergen sensitizations developed in 38% of the control patients and in 5.9% of the SLIT patients (P = .01).

SAFETY OF SUBCUTANEOUS AND SUBLINGUAL IMMUNOTHERAPY
Subcutaneous Immunotherapy

Adverse reactions associated with SCIT can be local or systemic. Local reactions, which can manifest as erythema, pruritus, and swelling at the injection site, are fairly common, with a frequency ranging from 26% to 82% of patients and 0.7% to 4% of injections.[70–72] Local reactions do not appear to be predictive of systemic reactions

Table 6
Efficacy of multiple allergen SCIT and SLIT immunotherapy for allergic rhinitis

SIT Method	Author, Year	Design	Subjects	Allergens	Findings Favoring Multiple Antigens
SCIT	Franklin and Lowell,[19] 1965	DBPC 8 months pre-ragweed season	24 adults Rhinoconjunctivitis	Pollen (trees, grass, plantain) with/without ragweed[a]	↓Symptoms medication scores in group with ragweed included
SCIT	Franklin and Lowell,[18] 1967	DBPC 5 months pre-ragweed season	24 adults Allergic rhinitis	Ragweed high or low dose + other allergens[a]	Ragweed high-dose group more effective
SLIT	Bousquet et al,[58] 1991	DBPC 3 day Rush 3 month pre-seasonal	70 adults (36 monosensitized to orchard) 34 polysensitized to orchard + other seasonal/perennial allergens, including other grasses[b] Allergic rhinitis ± mild Asthma	Orchard grass vs placebo (monosensitized) Orchard + 3 other relevant allergens vs placebo	Negative study Monosensitized treated patients improved. Polysensitized treated patients with multiple antigens were not significantly improved over placebo
SCIT ± SLIT	Cirla et al,[61] 2003	RCT Preseasonal grass and trees 2 years	36 adults Rhinoconjunctivitis ± mild asthma	SCIT: G5 grass mix (all pts) SLIT: birch/hazel or placebo	↓Conjunctivitis, cough for combined SIT, ↑nasal grass challenge (supports "priming" concept)

SCIT	Alvarez-Cuesta et al,[165] 2005	RT-DBPC 1 year		53 adults Seasonal allergic rhinitis	Orchard and Olive (polymerized) vs placebo (all negative to other allergens)	↓Symptoms and medication use, ↑ quality of life
SLIT	Marogna et al,[60] 2007	Open-label RCT 4 years		48 adults Rhinoconjunctivitis and mild asthma	Birch, grass, or both, or placebo (all negative to other allergens)	↓Symptoms & Medication scores, for all 3 treatment groups in both seasons. Grass alone = grass + birch in grass season but > birch alone. Birch alone = grass + birch in birch season but > grass alone. ↓ Nasal eosinophils

Table includes only trials with AR patients with results reported separately for multiple antigens (2 or more).

G5 = Timothy, orchard, rye, meadow, and fescue.

Abbreviation: AH, antihistamines.

[a] Subjects had remained symptomatic the prior ragweed season when on SCIT with ragweed and other allergens (details not given).

[b] Clinically patients only had seasonal AR.

Data from Nelson HS. Multiallergen immunotherapy for allergic rhinitis and asthma. J Allergy Clin Immunol 2009;123:763–9.

with subsequent injections,[72,73] although individuals with more frequent large local reactions may have a higher risk of future systemic reaction.[74]

SCIT systemic reactions (SRs) can range in severity from mild rhinitis to life-threatening anaphylaxis. SCIT SR rate varies greatly depending on several factors, including allergen dose, extract type, induction schedule, premeditation, and patient selection. A review of the SCIT SR rates reported in studies published between 1996 and 2010 found that the incidence of SRs with conventional build-up schedules was approximately 0.2% per injection and 2% to 7% of patients.[75] The SR rate with SCIT rush immunotherapy schedules ranged from 15% to 100% of patients who did not receive premedication to 3% to 79% of premedicated patients in one review.[76]

SCIT risk factors that have been identified from surveys and clinical trials include symptomatic or poorly controlled asthma. Delay in the administration of epinephrine was identified as a possible contributing factor in some of the immunotherapy fatalities. While it is recognized that progression of the systemic reaction from mild to severe can be very rapid, there are unfortunately no clear clinical predictors for when this will occur.

Fatal SCIT reactions are relatively rare but have been reported at a rate of approximately 1 in 2 to 2.5 million injections according to 3 surveys of American Academy of Allergy, Asthma and Immunology (AAAAI) members that span the period between 1945 and 2001.[77–79] In one of these surveys the incidence of unconfirmed near fatal reactions, which were defined as "respiratory compromise, hypotension, or both requiring emergency epinephrine," was 23 per year or 5.4 events per million injections.[80]

In a 3-year collaborative AAAAI/American College of Allergy, Asthma and Immunology (ACAAI) immunotherapy safety study, there were no fatalities reported in the approximately 8.1 million injections administered provided by 1922 SCIT prescribers in the time period from June 2008 to July 2009.[81] Eighty-two percent of 806 practices reported a total of 8502 SCIT SRs (SR rate: 10.2 SRs per 10,000 or 0.1% of injection visits). Most of these SRs were categorized as grade1 (74%) or grade 2 (23%). However, 3% of the reported SRs were grade 3, which was defined as "severe, life-threatening anaphylaxis: severe airway compromise due to severe bronchospasm or upper airway obstruction with stridor or hypotension." This figure would translate into 3 severe SRs per 100,000 injection visits. A multinational group emerged from the AAAAI/ACAAI coalition, composed of members of the academic, clinical, and research allergy community, to develop a universal grading system for immunotherapy SRs, the World Allergy Organization grading system for subcutaneous systemic reactions (**Table 7**).[75]

This grading system is composed of 5 grades, which are based on the organ system(s) involved and reaction severity. The organ systems are defined as cutaneous, conjunctival, upper respiratory, lower respiratory, gastrointestinal, cardiovascular, and other. The final grade is determined by the physician's clinical judgment after the event is over. In addition to facilitating comparison of outcomes from different clinical trials, consistent use of this uniform systemic reaction classification system will make it possible to collect better immunotherapy safety surveillance data and compare practice parameters with outcomes. These factors, in turn, may help determine the best approach to treat adverse reactions associated with immunotherapy, that is, when to administer epinephrine.

Sublingual Immunotherapy

Like SCIT, adverse reactions associated with SLIT can be either local or systemic. One consideration with the SLIT safety data reported in clinical trials and surveillance studies is that almost all doses are administered outside of the clinical setting with no direct medical supervision. Thus, the accuracy of the reporting of adverse events is dependent on the patient and/or family's interpretation and recall of the event.

The incidence of SRs appears to be significantly lower with SLIT, and severe systemic reactions are relatively uncommon. Conversely, local reactions, primarily oropharyngeal pruritus and/or swelling, are very common. In a study of 316 subjects receiving grass tablets, 46% reported oral pruritus and 18% mouth edema.[82] Most of the local symptoms were reported to be mild to moderate in severity, and generally resolved with continued treatment. In this study, fewer than 4% of subjects discontinued the study because of side effects. The findings in this study are fairly consistent with the safety outcomes reported in other SLIT clinical trials. In general, the withdrawal rate due to SLIT adverse reactions is low, and the majority of adverse events appear early in the treatment course and resolve with continued treatment.

Like SCIT, the SRs reported with SLIT range in severity, from mild reactions (eg, rhinitis or urticaria) to severe reactions (eg, asthma requiring hospitalization). In a comprehensive review of 104 SLIT studies published through October 2005, there were no fatalities in the 66 studies that provided some information on safety and tolerance, which included 4378 patients who received approximately 1,181,000 SLIT doses.[40] The amount of detail about the adverse events varied greatly in these studies, ranging from general summary statements, such as "no relevant side effects," to a detailed analysis of the adverse events. In the studies that specified the type of reaction, 169 of 314,959 were classified as SRs (0.056% of doses administered). There were 14 probable SLIT-related serious adverse events (SAE) in this review (1.4 SAE per 100,000 SLIT administered doses). The most common SAEs were asthma reactions, one of which required hospitalization. The other SLIT-related SAEs were abdominal pain/vomiting, uvula edema, and urticaria lasting for 48 hours.

Unlike SCIT, the incidence of SRs does not appear to be related to the induction schedule. Nor has a relationship been established between the allergen dose and adverse reaction rates associated with SLIT. Similar SR rates have been reported in the SLIT studies with no induction phase, as also with studies that employed buildup schedules that spanned 5 weeks.[83]

To date there have been no deaths reported with SLIT. However, systemic reactions of a severity to be categorized as anaphylaxis have been reported.[84–87] In a few of these cases of anaphylaxis the subject had experienced earlier systemic reactions related to SLIT.[84,87] In addition 2 subjects, who had to discontinue SCIT due to SRs, had anaphylactic reactions with their first SLIT dose.[88] Other investigators have reported systemic reactions to SLIT in patients who had not tolerated SCIT.[89] A review of comorbidities demonstrates that most of the patients with SLIT-related SAEs or anaphylaxis had asthma, which has been identified as a risk factor for SCIT SRs.[90]

In summary, while no clear predictors for SLIT adverse reactions have been identified, previous SRs to SLIT or SCIT and a history of asthma appear to be risk factors. Because this treatment is administered at home without direct medical supervision, patients prescribed SLIT should be provided with specific instructions on how to manage adverse reactions and unplanned treatment interruptions, as well as when to withhold SLIT administration. Consideration should also be given to the ability of patients and/or their family to adhere to these instructions and the treatment regimen.

In general, SLIT appears to be associated with fewer and less severe adverse reactions than SCIT. Oropharyngeal reactions are the most common SLIT adverse events but other reactions, such as asthma, urticaria, and gastrointestinal pain have been reported, as well as a few cases of anaphylaxis. Further studies are needed to identify and characterize SLIT risk factors, and to determine how to select the most appropriate patients to receive this treatment outside of a medically supervised setting.

Table 7
Subcutaneous systemic reaction grading system

	World Allergy Organization Subcutaneous Immunotherapy Systemic Reaction Grading System (See Text)[e]				
Grade 1	Grade 2	Grade 3	Grade 4	Grade 5
Symptom(s)/sign(s) of one organ system present[a]	*Symptom(s)/sign(s) of more than one organ system present*	*Lower respiratory*	*Lower or upper respiratory*	Death
Cutaneous	or	Asthma (eg, 40% PEF or FEV$_1$ drop NOT responding to an inhaled bronchodilator)	Respiratory failure with or without loss of consciousness	
Generalized pruritus, urticaria, flushing, or sensation of heat or warmth[b]	*Lower respiratory*		or	
or	Asthma: cough, wheezing, shortness of breath (eg, <40% PEF or FEV$_1$ drop, responding to an inhaled bronchodilator)	or	*Cardiovascular*	
Angioedema (not laryngeal, tongue, or uvular)		*Upper respiratory*	Hypotension with or without loss of consciousness	
or	or	Laryngeal, uvula, or tongue edema with or without stridor		
Upper respiratory	*Gastrointestinal*			
Rhinitis (eg, sneezing, rhinorrhea, nasal pruritus, and/or nasal congestion)	Abdominal cramps, vomiting, or diarrhea			
	or			
or	*Other*			
Throat-clearing (itchy throat)	Uterine cramps			
or				
Cough perceived to come from the upper airway, not the lung, larynx, or trachea				
or				
Conjunctival				
Conjunctival erythema, pruritus, or tearing				
or				
Other				
Nausea, metallic taste, or headache				

Patients may also have a feeling of impending doom, especially in grades 2, 3, or 4.
Note: children with anaphylaxis seldom convey a sense of impending doom and their behavior changes may be a sign of anaphylaxis, eg, becoming very quiet or irritable and cranky.

Scoring includes a suffix that denotes if and when epinephrine is or is not administered in relationship to symptom(s)/sign(s) of the SR: a, ≤5 minutes; b, >5 minutes to ≤10 minutes; c, >10 to ≤20 minutes; d, >20 minutes; z, epinephrine not administered.

The final grade of the reaction will not be determined until the event is over, regardless of the medication administered. The final report should include the first symptom(s)/sign(s) and the time of onset after the subcutaneous allergen immunotherapy injection[c] and a suffix reflecting if and when epinephrine was or was not administered, eg, Grade 2a; rhinitis:10 minutes.

Final report: Grade a–d, or z

Final report: Grade a-d, or z	First symptom	Time of onset of first symptom
Comments[iv]		

Abbreviations: FEV_1, forced expiratory volume in 1 second; PEF, peak expiratory flow. Comments.[d]

[a] Each Grade is based on organ system involved and severity. Organ systems are defined as: cutaneous, conjunctival, upper respiratory, lower respiratory, gastro-intestinal, cardiovascular and other. A reaction from a single organ system such as cutaneous, conjunctival, or upper respiratory, but not asthma, gastrointestinal, or cardiovascular is classified as a Grade 1. Symptom(s)/sign(s) from more than one organ system or asthma, gastrointestinal, or cardiovascular are classified as Grades 2 or 3. Respiratory failure or hypotension, with or without loss of consciousness, defines Grade 4 and death Grade 5. The Grade is determined by the physician's clinical judgment.

[b] This constellation of symptoms may rapidly progress to a more severe reaction.

[c] Symptoms occurring within the first minutes after the injection may be a sign of severe anaphylaxis. Mild symptoms may progress rapidly to severe anaphylaxis and death.

[d] If signs or symptoms are not included in the Table or the differentiation between an SR and vasovagal (vasodepressor) reaction, which may occur with any medical intervention, is difficult, please include comment, as appropriate.

[e] The World Allergy Organization Subcutaneous Systemic Reaction Grading System has been endorsed by the AAAAI and ACAAI.

From Cox L, Larenas-Linnemann D, Lockey RF, et al. Speaking the same language: the World Allergy Organization Subcutaneous Immunotherapy Systemic Reaction Grading System. J Allergy Clin Immunol 2010;125(3):569–74, 574. e1–7; with permission.

IMMUNOLOGIC MECHANISMS

The immunologic changes associated with SLIT and SCIT are complex, and the exact mechanism or mechanisms responsible for their clinical efficacy are still being elucidated (**Figs. 4** and **5**). In the past 20 years there have been considerable advancements in the understanding of the immunologic changes and the role they play in SCIT efficacy.[91–94] Compared with SCIT, the knowledge of the exact mechanism(s) of action of SLIT is at a more basic level, although it appears that the immunologic changes associated with the two methods are similar. Decreased response to allergen challenge accompanied by immunologic changes, such as increase in specific IgG, IgE-blocking antibodies, and specific IgE with blunting of further seasonal increases in IgE, has been demonstrated with both forms of SIT.[43,91] Early immunologic events seen with both methods include the generation of a population of T-regulatory cells, which may produce inhibitory cytokines such as interleukin (IL)-10, IL-12, transforming growth factor β, or both.[91,95,96] Interferon-γ production following Th1 cell stimulation has been demonstrated with both forms of SIT.[91,95,97,98] Nonreactivity and immune deviation of allergen-specific T cells are immunologic changes seen later in both forms of immunotherapy.[95,99] These time-related immunologic changes may be related to SCIT allergen dose.[91] Although the relationship between allergen dose and time-related immunologic changes has not been especially studied in SLIT, there does appear to be a relationship between SLIT allergen dose and the immunologic changes seen in effective immunotherapy.[41]

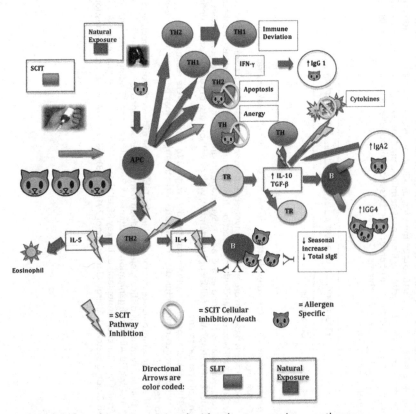

Fig. 4. Postulated mechanisms associated with subcutaneous immunotherapy.

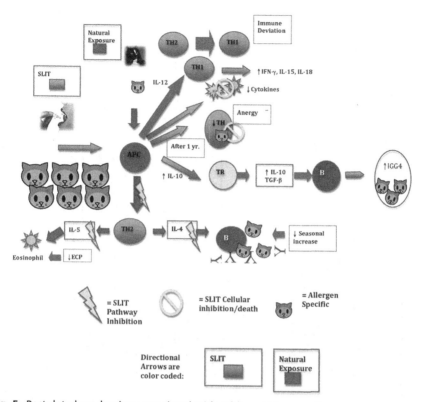

Fig. 5. Postulated mechanisms associated with sublingual immunotherapy.

Further studies aimed at better understanding of the immunologic mechanisms responsible for both form of immunotherapy are needed.

PRACTICAL CONSIDERATIONS OF ALLERGEN IMMUNOTHERAPY: COST AND COMPLIANCE

Direct health care expenditures attributable to allergic rhinitis are substantial. In 2002, the estimated direct health care costs in the United States were $7.3 billion.[100] Indirect costs due to loss of productivity, missed school, and other factors were estimated to be $4.28 billion, bringing the total costs up to $11.58 billion, the equivalent of $16.2 billion in 2010 dollars.

The cost-effectiveness of a particular treatment has begun to play an important role in determining health care coverage on both sides of the Atlantic. Although few studies have demonstrated the cost-effectiveness of pharmacotherapy for allergic rhinitis, the economic benefits of SLIT and SCIT has been examined in several studies. Various methods were employed to investigate the economic impact of SIT, including analyses based on prospective clinical trials, retrospective claims, and other data. Some studies included the economic impact of improved quality of life or the incremental cost-effectiveness ratio in the analysis. The incremental cost-effectiveness ratio (ICER), calculated as the cost difference between SIT and standard treatment divided by the difference in effect and Quality-Adjusted Life Years (QALY), is a measure of the patient's health-related quality of life on a scale from 0 (dead) to 1 (perfect

Table 8
Economic analysis of allergen immunotherapy

Study	Study Design	Results
PROSPECTIVE TRIALS		
Ariano et al,[155] 2006 Italy	Prospective, randomized, open, parallel-group trial SCIT vs ST alone for 3 years and then followed for 3 years after SCIT discontinued 30 adults with AR and/or asthma due to *Parietaria* SCIT (n = 20), pharmacotherapy alone (n = 10)	A significant cost reduction in favor of SCIT observed during treatment: 15% in second year, 48% in third year, and maintained through sixth year, with an 80% reduction 3 years after stopping SCIT. The net saving for each patient at the final evaluation corresponded to $830/year
RETROSPECTIVE ADMINISTRATIVE CLAIMS ANALYSES		

Donahue et al,[104] 1999 USA	Retrospective administrative claims analysis (HMO)
	
	SCIT completers vs discontinued SCIT
	
	603 adults and children with AR and/or asthma
	
	33% (n = 128) completed 3.5 years IT
		Overall cost of SCIT completers was nearly 3-fold greater than group that discontinued SCIT
		
		MCD = Completed SCIT minus Discontinued SCIT
		Annual cost difference for SCIT services: $698 − $508 = $190
		Annual cost difference non-SCIT costs: $421 − $247 = $174
		Total cost of SCIT + other health care costs:
		  • SCIT completers $698 + $508 = $1206
		  • SCIT discontinued:$247 + $421 =$668
		Note: AR and asthma costs before SCIT were 30% higher in the SCIT completed group, suggesting a greater disease burden than group that discontinued SCIT

Hankin et al,[106] 2008 USA	Retrospective administrative claims analysis 6 months pre SCIT initiation vs 6 months post SCIT discontinuation 354 children with AR with or without asthma	MCD = 6 months pre-IT minus 6 months post-IT Pharmacy: −$54, Outpatient: −$233, Inpatient: −$2316 Total: −$215 Mean weighted 6-month savings: $401

Study	Description	Results
Hankin et al,[105] 2010 USA	Retrospective administrative claims analysis. SCIT vs matched controls with no SCIT. 2771 children with AR who received SCIT vs 11,010 matched controls with AR who did not receive SCIT	18-month median per-patient health care costs: SCIT vs no SCIT. Inpatient costs: $3901 vs $4414 (P = .06). Outpatient costs: $1829 vs $2594 (P<.001). Outpatient costs excluding visits related to IT or the cost of IT: $1107 vs $2626 (P<.001). Pharmacy costs: $1108 vs $1316 (P<.001). Total health care costs: $3247 vs $4872 (P<.001)
Berto et al,[156] 2005 Italy	Retrospective administrative claims analysis (1 year pre SLIT initiation) vs (1 year post SLIT discontinuation). 135 children with AR and/or asthma receiving ≥3 years of sublingual IT at a single allergy clinic	MCD = Year before SLIT minus Year after SLIT. MCD (direct): $481 vs $213. MCD (indirect): $2,538 vs $598
ECONOMIC MODELS		
Bachert et al,[101] 2007 7 European countries	Economic Modeling Study. 634 adults with rhinoconjunctivitis due to grass pollen. SLIT tablet (n = 316) vs Placebo (n = 318)	From a Payer perspective, assuming an annual cost of IT of $1860, cost per QALY ranged from $16,033 in the Netherlands to $22,646 in Germany
Bernstein et al,[157] 2004 USA	Economic Modeling. SCIT vs ST. Hypothetical model 3 allergy treatment centers	5-year total costs IT: $4560-$4773. 5-year total costs drug therapy: $10,200
Berto et al,[158] 2006 Italy	Economic Modeling Study. Epidemiologic and resource use data from 2230 patients on SLIT vs ST. Outcome: improved symptoms and asthma avoided outcomes. 1000 adults treated with SLIT for 3 years and followed for 6 years vs SC for 6 years	SLIT was dominant over ST from both a payer and societal perspective. 6-year mean savings per patient who received SLIT vs ST: • $639 (payer perspective) • $2662 (societal perspective)

(continued on next page)

Table 8
(continued)

Study	Study Design	Results
Berto et al,[102] 2008 Italy	Economic Modeling Study 1-year observational study of 102 patients with grass pollen–induced AR with or without asthma SLIT (n = 54) vs ST (n = 48)	Overall yearly cost of treatment per patient was greater for SLIT (311.4 vs 179.8 €/patient, $P<.0001$), in the AR only subgroup (287.9 vs 115.8 €/patient, $P<.0001$), and in the AR plus asthma subgroup (362.4 vs 229.6 €/patient, $P<.0001$)
Brüggenjürgen et al,[159] 2008 Germany	Economic Modeling Study SCIT vs ST 1000 hypothetical patients with AR or allergic asthma who received either SCIT for 3 years or ST over a time horizon of 15 years	Total costs/patient @ 15 years: SCIT = €24,000; ST = €26,100 (annual cost savings ~€140 per SCIT-treated patient) From a third-party payer's perspective, a patient treated with SCIT + ST incurred annual costs of approximately €750 compared with €690 of those receiving only ST The resulting ICER was positive for all patients (€8308 per QALY), and demonstrated that SCIT was a cost-effective treatment
Keiding and Jorgensen,[160] 2007 6 European countries	Economic Modeling Study 410 adults with seasonal rhinoconjunctivitis due to grass pollen SCIT (n = 307) vs placebo (n = 103)	From a payer perspective, the ICER for SCIT vs ST per symptom-free day and well day ranged from $32 (Austria) to $84 (Netherlands) and from $30 (Austria) to $76 (Netherlands), respectively When indirect costs were included, SCIT dominated ST in 4 of the 6 countries for both variables. Cost-effectiveness differences by country were largely a differences due to up-dosing practices
Nasser et al,[161] 2008 UK	Economic modeling study Hypothetical adult patients with rhinoconjunctivitis and asthma SLIT tablet (n = 79) vs Placebo (n = 72)	QALY gained @ 9 years = 0.197, equivalent to an extra 72 days of perfect health for patients treated with SLIT when compared with those receiving placebo

Omnes et al,[103] 2007 France	Economic Modeling Study SCIT vs SLIT vs ST 1000 hypothetical adults and children with AR who received SCIT, SLIT (3–4 years), or ST Outcome: patients improved and asthma cases avoided over time horizon of 7–8 years	ST least expensive but both forms of SIT found to be more effective both in terms of the number of patients with improved symptoms and asthma cases avoided SCIT was more cost-effective than SLIT in terms of both parameters
Pokladnikova et al,[162] 2008 Czech Republic	Economic Modeling Study SCIT vs SLIT vs ST 64 patients with allergic rhinoconjunctivitis who received SLIT (n = 19), SCIT (n = 23), or standard symptomatic treatment (n = 22) over 3 years	Payer perspective, the total average direct medical cost per patient of 3-year SIT was: • ~SLIT €416 vs SCIT €482, patient perspective: • All out-of-pocket costs: SLIT €176 vs €255 for SCIT • Allergen extract costs: SLIT €72 vs SCIT €55 • Direct and indirect costs over 3-year SIT costs per patient: SLIT €684 vs SCIT €1004
Schadlich and Brech,[163] 2000 Germany	Economic Modeling Study SCIT vs ST 1000 hypothetical adults with AR receiving SCIT for 3 years vs ST and followed for 10 years	Break-even point (cumulative costs) reached between years 6 and 8 After 10 years, SCIT led to net savings from the perspectives of society, the health care system, and third-party payer Net savings of $377 (payer) to $690 (societal) per patient over 10 years

Abbreviations: AR, allergic rhinitis; ICER, incremental cost-effectiveness ratio, calculated as the cost difference between SIT and ST divided by the difference in effect; MCD, mean cost difference per patient; NS, not significant; QALY, quality-adjusted life year, measure of health-related quality of life on a scale from 0 (dead) to 1 (perfect health); ST, standard treatment, ie, pharmacotherapy.

health). In the United Kingdom, the National Institute for Health and Clinical Excellence considers a drug cost-effective if it can generate one QALY for less than €29,200 compared with an alternative.[101] A medication that is considered cost-effective is more than twice as likely to be recommended by the National Institute for Health and Clinical Excellence.

It is likely that most of the SLIT studies that have examined and demonstrated cost-effectiveness have employed single-allergen treatment (see **Table 8** for SIT economic analysis).[101–103] The cost-effectiveness of multiallergen SLIT may not be as favorable. Most studies compared the costs of SLIT with pharmacotherapy alone, and none have prospectively compared the cost-effectiveness of SLIT and SCIT. One cost-effectiveness analysis from a health insurance perspective compared SCIT, SLIT, and symptomatic treatment in pollen-allergic or dust mite–allergic patients using a decision tree model defined by an expert panel.[103] Efficacy was measured by the number of improved patients and "... asthma cases avoided" (ie, new onset asthma) and resource use (eg, clinic visits, laboratory tests, medications, and SIT but not hospitalization costs). The model time horizon was 6 years and patients were assumed to have received SIT for 3 or 4 years. Although standard therapy was the least expensive treatment, both forms of SIT were more effective in terms of the number of patients with improved symptoms and asthma cases avoided. SCIT was more cost-effective than SLIT. Compared with standard therapy, the ICER per additional improved patient for SCIT ranged from €349 (children with dust mite allergy) to €722 (adults with pollen allergy) versus SLIT from €630 (children with pollen allergy) to €2371 (children with dust mite allergy).[103]

To date, only 3 studies have examined the cost-effectiveness of SCIT in the United States, where multiallergen therapy is the standard practice.[104–106] One United States retrospective claims analysis published in 1999 found that adults and children who completed 3.5 years of SCIT had 55% higher medical costs compared with patients who completed IT of shorter duration.[104] However, those who completed the longer course of SCIT treatment also had 30% higher medical costs during the year before starting SIT, suggesting a higher disease burden, a potential confounding variable.

More recently, two large-scale, retrospective, United States-based studies have examined whether SCIT confers economic benefits among children with allergic rhinitis.[105,106] In the first study, researchers conducted a 7-year (1997–2004) retrospective claims analysis of Florida Medicaid-enrolled children with newly diagnosed allergic rhinitis to examine short-term (6-month) pre-SCIT versus post-SCIT health care costs.[106] There were significant reductions in the use of outpatient, pharmacy, and inpatient services in the 6 months after SCIT compared with 6 months pre-SCIT. This reduction in health care use resulted in a 6-month total cost saving of $401, which offset the average total cost of immunotherapy ($424 per patient).

In the second study, these investigators examined 10 years (1997–2007) of Florida Medicaid data to compare health care costs between children with newly diagnosed allergic rhinitis, who subsequently received SCIT, with a control group of patients with newly diagnosed allergic rhinitis who did not receive SCIT.[105] The groups were matched by age at first allergic rhinitis diagnosis, sex, race/ethnicity, and diagnosis of asthma, conjunctivitis, and atopic dermatitis. SCIT-treated patients had significantly lower 18-month median per-patient total health care costs ($3247 vs $4872), outpatient costs exclusive of SCIT-related care ($1107 vs $2626), and pharmacy costs ($1108 vs $1316) compared with matched controls (P<.001 for all). The significant difference in total health care costs was evident 3 months after initiating SCIT and progressively increased through to the end of the study.

Collectively, these studies provide considerable support for the cost-effectiveness of SIT compared with pharmacotherapy during treatment. This effect is even greater when one considers the persistent clinical benefits of SIT after discontinuation of treatment, an effect not seen with pharmacotherapy.[107,108]

Adherence/Compliance

Adherence to the immunotherapy regimen is a key component of successful treatment. Adherence (also known as compliance) and reasons for noncompliance with SIT regimens has been assessed in several studies. Noncompliance was defined in most studies as stopping the immunotherapy program without the approval of the prescribing physician. Three retrospective SCIT studies performed in United States reported noncompliance rates ranging from 33% to 54% of patients, with inconvenience cited as one of the main reasons for discontinuation.[109–111] Another retrospective United States SCIT study reported a much higher rate of noncompliance in those who received their injections in facilities outside the allergist's office compared with in the prescribing allergist's office.[112] In the aforementioned 7-year retrospective claims analysis of Florida Medicaid-enrolled children, only 16% of the patients who were prescribed SCIT completed a 3-year course of treatment.[106]

Three studies in a mixed-age population assessed SLIT compliance with either unscheduled telephone requests to count remaining tablets[69,113] or measurement of remaining extract on clinic visits.[114] High compliance, defined as taking medications greater than 80% of the time, was reported in 72% to 97% of patients. One study prospectively investigated the compliance with 3 immunotherapy methods, SLIT, SCIT, and nasal immunotherapy, in 2774 children (aged 6–15 years).[115] The highest noncompliance rate was seen in the nasal immunotherapy group (73.2% of patients) followed by SLIT (21.5% of patients) and SCIT (10.9 % of patients). Expense was the most frequently cited reason for discontinuation in the SLIT and SCIT groups (36.4% and 39.6%, respectively). The second most common reason was "too time consuming" for SCIT (24.2 %) and "ineffective" for SLIT (24.9%).

Although these studies show that noncompliance can be relatively high for both SCIT and SLIT, it is less so than that associated with taking topical (eg, inhaled or intranasal) medications. Furthermore, the degree of compliance with SIT can be monitored with more accuracy.

SUMMARY

Specific allergen immunotherapy, via both the subcutaneous and sublingual routes, has been shown in numerous clinical trials to be effective in reducing the clinical symptoms associated with allergic rhinitis. In addition, both methods provide persistent clinical efficacy after treatment discontinuation and may prevent the progression of the allergic disease. SLIT appears to have a better safety profile and may be associated with better adherence. Both methods have been found to be cost-effective when compared with pharmacotherapy alone, but no cost-effectiveness studies employing multiple allergens with SLIT have been performed. On the other hand, two United States studies that primarily used multiallergen SCIT demonstrated significant cost reductions compared with pre-SCIT costs and a matched control population. The immunologic mechanisms associated with both methods are still being elucidated. Although considerably more is known about the immunologic changes associated with SCIT, it appears that the mechanisms of SLIT and SCIT may be similar. At present, SCIT is the only method with an FDA-approved formulation in the United States.

ACKNOWLEDGMENTS

The authors would like to acknowledge Cheryl Hankin, PhD with assistance SIT pharmoeconmic section.

REFERENCES

1. Cox L, Jacobsen L. Comparison of allergen immunotherapy practice patterns in the United States and Europe. Ann Allergy Asthma Immunol 2009;103(6):451–9 [quiz: 459–61, 495].
2. Tucker MH, Tankersley MS. Perception and practice of sublingual immunotherapy among practicing allergists. Ann Allergy Asthma Immunol 2008; 101(4):419–25.
3. Freeman J. Further observations of the treatment of hay fever by hypodermic inoculations of pollen vaccine. Lancet 1911;2:814–7.
4. Freeman J. "Rush inoculation", with special reference to hay fever treatment. Lancet 1930;1:744–7.
5. Noon L. Prophylactic inoculation against hay fever. Lancet 1911;1:1572–3.
6. Durham SR, Walker SM, Varga EM, et al. Long-term clinical efficacy of grass-pollen immunotherapy. N Engl J Med 1999;341:468–75.
7. Jacobsen L, Niggemann B, Dreborg S, et al. Specific immunotherapy has long-term preventive effect of seasonal and perennial asthma: 10-year follow-up on the PAT study. Allergy 2007;62(8):943–8.
8. Polosa R, Al-Delaimy WK, Russo C, et al. Greater risk of incident asthma cases in adults with allergic rhinitis and effect of allergen immunotherapy: a retrospective cohort study. Respir Res 2005;6:153.
9. Purello-D'Ambrosio F, Gangemi S, Merendino RA, et al. Prevention of new sensitizations in monosensitized subjects submitted to specific immunotherapy or not. A retrospective study. Clin Exp Allergy 2001;31(8):1295–302.
10. Inal A, Altintas DU, Yilmaz M, et al. Prevention of new sensitizations by specific immunotherapy in children with rhinitis and/or asthma monosensitized to house dust mite. J Investig Allergol Clin Immunol 2007;17(2):85–91.
11. Pajno GB, Barberio G, De Luca F, et al. Prevention of new sensitizations in asthmatic children monosensitized to house dust mite by specific immunotherapy. A six-year follow-up study. Clin Exp Allergy 2001;31(9):1392–7.
12. Des Roches A, Paradis L, Menardo JL, et al. Immunotherapy with a standardized *Dermatophagoides pteronyssinus* extract. VI. Specific immunotherapy prevents the onset of new sensitizations in children. J Allergy Clin Immunol 1997;99(4): 450–3.
13. Oppenheimer J, Areson JG, Nelson HS. Safety and efficacy of oral immunotherapy with standardized cat extract. J Allergy Clin Immunol 1994;93(1 Pt 1): 61–7.
14. Buchanan AD, Green TD, Jones SM, et al. Egg oral immunotherapy in nonanaphylactic children with egg allergy. J Allergy Clin Immunol 2007;119(1): 199–205.
15. Jones SM, Pons L, Roberts JL, et al. Clinical efficacy and immune regulation with peanut oral immunotherapy. J Allergy Clin Immunol 2009;124(2):292–300, 300.e1–97.e1.
16. Staden U, Rolinck-Werninghaus C, Brewe F, et al. Specific oral tolerance induction in food allergy in children: efficacy and clinical patterns of reaction. Allergy 2007;62(11):1261–9.

17. Frankland AW, Augustin R. Prophylaxis of summer hay-fever and asthma: a controlled trial comparing crude grass-pollen extract with isolated main protein component. Lancet 1954;1:1055–7.

18. Lowell FC, Franklin W. A double-blind study of the effectiveness and specificity of injection therapy in ragweed hay fever. N Engl J Med 1965;273(13): 675–9.

19. Franklin W, Lowell FC. Comparison of two dosages of ragweed extract in the treatment of pollenosis. JAMA 1967;201(12):915–7.

20. Johnstone DE, Dutton A. The value of hyposensitization therapy for bronchial asthma in children—a 14-year study. Pediatrics 1968;42(5):793–802.

21. Creticos PS, Marsh DG, Proud D, et al. Responses to ragweed-pollen nasal challenge before and after immunotherapy. J Allergy Clin Immunol 1989;84(2): 197–205.

22. Creticos PS, Van Metre TE, Mardiney MR, et al. Dose response of IgE and IgG antibodies during ragweed immunotherapy. J Allergy Clin Immunol 1984;73(1 Pt 1): 94–104.

23. Frew AJ, Powell RJ, Corrigan CJ, et al. Efficacy and safety of specific immunotherapy with SQ allergen extract in treatment-resistant seasonal allergic rhinoconjunctivitis. J Allergy Clin Immunol 2006;117(2):319–25.

24. Lent AM, Harbeck R, Strand M, et al. Immunologic response to administration of standardized dog allergen extract at differing doses. J Allergy Clin Immunol 2006;118(6):1249–56.

25. Nanda A, O'connor M, Anand M, et al. Dose dependence and time course of the immunologic response to administration of standardized cat allergen extract. J Allergy Clin Immunol 2004;114(6):1339–44.

26. Des Roches A, Paradis L, Knani J, et al. Immunotherapy with a standardized *Dermatophagoides pteronyssinus* extract. V. Duration of the efficacy of immunotherapy after its cessation. Allergy 1996;51(6):430–3.

27. Joint Task Force on Practice Parameters; American Academy of Allergy, Asthma and Immunology; American College of Allergy, Asthma and Immunology; et al. Allergen immunotherapy: a practice parameter second update. J Allergy Clin Immunol 2007;120(3 Suppl):S25–85.

28. Calderon MA, Alves B, Jacobson M, et al. Allergen injection immunotherapy for seasonal allergic rhinitis. Cochrane Database Syst Rev 2007;1:CD001936.

29. Horst M, Hejjaoui A, Horst V, et al. Double-blind, placebo-controlled rush immunotherapy with a standardized Alternaria extract. J Allergy Clin Immunol 1990; 85(2):460–72.

30. Varney VA, Edwards J, Tabbah K, et al. Clinical efficacy of specific immunotherapy to cat dander: a double-blind placebo-controlled trial. Clin Exp Allergy 1997;27(8):860–7.

31. Kohno Y, Minoguchi K, Oda N, et al. Effect of rush immunotherapy on airway inflammation and airway hyperresponsiveness after bronchoprovocation with allergen in asthma. J Allergy Clin Immunol 1998;102(6 Pt 1):927–34.

32. Eng PA, Borer-Reinhold M, Heijnen IA, et al. Twelve-year follow-up after discontinuation of preseasonal grass pollen immunotherapy in childhood. Allergy 2006;61(2):198–201.

33. Jacobsen L, Nüchel Petersen B, Wihl JA, et al. Immunotherapy with partially purified and standardized tree pollen extracts. IV. Results from long-term (6-year) follow-up. Allergy 1997;52(9):914–20.

34. Wilson DR, Lima MT, Durham SR. Sublingual immunotherapy for allergic rhinitis: systematic review and meta-analysis. Allergy 2005;60(1):4–12.

35. Halken S, Agertoft L, Seidenberg J, et al. Five-grass pollen 300IR SLIT tablets: efficacy and safety in children and adolescents. Pediatr Allergy Immunol 2010; 21(6):970–6.

36. Wahn U, Tabar A, Kuna P, et al. Efficacy and safety of 5-grass-pollen sublingual immunotherapy tablets in pediatric allergic rhinoconjunctivitis. J Allergy Clin Immunol 2009;123(1):160–6.e3.

37. Penagos M, Compalati E, Tarantini F, et al. Efficacy of sublingual immunotherapy in the treatment of allergic rhinitis in pediatric patients 3 to 18 years of age: a meta-analysis of randomized, placebo-controlled, double-blind trials. Ann Allergy Asthma Immunol 2006;97(2):141–8.

38. Sanchez Palacios A, Schamann F, Garcia JA. [Sublingual immunotherapy with cat epithelial extract. Personal experience]. Allergol Immunopathol (Madr) 2001;29(2):60–5 [in Spanish].

39. Andre C, Perrin-Fayolle M, Grosclaude M, et al. A double-blind placebo-controlled evaluation of sublingual immunotherapy with a standardized ragweed extract in patients with seasonal rhinitis. Evidence for a dose-response relationship. Int Arch Allergy Immunol 2003;131(2):111–8.

40. Cox LS, Larenas Linnemann D, Nolte H, et al. Sublingual immunotherapy: a comprehensive review. J Allergy Clin Immunol 2006;117(5):1021–35.

41. Durham SR, Yang WH, Pedersen MR, et al. Sublingual immunotherapy with once-daily grass allergen tablets: a randomized controlled trial in seasonal allergic rhinoconjunctivitis. J Allergy Clin Immunol 2006;117(4):802–9.

42. Didier A, Malling HJ, Worm M, et al. Optimal dose, efficacy, and safety of once-daily sublingual immunotherapy with a 5-grass pollen tablet for seasonal allergic rhinitis. J Allergy Clin Immunol 2007;120:1338–45.

43. Dahl R, Kapp A, Colombo G, et al. Sublingual grass allergen tablet immunotherapy provides sustained clinical benefit with progressive immunologic changes over 2 years. J Allergy Clin Immunol 2008;121(2):512–8.e2.

44. Durham SR, Emminger W, Kapp A, et al. Long-term clinical efficacy in grass pollen-induced rhinoconjunctivitis after treatment with SQ-standardized grass allergy immunotherapy tablet. J Allergy Clin Immunol 2010;125(1):131–8.e1–7.

45. Horak F, Zieglmayer P, Zieglmayer R, et al. Early onset of action of a 5-grass-pollen 300-IR sublingual immunotherapy tablet evaluated in an allergen challenge chamber. J Allergy Clin Immunol 2009;124(3):471–7, 477.e1.

46. Arbes SJ Jr, Gergen PJ, Elliott L, et al. Prevalences of positive skin test responses to 10 common allergens in the US population: results from the third National Health and Nutrition Examination Survey. J Allergy Clin Immunol 2005;116(2):377–83.

47. Craig TJ, King TS, Lemanske RF Jr, et al. Aeroallergen sensitization correlates with PC(20) and exhaled nitric oxide in subjects with mild-to-moderate asthma. J Allergy Clin Immunol 2008;121(3):671–7.

48. Ciprandi G, Cadario G, Di Gioacchino GM, et al. Sublingual immunotherapy in children with allergic polysensitization. Allergy Asthma Proc 2010;31(3): 227–31.

49. Ciprandi G, Incorvaia C, Puccinelli P, et al. The POLISMAIL lesson: sublingual immunotherapy may be prescribed also in polysensitized patients. Int J Immunopathol Pharmacol 2010;23(2):637–40.

50. Malling HJ, Montagut A, Melac M, et al. Efficacy and safety of 5-grass pollen sublingual immunotherapy tablets in patients with different clinical profiles of allergic rhinoconjunctivitis. Clin Exp Allergy 2009;39(3):387–93.

51. Haugaard L, Dahl R, Jacobsen L. A controlled dose-response study of immunotherapy with standardized, partially purified extract of house dust mite: clinical efficacy and side effects. J Allergy Clin Immunol 1993;91(3):709–22.
52. Nelson HS. Multiallergen immunotherapy for allergic rhinitis and asthma. J Allergy Clin Immunol 2009;123(4):763–9.
53. Moller C, Dreborg S, Ferdousi HA, et al. Pollen immunotherapy reduces the development of asthma in children with seasonal rhinoconjunctivitis (the PAT-study). J Allergy Clin Immunol 2002;109(2):251–6.
54. Haugaard L, Dahl R. Immunotherapy in patients allergic to cat and dog dander. I. Clinical results. Allergy 1992;47(3):249–54.
55. Moncayo Coello CV, Rosas Vargas MA, del Rio Navarro BE, et al. [Quality of life in children with allergic rhinitis before and after being treated with specific immunotherapy (cases and controls)]. Rev Alerg Mex 2003;50(5):170–5 [in Spanish].
56. Guardia P, Moreno C, Justicia JL, et al. Tolerance and short-term effect of a cluster schedule with pollen-extracts quantified in mass-units. Allergol Immunopathol (Madr) 2004;32(5):271–7.
57. Adkinson NF Jr, Eggleston PA, Eney D, et al. A controlled trial of immunotherapy for asthma in allergic children. N Engl J Med 1997;336(5):324–31.
58. Bousquet J, Becker WM, Hejjaoui A, et al. Differences in clinical and immunologic reactivity of patients allergic to grass pollens and to multiple-pollen species. II. Efficacy of a double-blind, placebo-controlled, specific immunotherapy with standardized extracts. J Allergy Clin Immunol 1991;88(1):43–53.
59. Rosenstreich DL, Eggleston P, Kattan M, et al. The role of cockroach allergy and exposure to cockroach allergen in causing morbidity among inner-city children with asthma. N Engl J Med 1997;336(19):1356–63.
60. Marogna M, Spadolini I, Massolo A, et al. Effects of sublingual immunotherapy for multiple or single allergens in polysensitized patients. Ann Allergy Asthma Immunol 2007;98(3):274–80.
61. Cirla AM, Cirla PE, Parmiani S, et al. A pre-seasonal birch/hazel sublingual immunotherapy can improve the outcome of grass pollen injective treatment in bisensitized individuals. A case-referent, two-year controlled study. Allergol Immunopathol (Madr) 2003;31(1):31–43.
62. Amar SM, Harbeck RJ, Sills M, et al. Response to sublingual immunotherapy with grass pollen extract: monotherapy versus combination in a multiallergen extract. J Allergy Clin Immunol 2009;124(1):150–6. e1–5.
63. Guerra S, Sherrill DL, Baldacci S, et al. Rhinitis is an independent risk factor for developing cough apart from colds among adults. Allergy 2005;60(3):343–9.
64. Lombardi C, Passalacqua G, Gargioni S, et al. The natural history of respiratory allergy: a follow-up study of 99 patients up to 10 years. Respir Med 2001;95(1):9–12.
65. Leynaert B, Neukirch C, Kony S, et al. Association between asthma and rhinitis according to atopic sensitization in a population-based study. J Allergy Clin Immunol 2004;113(1):86–93.
66. Torén K, Olin AC, Hellgren J, et al. Rhinitis increase the risk for adult-onset asthma—a Swedish population-based case-control study (MAP-study). Respir Med 2002;96(8):635–41.
67. Marogna M, Tomassetti D, Bernasconi A, et al. Preventive effects of sublingual immunotherapy in childhood: an open randomized controlled study. Ann Allergy Asthma Immunol 2008;101(2):206–11.

68. Novembre E, Galli E, Landi F, et al. Coseasonal sublingual immunotherapy reduces the development of asthma in children with allergic rhinoconjunctivitis. J Allergy Clin Immunol 2004;114(4):851–7.
69. Marogna M, Spadolini I, Massolo A, et al. Randomized controlled open study of sublingual immunotherapy for respiratory allergy in real-life: clinical efficacy and more. Allergy 2004;59(11):1205–10.
70. Nelson BL, Dupont LA, Reid MJ. Prospective survey of local and systemic reactions to immunotherapy with pollen extracts. Ann Allergy 1986;56(4): 331–4.
71. Prigal SJ. A ten-year study of repository injections of allergens: local reactions and their management. Ann Allergy 1972;30(9):529–35.
72. Tankersley MS, Butler KK, Butler WK, et al. Local reactions during allergen immunotherapy do not require dose adjustment. J Allergy Clin Immunol 2000; 106(5):840–3.
73. Kelso JM. The rate of systemic reactions to immunotherapy injections is the same whether or not the dose is reduced after a local reaction. Ann Allergy Asthma Immunol 2004;92(2):225–7.
74. Roy SR, Sigmon JR, Olivier J, et al. Increased frequency of large local reactions among systemic reactors during subcutaneous allergen immunotherapy. Ann Allergy Asthma Immunol 2007;99(1):82–6.
75. Cox L, Larenas-Linnemann D, Lockey RF, et al. Speaking the same language: the World Allergy Organization subcutaneous immunotherapy systemic reaction grading system. J Allergy Clin Immunol 2010;125(3):569–74, 574.e1–574.e7.
76. Cox L. Advantages and disadvantages of accelerated immunotherapy schedules. J Allergy Clin Immunol 2008;122(2):432–4.
77. Reid MJ, Lockey RF, Turkeltaub PC, et al. Survey of fatalities from skin testing and immunotherapy 1985–1989. J Allergy Clin Immunol 1993;92(1 Pt 1):6–15.
78. Lockey RF, Benedict LM, Turkeltaub PC, et al. Fatalities from immunotherapy (IT) and skin testing (ST). J Allergy Clin Immunol 1987;79(4):660–77.
79. Bernstein DI, Wanner M, Borish L, et al. Twelve-year survey of fatal reactions to allergen injections and skin testing: 1990–2001. J Allergy Clin Immunol 2004; 113(6):1129–36.
80. Amin HS, Liss GM, Bernstein DI. Evaluation of near-fatal reactions to allergen immunotherapy injections. J Allergy Clin Immunol 2006;117(1):169–75.
81. Bernstein DI, Wanner M, Borish L, et al. Surveillance of systemic reactions to subcutaneous immunotherapy injections: year 1 outcomes of the ACAAI and AAAAI collaborative study. Ann Allergy Asthma Immunol 2010;104(6):530–5.
82. Dahl R, Kapp A, Colombo G, et al. Efficacy and safety of sublingual immunotherapy with grass allergen tablets for seasonal allergic rhinoconjunctivitis. J Allergy Clin Immunol 2006;118(2):434–40.
83. Cox L. Sublingual immunotherapy in pediatric allergic rhinitis and asthma: efficacy, safety, and practical considerations. Curr Allergy Asthma Rep 2007;7(6): 410–20.
84. Blazowski L. Anaphylactic shock because of sublingual immunotherapy overdose during third year of maintenance dose. Allergy 2008;63(3):374.
85. Antico A, Pagani M, Crema A. Anaphylaxis by latex sublingual immunotherapy. Allergy 2006;61(10):1236–7.
86. Eifan AO, Keles S, Bahceciler NN, et al. Anaphylaxis to multiple pollen allergen sublingual immunotherapy. Allergy 2007;62(5):567–8.
87. Dunsky EH, Goldstein MF, Dvorin DJ, et al. Anaphylaxis to sublingual immunotherapy. Allergy 2006;61(10):1235.

88. de Groot H, Bijl A. Anaphylactic reaction after the first dose of sublingual immunotherapy with grass pollen tablet. Allergy 2009;64(6):963–4.
89. Cochard MM, Eigenmann PA. Sublingual immunotherapy is not always a safe alternative to subcutaneous immunotherapy. J Allergy Clin Immunol 2009; 124(2):378–9.
90. Simons FE, Frew AJ, Ansotegui IJ, et al. Risk assessment in anaphylaxis: current and future approaches. J Allergy Clin Immunol 2007;120(1):S2–24.
91. Francis J, James LK, Paraskevopoulos G, et al. Grass pollen immunotherapy: IL-10 induction and suppression of late responses precedes IgG4 inhibitory antibody activity. J Allergy Clin Immunol 2008;121(5):1120–5.e2.
92. Francis JN, Lloyd CM, Sabroe I, et al. T lymphocytes expressing CCR3 are increased in allergic rhinitis compared with non-allergic controls and following allergen immunotherapy. Allergy 2007;62(1):59–65.
93. Francis JN, Till SJ, Durham SR. Induction of IL-10+CD4+CD25+ T cells by grass pollen immunotherapy. J Allergy Clin Immunol 2003;111(6):1255–61.
94. Till SJ, Durham SR. Immunological responses to allergen immunotherapy. Clin Allergy Immunol 2004;18:85–104.
95. Bohle B, Kinaciyan T, Gerstmayr M, et al. Sublingual immunotherapy induces IL-10-producing T regulatory cells, allergen-specific T-cell tolerance, and immune deviation. J Allergy Clin Immunol 2007;120(3):707–13.
96. O'Hehir RE, Gardner LM, de Leon MP, et al. House dust mite sublingual immunotherapy: the role for transforming growth factor-beta and functional regulatory T cells. Am J Respir Crit Care Med 2009;180(10):936–47.
97. Jutel M, Akdis M, Budak F, et al. IL-10 and TGF-beta cooperate in the regulatory T cell response to mucosal allergens in normal immunity and specific immunotherapy. Eur J Immunol 2003;33(5):1205–14.
98. Durham SR, Till SJ. Immunologic changes associated with allergen immunotherapy. J Allergy Clin Immunol 1998;102(2):157–64.
99. Till SJ, Francis JN, Nouri-Aria K, et al. Mechanisms of immunotherapy. J Allergy Clin Immunol 2004;113(6):1025–34 [quiz: 1035].
100. Wallace D, Dykewicz MS, Bernstein DI, et al. The diagnosis and management of rhinitis: an updated practice parameter. J Allergy Clin Immunol 2008;122(2):S1–84.
101. Bachert C, Vestenbaek U, Christensen J, et al. Cost-effectiveness of grass allergen tablet (GRAZAX(R)) for the prevention of seasonal grass pollen induced rhinoconjunctivitis - a Northern European perspective. Clin Exp Allergy 2007;37(5):772–9.
102. Berto P, Frati F, Incorvaia C, et al. Comparison of costs of sublingual immunotherapy and drug treatment in grass-pollen induced allergy: results from the SIMAP database study. Curr Med Res Opin 2008;24(1):261–6.
103. Omnes LF, Bousquet J, Scheinmann P, et al. Pharmacoeconomic assessment of specific immunotherapy versus current symptomatic treatment for allergic rhinitis and asthma in France. Eur Ann Allergy Clin Immunol 2007;39(5):148–56.
104. Donahue JG, Greineder DK, Connor-Lacke L, et al. Utilization and cost of immunotherapy for allergic asthma and rhinitis. Ann Allergy Asthma Immunol 1999; 82(4):339–47.
105. Hankin CS, Cox L, Lang D, et al. Allergen immunotherapy and health care cost benefits for children with allergic rhinitis: a large-scale, retrospective, matched cohort study. Ann Allergy Asthma Immunol 2010;104(1):79–85.
106. Hankin CS, Cox L, Lang D, et al. Allergy immunotherapy among Medicaid-enrolled children with allergic rhinitis: patterns of care, resource use, and costs. J Allergy Clin Immunol 2008;121(1):227–32.

107. Guilbert TW, Morgan WJ, Zeiger RS, et al. Long-term inhaled corticosteroids in preschool children at high risk for asthma. N Engl J Med 2006;354(19): 1985–97.

108. Strunk RC, Sternberg AL, Szefler SJ, et al. Long-term budesonide or nedocromil treatment, once discontinued, does not alter the course of mild to moderate asthma in children and adolescents. J Pediatr 2009;154(5):682–7.

109. More DR, Hagan LL. Factors affecting compliance with allergen immunotherapy at a military medical center. Ann Allergy Asthma Immunol 2002;88(4):391–4.

110. Lower T, Henry J, Mandik L, et al. Compliance with allergen immunotherapy. Ann Allergy 1993;70(6):480–2.

111. Cohn JR, Pizzi A. Determinants of patient compliance with allergen immunotherapy. J Allergy Clin Immunol 1993;91(3):734–7.

112. Tinkelman D, Smith F, Cole WQ, et al. Compliance with an allergen immunotherapy regime. Ann Allergy Asthma Immunol 1995;74(3):241–6.

113. Lombardi C, Gani F, Landi M, et al. Quantitative assessment of the adherence to sublingual immunotherapy. J Allergy Clin Immunol 2004;113(6):1219–20.

114. Passalacqua G, Musarra A, Pecora S, et al. Quantitative assessment of the compliance with a once-daily sublingual immunotherapy regimen in real life (EASY Project: Evaluation of a novel SLIT formulation during a Year). J Allergy Clin Immunol 2006;117(4):946–8.

115. Pajno GB, Vita D, Caminiti L, et al. Children's compliance with allergen immunotherapy according to administration routes. J Allergy Clin Immunol 2005;116(6): 1380–1.

116. Niggemann B, Jacobsen L, Dreborg S, et al. Five-year follow-up on the PAT study: specific immunotherapy and long-term prevention of asthma in children. Allergy 2006;61(7):855–9.

117. Polosa R, Li Gotti F, Mangano G, et al. Effect of immunotherapy on asthma progression, BHR and sputum eosinophils in allergic rhinitis. Allergy 2004; 59(11):1224–8.

118. Limb SL, Brown KC, Wood RA, et al. Long-term immunologic effects of broad-spectrum aeroallergen immunotherapy. Int Arch Allergy Immunol 2006;140: 245–51.

119. Eng PA, Reinhold M, Gnehm HP. Long-term efficacy of preseasonal grass pollen immunotherapy in children. Allergy 2002;57(4):306–12.

120. Balda BR, Wolf H, Baumgarten C, et al. Tree-pollen allergy is efficiently treated by short-term immunotherapy (STI) with seven preseasonal injections of molecular standardized allergens. Allergy 1998;53(8):740–8.

121. Jutel M, Jaeger L, Suck R, et al. Allergen-specific immunotherapy with recombinant grass pollen allergens. J Allergy Clin Immunol 2005;116(3):608–13.

122. Corrigan CJ, Kettner J, Doemer C, et al. Efficacy and safety of preseasonal-specific immunotherapy with an aluminium-adsorbed six-grass pollen allergoid. Allergy 2005;60(6):801–7.

123. Colás C, Monzón S, Venturini M, et al. Double-blind, placebo-controlled study with a modified therapeutic vaccine of Salsola kali (Russian thistle) administered through use of a cluster schedule. J Allergy Clin Immunol 2006;117(4):810–6.

124. Pauli G, Larsen TH, Rak S, et al. Efficacy of recombinant birch pollen vaccine for the treatment of birch-allergic rhinoconjunctivitis. J Allergy Clin Immunol 2008; 122(5):951–60.

125. Dahl R, Stender A, Rak S. Specific immunotherapy with SQ standardized grass allergen tablets in asthmatics with rhinoconjunctivitis. Allergy 2006;61(2): 185–90.

126. Roder E, Moed H, Berger MY, et al. Sublingual immunotherapy with grass pollen is not effective in symptomatic youngsters in primary care. J Allergy Clin Immunol 2007;119(4):892–8.

127. de Blay F, Barnig C, Kanny G, et al. Sublingual-swallow immunotherapy with standardized 3-grass pollen extract: a double-blind, placebo-controlled study. Ann Allergy Asthma Immunol 2007;99(5):453–61.

128. Pfaar O, Klimek L. Efficacy and safety of specific immunotherapy with a high-dose sublingual grass pollen preparation: a double-blind, placebo-controlled trial. Ann Allergy Asthma Immunol 2008;100(3):256–63.

129. Ott H, Sieber J, Brehler R, et al. Efficacy of grass pollen sublingual immunotherapy for three consecutive seasons and after cessation of treatment: the ECRIT study. Allergy 2009;64(1):179–86.

130. Bufe A, Eberle P, Franke-Beckmann E, et al. Safety and efficacy in children of an SQ-standardized grass allergen tablet for sublingual immunotherapy. J Allergy Clin Immunol 2009;123:167–73.e7.

131. Skoner D, Gentile D, Bush R, et al. Sublingual immunotherapy in patients with allergic rhinoconjunctivitis caused by ragweed pollen. J Allergy Clin Immunol 2010;125(3):660–6, 666.e1–666.e4.

132. Olsen OT, Larsen KR, Jacobsan L, et al. A 1-year, placebo-controlled, double-blind house-dust-mite immunotherapy study in asthmatic adults. Allergy 1997; 52(8):853–9.

133. Ewan PW, Alexander MM, Snape C, et al. Effective hyposensitization in allergic rhinitis using a potent partially purified extract of house dust mite. Clin Allergy 1988;18(5):501–8.

134. Niu CK, Chen WY, Huang JL, et al. Efficacy of sublingual immunotherapy with high-dose mite extracts in asthma: a multi-center, double-blind, randomized, and placebo-controlled study in Taiwan. Respir Med 2006;100(8):1374–83.

135. Ippoliti F, De Santis W, Volterrani A, et al. Immunomodulation during sublingual therapy in allergic children. Pediatr Allergy Immunol 2003;14(3):216–21.

136. Hirsch T, Sahn M, Leupold W. Double-blind placebo-controlled study of sublingual immunotherapy with house dust mite extract (D.pt.) in children. Pediatr Allergy Immunol 1997;8(1):21–7.

137. Passalacqua G, Pasquali M, Ariano R, et al. Randomized double-blind controlled study with sublingual carbamylated allergoid immunotherapy in mild rhinitis due to mites. Allergy 2006;61(7):849–54.

138. Pham-Thi N, de Blic J, Scheinmann P. Sublingual immunotherapy in the treatment of children. Allergy 2006;61(Suppl 81):7–10.

139. Lue KH, Lin YH, Sun HL, et al. Clinical and immunologic effects of sublingual immunotherapy in asthmatic children sensitized to mites: a double-blind, randomized, placebo-controlled study. Pediatr Allergy Immunol 2006;17(6): 408–15.

140. Guez S, Vatrinet C, Fadel R, et al. House-dust-mite sublingual-swallow immunotherapy (SLIT) in perennial rhinitis: a double-blind, placebo-controlled study. Allergy 2000;55(4):369–75.

141. Mirone C, Albert F, Tosi A, et al. Efficacy and safety of subcutaneous immunotherapy with a biologically standardized extract of Ambrosia artemisiifolia pollen: a double-blind, placebo-controlled study. Clin Exp Allergy 2004;34(9): 1408–14.

142. Creticos P, Adkinson NF Jr, Kagey-Sobotka A, et al. Nasal challenge with ragweed pollen in hay fever patients: effect of immunotherapy. J Clin Invest 1985;76:2247–53.

143. Bowen T, Greenbaum J, Charbonneau Y, et al. Canadian trial of sublingual swallow immunotherapy for ragweed rhinoconjunctivitis. Ann Allergy Asthma Immunol 2004;93(5):425–30.

144. Varney VA, Gaga M, Frew AJ, et al. Usefulness of immunotherapy in patients with severe summer hay fever uncontrolled by antiallergic drugs. BMJ 1991; 302(6771):265–9.

145. Dolz I, Martínez-Cócera C, Bartolomé JM, et al. A double-blind, placebo-controlled study of immunotherapy with grass-pollen extract Alutard SQ during a 3-year period with initial rush immunotherapy. Allergy 1996;51(7):489–500.

146. Walker SM, Pajno GB, Lima MT, et al. Grass pollen immunotherapy for seasonal rhinitis and asthma: a randomized, controlled trial. J Allergy Clin Immunol 2001; 107(1):87–93.

147. Leynadier F, Banoun L, Dollois B, et al. Immunotherapy with a calcium phosphate-adsorbed five-grass-pollen extract in seasonal rhinoconjunctivitis: a double-blind, placebo-controlled study. Clin Exp Allergy 2001;31(7):988–96.

148. Larenas Linnemann D, Guidos Fogelbach GA, Arias Cruz A. [Practice patterns in Mexican allergologists about specific immunotherapy with allergens]. Rev Alerg Mex 2008;55(2):53–61 [in Spanish].

149. Pfaar O, Anders C, Klimek L. Clinical outcome measures of specific immunotherapy. Curr Opin Allergy Clin Immunol 2009;9(3):208–13.

150. Khinchi MS, Poulsen LK, Carat F, et al. Clinical efficacy of sublingual and subcutaneous birch pollen allergen-specific immunotherapy: a randomized, placebo-controlled, double-blind, double-dummy study. Allergy 2004;59(1):45–53.

151. Bodtger U, Poulsen LK, Jacobi HH, et al. The safety and efficacy of subcutaneous birch pollen immunotherapy—a one-year, randomised, double-blind, placebo-controlled study. Allergy 2002;57(4):297–305.

152. Horak F, Stübner P, Berger UE, et al. Immunotherapy with sublingual birch pollen extract. A short-term double-blind placebo study. J Investig Allergol Clin Immunol 1998;8(3):165–71.

153. Voltolini S, Modena P, Minale P, et al. Sublingual immunotherapy in tree pollen allergy. Double-blind, placebo-controlled study with a biologically standardised extract of three pollens (alder, birch and hazel) administered by a rush schedule. Allergol Immunopathol (Madr) 2001;29(4):103–10.

154. Valovirta E, Jacobsen L, Ljørring C, et al. Clinical efficacy and safety of sublingual immunotherapy with tree pollen extract in children. Allergy 2006;61(10): 1177–83.

155. Ariano R, Berto P, Tracci D, et al. Pharmacoeconomics of allergen immunotherapy compared with symptomatic drug treatment in patients with allergic rhinitis and asthma. Allergy Asthma Proc 2006;27(2):159–63.

156. Berto P, Bassi M, Incorvaia C, et al. Cost effectiveness of sublingual immunotherapy in children with allergic rhinitis and asthma. Eur Ann Allergy Clin Immunol 2005;37(8):303–8.

157. Bernstein JA. Pharmacoeconomic considerations for allergen immunotherapy. Clin Allergy Immunol 2004;18:151–64.

158. Berto P, Passalacqua G, Crimi N, et al. Economic evaluation of sublingual immunotherapy vs symptomatic treatment in adults with pollen-induced respiratory allergy: the Sublingual Immunotherapy Pollen Allergy Italy (SPAI) study. Ann Allergy Asthma Immunol 2006;97(5):615–21.

159. Bruggenjurgen B, Reinhold T, Brehler R, et al. Cost-effectiveness of specific subcutaneous immunotherapy in patients with allergic rhinitis and allergic asthma. Ann Allergy Asthma Immunol 2008;101(3):316–24.

160. Keiding H, Jorgensen KP. A cost-effectiveness analysis of immunotherapy with SQ allergen extract for patients with seasonal allergic rhinoconjunctivitis in selected European countries. Curr Med Res Opin 2007;23(5):1113–20.

161. Nasser S, Vestenbaek U, Beriot-Mathiot A, et al. Cost-effectiveness of specific immunotherapy with Grazax in allergic rhinitis co-existing with asthma. Allergy 2008;63(12):1624–9.

162. Pokladnikova J, Krcmova I, Vlcek J. Economic evaluation of sublingual vs subcutaneous allergen immunotherapy. Ann Allergy Asthma Immunol 2008; 100(5):482–9.

163. Schadlich PK, Brecht JG. Economic evaluation of specific immunotherapy versus symptomatic treatment of allergic rhinitis in Germany. Pharmacoeconomics 2000;17(1):37–52.

164. Radulovic S, Calderon MA, Wilson D, et al. Sublingual immunotherapy for allergic rhinitis. Cochrane Database Syst Rev 2010;12:CD002893.

165. Alvarez-Cuesta E, Aragoneses-Gilsanz E, Martin-Garcia C, et al. Immunotherapy with depigmented glutaraldehyde-polymerized extracts: changes in quality of life. Clin Exp Allergy 2005;35:572–8.

The Role of Decongestants, Cromolyn, Guafenesin, Saline Washes, Capsaicin, Leukotriene Antagonists, and Other Treatments on Rhinitis

Nataliya M. Kushnir, MD

KEYWORDS

• Decongestants • Rhinitis • Saline wash • Allergy
• Alternative treatment • Herbal treatment • Acupuncture
• Leukotriene antagonist

Treatment of rhinitis should be selected based on careful diagnosis.[1] Clinical symptoms of allergic and nonallergic rhinitis are similar despite the significant difference in underlying mechanisms.[2,3] Most of the treatments reviewed in this article are available over the counter (OTC) and thus are a likely choice of patients suffering from acute or chronic rhinitis. Patients seek OTC medications to relieve their symptoms, such as congestion, rhinorrhea, and nasal pruritus, regardless of cause, which is sometimes difficult to establish.[4] Primary care physicians are more likely to recommend OTC products for mild symptoms of rhinitis.[5] According to surveys in chronic rhinitis, sufferers' dissatisfaction with prescribed treatments leads to decreased compliance and an increased reliance on multiple alternative options and OTC products.[6] Combination and single-ingredient nonprescription medications that are approved by the US Food and Drug Administration (FDA) as generally safe, although they do have side effects and, if used inappropriately, can cause worsening of the condition. Primary care physicians and subspecialists (eg, allergists, ear, nose, and

Allergy and Immunology Clinic of East Bay, 2320 Woolsey Street #314, Berkeley, CA 94705, USA
E-mail address: allergynk@gmail.com

Immunol Allergy Clin N Am 31 (2011) 601–617
doi:10.1016/j.iac.2011.05.008
0889-8561/11/$ – see front matter © 2011 Elsevier Inc. All rights reserved.
immunology.theclinics.com

throat specialists) face the issue of self-treatment, overdose, and related complications such as rhinitis medicamentosa,[7] atrophic rhinitis,[8] and septal perforation.[9]

OTC treatments can be used as effective and affordable therapeutic modalities when recommended by a physician. Adjunct treatments, such as herbal medicine, acupuncture and homeopathy, have become increasingly popular.[10] This article provides an overview of treatment suggestions, benefits, and side effects for available OTC, prescription drug, and alternative choices in addition to the therapies described in other articles.

DECONGESTANTS AND GUAIFENESIN

Decongestants and guaifenesin are most frequently used as symptomatic relief in acute viral and bacterial rhinosinusitis, and for congestion associated with chronic rhinitis or sinusitis.[11] Topical preparations such as sprays, drops, and mist produce immediate relief that usually lasts 12 to 24 hours. Oral preparations have delayed onset of action, last 12 to 24 hours, and are almost universally manufactured as ingredients of combination pills marketed for cold, sinus pressure, or sinus headache relief. Decongestants are indicated for treatment of vasomotor rhinitis, and as an add-on therapy in the optimum management of allergic rhinitis, viral illness, sinusitis, otitis media, and eustachian tube dysfunction.[12] It is important to remind patients that decongestants do not treat underlying cause, and thus should be only considered as adjunct and temporary options.

The desired intranasal effect of decongestants occurs through direct and indirect activation of postsynaptic α-adrenergic receptors located on the muscles lining the walls of blood vessels on nasal mucosa.[13] When activated through sympathomimetic mechanisms, the muscles contract, causing vasoconstriction. The constricted blood vessels now allow less fluid extravasation, which results in decreased edema of nasal tissues, as well as decreased mucus production, which in turn decreases airflow resistance.

A major limitation of the topical decongestants is rebound hyperemia and worsening of the symptoms that occur with chronic use (rhinitis medicamentosa).[14] Therefore, topical decongestants generally are used on a short-term basis for less than 5 days. Patients who continue to use nasal decongestant sprays beyond this point may become reliant on the medication to relieve their chronic congestion. If long-term therapy is needed, oral agents should be recommended.[15]

Systemic effects are unavoidable and undesirable. Because of nonselective activation of sympathetic systems, the most common side effects include hypertension, central nervous system (CNS) stimulation, sleepiness, nervousness, excitability, dizziness, and anxiety.[16] Infrequent adverse reactions include tachycardia and/or palpitations. Rarely, therapy may be associated with hallucinations, arrhythmias, seizures, and ischemic colitis.[17–20]

Decongestants are not indicated, or should be used with extreme caution, in diabetes mellitus, cardiovascular disease, hypertension, prostatic hypertrophy, hyperthyroidism, closed angle glaucoma, or those who are pregnant. Most decongestants are pregnancy category C.[21]

OTC cold and cough medicines do not work for children less than 6 years of age, and giving these medicines to young children cannot be recommended according to the recent ruling of the FDA committee.[22] Significant concern caused several fatalities associated with OTC decongestant use in children who are younger than 2 years, who are at the highest risk for toxicity and for whom safe dosing recommendations are lacking. Concerning patterns of use include taking more than 1 decongestant-containing product concurrently, using decongestant for extended periods, and using adult medicines for children.[23,24] Combination products can be particularly susceptible to problems with overdosing, because parents sometimes do not realize they are duplicating ingredients (**Table 1**).

Pseudoephedrine is a diastereomer of ephedrine and a precursor of methamphetamine and methcathinone. Pseudoephedrine is a chiral molecule, meaning it occurs in both left-handed and right-handed configurations, which can not be superimposed.[25] It causes the release of endogenous norepinephrine (noradrenaline) from storage vesicles in presynaptic neurons. The displaced noradrenaline is released into the neuronal synapse where it is free to activate the postsynaptic adrenergic receptors located on the smooth muscle lining the walls of blood vessels. When activated by pseudoephedrine, the muscles contract, causing the blood vessels to constrict (vasoconstriction).[26] The constricted blood vessels now allow less fluid to leave the blood vessels and enter the nose, throat, and sinus linings, which results in decreased inflammation of nasal membranes as well as decreased mucus production. The same vasoconstriction action can also result in hypertension, which is a noted side effect of pseudoephedrine.

The advantage of oral pseudoephedrine compared with topical nasal preparations, such as oxymetazoline, is that it does not cause rebound congestion (rhinitis medicamentosa). However, it is more likely to cause adverse effects, including hypertension, sweating, and anxiety. Pseudoephedrine should not be used if the patient has taken any monoamine oxidase inhibitors such as isocarboxazid (Marplan), phenelzine (Nardil), rasagiline (Azilect), selegiline (Eldepryl, Emsam), or tranylcypromine (Parnate) within at least 14 days. Serious, life-threatening side effects can occur.[16] Pseudoephedrine should be used with caution in patients with heart disease, high blood pressure, diabetes, or thyroid disorder.

Some brand names of medications that contain pseudoephedrine are found in **Box 1**.

The United States Congress has recognized that pseudoephedrine is used in the illegal manufacture of methamphetamine. Congress passed the Combat Methamphetamine Epidemic Act of 2005 (CMEA). The law was mainly directed at pseudoephedrine products, but it also applies to all OTC products containing ephedrine, pseudoephedrine, and phenylpropanolamine, as well as their salts, optical isomers, and salts of optical isomers. Pseudoephedrine was defined as a scheduled listed chemical product, and the products were taken off the shelves and sold only by pharmacists with certain regulations and personal identification checks.

Phenylephrine, or Neo-Synephrine, is used as a decongestant and sold as an oral medicine, as a nasal spray, or as eye drops. Phenylephrine is now the most common OTC decongestant in the United States, surpassing pseudoephedrine; oxymetazoline is a more common nasal spray. Phenylephrine has recently been marketed as a substitute for pseudoephedrine (eg, Sudafed, original formulation), although some research suggests that oral phenylephrine may be no more effective as a decongestant than a placebo[1] because it is extensively metabolized by monoamine oxidase.[2] It was believed to decrease objective signs of respiratory distress in infants with bronchiolitis. A large controlled study did not show any changes in the clinical course.[27] Phenylephrine is a direct selective α-adrenergic receptor agonist, and is less likely to cause side effects such as CNS stimulation, insomnia, anxiety, irritability, and restlessness. The primary side effect of phenylephrine is hypertension. As a nasal spray, phenylephrine is available in 1% and 0.5% concentrations. It causes some rebound congestion effects, similar to oxymetazoline.

Some examples of products available in the United States that contain phenylephrine are listed in **Box 2**.

Table 1
Decongestants

Decongestant	Mode of Action	Local Side Effects (Topical Preparations)	Systemic Side Effects (Oral Preparations)	OTC Preparation
Pseudoephedrine	Release of endogenous norepinephrine		Hypertension, sweating, anxiety, insomnia, headache. Pregnancy category C, found in breastmilk	Afrinol, Novafed, Sudafed (Johnson & Johnson [formerly Pfizer]) Actifed, Contac, Dimetapp® Decongestant, Dimetapp® 12-Hour Non-Drowsy®, Triaminic® Allergy Congestion Mucinex D, Eltor, ChlorTrimeton Nasal Decongestant, Contac Cold, Drixoral Decongestant
Phenylephrine	Direct selective α-adrenergic receptor agonist	Stinging, burning, sneezing, increased nasal discharge, drying of the nostrils, and altered taste. Rhinitis medicamentosa with prolonged use	Dizziness, rapid or pounding heartbeat, trouble sleeping, shaking of the hands, tremors, unusual weakness, hypertension, headache. Pregnanacy category C	Ah-Chew D, Dimetapp Cold Drops, Lusonal, Nasop, Nasop12, PediaCare Children's Decongestant, Phenyl-T, Sudafed PE, Sudogest PE, Triaminic Thin Strips Cold, Neo-Synephrine, Despec-SF, Sudafed PE Extra Strength, Triaminic Thin Strips Nasal Congestion, Dime
Oxymetazoline	Nonselectively agonizes α1 and α2 adrenergic receptors	Rhinitis medicamentosa with prolonged use. Burning, stinging, increased nasal discharge, dryness inside the nose, sneezing	Nervousness, nausea, dizziness, headache, difficulty falling asleep or staying asleep, fast or slow heartbeat	Afrin, Sudafed OM, Dristan, Vicks Sinex, Mucinex Full Force, Allerest 12 Hour Nasal Spray, Duramist Plus, Duration, Four-Way Nasal Spray, Genasal, Neo-Synephrine 12 Hour, Nostrilla, NRS Nasal, NTZ Long Acting Nasal, Oxyfrin, Oxymeta-12, Sinarest Nasal, Si
Guaifenesin	Acts as an expectorant by increasing the volume and reducing the viscosity of secretions		Dizziness, nausea, vomiting	Anti-Tuss, Bidex, Breonesin, Duratuss G, Fenesin, Ganidin NR, GG 200 NR, Guaifenesin LA, Guaifenex G, Guaifenex LA, Humibid LA, Humibid Pediatric, Liquibid, Muco-Fen 1200, Muco-Fen 800, Muco-Fen LA, Naldecon-EX Senior, Organidin NR, Pneumomist, Q-Bid LA

Box 1
Medications that contain pseudoephedrine

Sudafed (Johnson & Johnson [formerly Pfizer])

Actifed (Burroughs Wellcome)

Contac (GlaxoSmithKline)

Dimetapp Decongestant, Dimetapp 12-Hour Non-Drowsy (Wyeth)

Triaminic Allergy Congestion

Claritin-D (loratadine + pseudoephedrine)

Zyrtec-D 12 Hour (pseudoephedrine hydrochloride + cetirizine hydrochloride)

Mucinex D (Reckitt Benckiser)

Eltor (Sanofi-Adventis)

Oxymetazoline is an adrenomimetic that nonselectively agonizes $\alpha 1$ and $\alpha 2$ adrenergic receptors.[28] Because vascular beds widely express $\alpha 1$ receptors, the action of oxymetazoline results in vasoconstriction. In addition, the local application of the drug also results in vasoconstriction because of its action on endothelial postsynaptic $\alpha 2$ receptors. As a result, it increases the diameter of the airway lumen and reduces fluid exudation from postcapillary venules.[25] Patients who continue to use oxymetazoline beyond this point may become reliant on the medication to relieve their chronic congestion.[29]

Examples of US products that contain oxymetazoline are found in **Box 3**.

Guaifenesin, or guaiphenesin (formerly BAN), also known as glycerol guaiacolate, is derived from guaiacol, a component of creosote. The efficient flow of respiratory mucus is a first level of immune defense that requires an appropriate viscosity and elasticity for optimal barrier and ciliary functions. In rhinitis, increased thick mucus is a common symptom that is difficult to manage. Guaifenesin is believed to act as an expectorant by increasing the volume and reducing the viscosity of secretions. Although there are subjective improvements, there is only partial evidence that the improvement is associated with changes in the characteristics and volume of the sputum.[30] When given in high doses, guaifenesin acts as an emetic.

Box 2
Products that contain phenylephrine

Alka-Seltzer Cold Formula Effervescent (Bayer)

Sudafed PE Non-Drowsy Nasal Decongestant (Pfizer)

Robitussin CF (Wyeth)

Tylenol Sinus, Tylenol Sinus Congestion & Pain (McNeil-PPC)

DayQuil Capsules (Procter & Gamble)

Dristan (Wyeth)

Theraflu (Novartis)

Benadryl Allergy & Sinus Headache (Warner-Lambert)

Excedrin Sinus Headache (Acme United Corporation)

Box 3
Products that contain oxymetazoline

Afrin

Sudafed OM (Pfizer)

Dristan (Wyeth)

Vicks Sinex (Procter & Gamble)

Mucinex Full Force (Reckitt Benckiser Pharmaceuticals, Inc.)

There have been few recent studies on the use of guaifenesin as decongestant. In patients infected with rhinovirus, guaifenesin leads to a subjective thinning of mucus quality.[31] In patients with human immunodeficiency virus (HIV) with chronic nasal congestion and postnasal drip, 1200 mg of guaifenesin twice daily led to a significant decrease in nasal congestion and a thinning of postnasal drainage compared with placebo.[32] The thinning of postnasal secretions seems to be the one consistently reported benefit of guaifenesin, although the effect is rarely profound and other nasal symptoms are not altered.

Guaifenesin is included in more than 100 products, such as:

Mucinex (Reckitt Benckiser Pharmaceuticals, Inc.)
Robitussin DAC, Robitussin AC (Wyeth)
Cheratussin DAC, Cheratussin AC (Qualitest)
Bidex 400 (Stewart-Jackson Pharmacal Inc.).

LEUKOTRIENE ANTAGONISTS

Cysteinyl leukotrienes (CysLTs) are a family of inflammatory lipid mediators synthesized from arachidonic acid by a variety of cells, including mast cells, eosinophils, basophils, and macrophages. CysLTs are increased in patients with allergic rhinitis and are released following allergen exposure.[33] The corticosteroid-resistant leukotriene pathway may contribute to the development of inflammation in allergic diseases that do not respond to the introduction of corticosteroids. Inhibition of this pathway has potential therapeutic benefit in various allergic diseases that have involvement of corticosteroid insensitivity.[34]

Two cysteinyl leukotriene receptor antagonists (LTRA) are available in the United States. Zafirlukast (Accolate, AstraZeneca, Wilmington, DE, USA) and montelukast (Singulair, Merck Co., Inc., Whitehouse Station, NJ, USA) were initially approved as chronic controlling therapies for asthma. Studies have shown both to be effective in treating patients with allergic rhinitis, and montelukast has an indication for seasonal allergic rhinitis. Two-week trials using zafirlukast for allergic rhinitis showed a significant reduction in nasal congestion, sneezing, and rhinorrhea compared with placebo.[35] Montelukast has been shown to improve multiple allergic rhinitis parameters including both allergen-induced nasal and ocular symptoms as well as rhinitis symptom scores. Published clinical evidence undoubtedly establishes montelukast as a viable alternative for the treatment of seasonal allergic rhinitis. Its benefits are equivalent to antihistamines when used as monotherapy, but less than intranasal corticosteroids. The addition of an antihistamine to montelukast does seem to have added benefits and, at times, is reported to be equivalent to intranasal corticosteroids.[36]

Leukotriene receptor antagonists (LTRA) tend to be well tolerated with few side effects. Zafirlukast can cause transaminitis. Both zafirlukast and montelukast are pregnancy category B, and montelukast is frequently used in young children. Their effect is roughly equivalent to nonsedating antihistamines in some patients, and LTRAs tend to provide more relief of congestion and less relief of itch and rhinnorhea.[37] LTRAs have never been shown to be superior to, or even comparable with, intranasal corticosteroids. Objective and subjective evidence suggests that leukotriene receptor antagonist–antihistamine combination therapy is more effective than antihistamine alone in the control of allergic rhinitis symptoms.[38] However, they are often considered as single-agent therapy to treat patients with both mild allergic rhinitis and asthma. These agents have been found to be safe and effective in reducing symptoms associated with allergic rhinitis in children. Alternative forms such as liquids or oral disintegrating tablets are available for most agents, allowing ease of administration to most young children and infants.[39]

CROMOLYN

Cromolyn (also referred to as cromoglicic acid, cromoglycate, or cromoglicate) is traditionally described as a mast cell stabilizer, and is commonly marketed as the sodium salt sodium cromoglicate or cromolyn sodium. This drug prevents the release of inflammatory chemicals such as histamine from mast cells. It has no intrinsic bronchodilator, antihistaminic, or antiinflammatory activity but can be added to the treatment regimens as a mast cell stabilizer.[40]

In vitro and in vivo animal studies have shown that cromolyn sodium inhibits the degranulation of sensitized mast cells that occurs after exposure to specific antigens. Cromolyn sodium inhibits the release of histamine and the slow-acting substance of anaphylaxis (SRS-A).[41] Rhinitis induced by the inhalation of specific antigens can be inhibited to varying degrees by pretreatment with cromolyn sodium nasal solution. Another activity shown in vitro is the capacity of cromolyn sodium to inhibit the degranulation of nonsensitized rat mast cells by phospholipase A and the subsequent release of chemical mediators. Cromolyn sodium is poorly absorbed and thus considered safe.[42] Its clinical efficacy in patients with mild or moderate persistent asthma and allergic rhinitis is well documented.[40,43] There is no clinical evidence that cromolyn can be overdosed. It can be used during pregnancy and in children.[44,45] However, it is not effective if used less then 4 times a day and may take up to 1 to 4 weeks to produce noticeable effect. Thus it is not effective for immediate relief of symptoms and is considered more useful as preventive treatment of allergic rhinitis. It represents a good choice when other nasal sprays are contraindicated or not tolerated.

Available forms include Nasalcrom (United States), Prevalin (Netherlands), and Rynacrom (United Kingdom).

NASAL WASH

Nasal irrigation (wash) has been practiced in India for centuries as one of the disciplines of yoga; it is believed to promote good nasal health and healthy breathing. This technique was adapted by modern medicine and now widely used by allergists and otolaryngologists in the treatment of sinus and nasal problems in patients with acute and chronic rhinosinusitis including symptoms of facial pain, headache, halitosis, cough, anterior rhinorrhea (watery discharge), and nasal congestion.[46,47] Various devices are available on market, such as neti pot, saline nasal spray, and pressure rinse bottles. Neti pots are more traditional devices used for yoga practices. They can be made of metal, glass, or ceramic, and rely on gravity alone, along with head positioning and repeated practice, to rinse the outer sinus cavities. Nasal irrigation or nasal lavage or nose douche is the personal hygiene practice in which the nasal cavity is washed to flush out excess mucus and debris from the nose and sinuses. A more advanced yoga exercise, vyutkrama kapalbhati, involves pouring the same salt water solution into one nostril while the other is held closed, so that the solution runs out of the mouth. It allows more thorough irrigation of the nasal cavity and the sinuses. The irrigation bottle made by Neilmed allows any nonsophisticated user to perform the irrigation with excellent results; the squeeze bottle delivers user-controlled pressure to create turbulent solution flow in the nasal cavity. A typical home recipe for an isotonic solution varies and consists of 1 cup of water (240 mL), one-quarter of a teaspoon of salt, and a pinch of baking soda for an isotonic solution. For a hypertonic solution, the amount of salt would be doubled or tripled (**Fig. 1**).

As a treatment modality in rhinitis or sinusitis, nasal irrigation achieves 3 goals: it removes the allergen, shortening exposure during pollen seasons; it removes pollutants that are otherwise deposited on the mucus membranes; and it reduces the amount of mucus, thus helping with reduction of postnasal drip. Hypertonic solutions also work as decongestants, reducing swelling by natural osmosis. Therefore, although isotonic solution is recommended for daily use, hypertonic solution can be used in conditions accompanied by congestion. A small amount of baking soda is used as an optional buffering ingredient to adjust the pH value to that of the body.

Spraying the solution into the nostrils is more convenient but also less effective. The most effective methods ensure that the liquid enters through one nostril and then either runs out of the other nostril or goes through the nasal cavity to the back of the throat from where it may be spat out. The necessary pressure comes from gravity, from squeezing a plastic bottle or a syringe, or from an electrical pump.

Physicians generally agree that iodized table salt is not acceptable, and that pickling salt or sea salt is preferred because it also does not contain any other additives such as anticaking agents. Most sources advise that tap water should be boiled for several minutes to ensure sterility before it is cooled and used, but it is not clear whether this is really necessary. Nasal saline irrigation can be considered as a good adjunctive

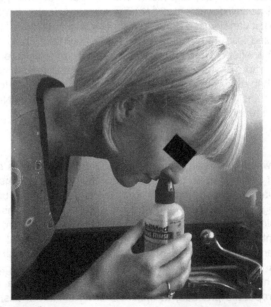

Fig. 1. Nasal wash procedure.

treatment option for allergic rhinitis. It permitted the use of less topical steroids for controlling allergic rhinitis in children, which contributes to fewer side effects and less economic burden. However, these solutions should be selectively prescribed rather than used based on anecdotal evidence. Further studies should be conducted to develop a protocol for standardized use of saline solution irrigation in various nasal pathologies.

CAPSAICIN

Capsaicin was first isolated in impure form as the active component of chili peppers, which are plants belonging to the genus *Capsicum*. The compound was first isolated in pure, crystalline form in the eighteenth century by John Clough Thresh, who gave it the name capsaicin. Pure capsaicin is a hydrophobic, colorless, odorless, crystalline to waxy compound. Later, German pharmacologist Rudolf Buchheim and, in 1878, the Hungarian doctor Endre Hőgyes, stated that capsicol (partially purified capsaicin) caused the burning feeling when in contact with mucous membranes and increased secretion of gastric juices. Similar substances were isolated from chili peppers by the Japanese chemists Kosuge and Inagaki, who named them capsaicinoids. Capsaicin is a phenolic chemical contained within the oil of the *Capsicum* pepper.[48] Capsaicin is initially irritating to its targeted area. However, the area becomes desensitized to the irritation after repeated use. Nerve endings responsible for rhinorrhea, sneezing, and congestion become desensitized when capsaicin is applied to the nasal mucosa.[49] Beneficial effects of drug treatment may be caused by its specific action on the peripheral endings of primary sensory neurons leading to their functional blockade.[50]

Capsaicin is used as a pharmacologic agent in research studies in mice and rats. An intranasal spray of capsaicin was evaluated in many clinical studies.[50–54] In one such study, capsaicin nasal spray was used as a once-weekly treatment for 5 weeks. The subjective intensity of their nasal obstruction, rhinorrhea, and sneezing frequency were evaluated throughout the study and the vascular effects of capsaicin on the nasal mucosa were recorded by anterior rhinomanometry and laser Doppler flowmetry. Intranasal capsaicin application evoked a larger vascular response in patients with rhinitis than in controls. Both nasal vascular responses and subjective discomfort following capsaicin were markedly reduced after the fifth application. All symptoms were significantly improved throughout a 6-month follow-up period. No significant side effects occurred and weaning from nasal vasoconstrictor agents was possible. Both the subjective symptom score and objective measurements of vascular reactivity suggest that repeated intranasal capsaicin application could be beneficial for patients with chronic rhinitis, possibly by reducing hyperreactive nasal reflexes.[55] Capsaicin use has been targeted to patients presenting with congestion, rhinorrhea, sneezing, or a combination of these symptoms. No consensus is reported for dosages of capsaicin. Suggested regimens range from 3.3×10^{-3} mol capsaicin dissolved in 70% ethanol sprayed into each nostril once a week for 5 weeks to a solution containing capsaicin 0.15 mg/0.5 mL applied to each nostril every 2 or 3 days for 7 treatments.[54] A capsaicin formulation called Sinol Nasal Spray is available OTC at pharmacies.

OTHER TREATMENTS

Menthol is a compound obtained from peppermint or other mint oils. It is marketed for many different conditions such as muscle aches, sore throat, and congestion. It is available in lozenges, nasal sprays, vaporubs, inhalers, and cough syrups, and is widely used as a treatment of rhinitis that is associated with acute upper respiratory tract infection and allergy. Menthol as a plant extract has been used in traditional medicine in Asia for the treatment of respiratory diseases for hundreds of years, but it was only introduced to the West as a medicine at the end of the nineteenth century. With the recent discovery of a menthol receptor on the sensory nerves that modulate the cool sensation, menthol has graduated from the realms of herbal medicine into molecular pharmacology.[56] Menthol is not known to cause any significant side effects but should be discontinued if there are any signs of personal hypersensitivity.

Herbs and Alternative Treatments

For centuries, herbs were used to treat rhinitis, and most of the modern drugs are isolates of active herbal ingredients. The specialty of allergy and immunology has seen the second largest increase in the popularity of complementary and alternative medicine (second only to practitioners who treat lower back pain).[10] However, herbs can trigger side effects and can interact with other herbs, supplements, or medications. For these reasons, herbs should only be taken under the supervision of a health care practitioner trained in their use. Pregnant women and young children should not use herbal preparation because safety studies are not available and toxic levels may be easily reached because of higher absorption rates in these patients.

Ephedrine is an alkaloid derived from various plants in the genus *Ephedra* (family Ephedraceae). It is most usually marketed in the hydrochloride and sulfate forms. Ephedrine is a sympathomimetic amine commonly used as a decongestant, but it is also a stimulant, appetite suppressant, concentration aid, and is used in some countries to treat hypotension. Ephedrine is similar in structure to the semisynthetic derivatives amphetamine and methamphetamine. Ephedrine is not sold as part of OTC cold or decongestant medications, but is available in health stores outside the United States as diet or weight-loss pills, or as a herb. On February 6, 2004, the FDA issued a final rule prohibiting the sale of dietary supplements containing ephedrine alkaloids (ephedra) because such supplements present an unreasonable risk of illness or injury. Major safety concerns have been associated with ephedra or ephedrine use, including hypertension (high blood pressure), tachycardia, CNS excitation, arrhythmia, myocardial infarction (heart attack), and stroke (**Fig. 2**).

In traditional Chinese medicines, the herb má huáng (*Ephedra sinica*) contains ephedrine and pseudoephedrine as its principal active constituents.

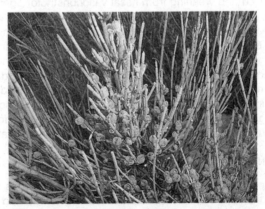

Fig. 2. *Ephedra fragilis.* (*From* Wikipedia, The Free Encyclopedia. February 26, 2011. Available at: http://en.wikipedia.org/wiki/Ephedra_fragilis. Accessed June 15, 2011.)

Butterbur (*Petasites hybridus*, 500 mg per day) has traditionally been used to treat asthma and bronchitis and to reduce mucus, and several scientific studies show that it can be helpful. One study of 125 people with hay fever found that an extract of butterbur was as effective as cetirizine. Another study compared butterbur with phenofexadine, with similar findings. One of the mechanisms of action is protection against AMP-induced nasal responsiveness during the grass pollen season in sensitized patients.[57] It has not been established whether taking butterbur for longer than 12 to 16 weeks is safe. Butterbur can cause stomach upset, headache, and drowsiness (**Fig. 3**).

Goldenseal (*Hydrastis canadensis*) is sometimes included in herbal remedies for allergic rhinitis. Laboratory studies suggest that berberine, the active ingredient in goldenseal, has antibacterial and immune-enhancing properties,[58] but there is no evidence that it is effective specifically for allergic rhinitis (**Fig. 4**).

Stinging nettle (*Urtica dioica*, 600 mg per day for 1 week) is indicated for the treatment of multiple conditions, including allergic rhinitis.[59] It is commonly used as freeze-dried leaves. Studies so far are lacking. Only 1 small study suggested that stinging nettle might help relieve symptoms of allergic rhinitis (**Fig. 5**).

Sho seiryu to, also known as TJ-19, is a Japanese herbal formula often used for short periods of time to ward off, and help a patient recover from, colds in the absence of fever. In Chinese, this same herbal formula is known as xiao qing long tang, and the indications are identical to those of sho seiryu to. The ingredients are equal proportions of licorice root, schizandra fruit, ephedra, cinnamon twig, ginger root, peony root, asarum herb, and pinella. Traditionally, 1 dose of sho seiryu to contains 9 g of each ingredient. This formula is not recommended for prolonged use and may be used in combination with acupuncture. The mechanism of action of sho seiryu to was studied extensively. It was found to inhibit allergen-induced synthesis of tumor necrosis factor α by peripheral blood mononuclear cells in patients with perennial allergic rhinitis,[60] and to suppress histamine signaling at the transcriptional level.[61]

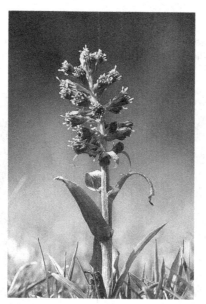

Fig. 3. *Petasites hybridus.* (Photo by Richard Bartz, Munich, Germany.)

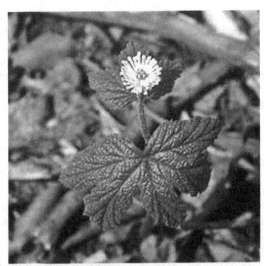

Fig. 4. *Hydrastis canadensis.* (*From* Wikipedia, The Free Encyclopedia. May 18, 2009. Available at: http://commons.wikimedia.org/wiki/Hydrastis_canadensis. Accessed June 15, 2011.)

Biminne is another Chinese herbal formula used to treat allergic rhinitis. It is not known how biminne works, or whether it is safe to use for extended periods. In a study of 58 people with year-round allergic rhinitis, biminne relieved at least some symptoms in most of the participants. People in the study took the formula 5 times a day for 12 weeks, and they still showed the benefit of biminne even after 1 year. Biminne contains Chinese skullcap (*Scutellaria baicalensis*), *Ginkgo biloba*, horny goat weed (*Epimedium sagittatum*), *Schizandra chinensis*, Japanese apricot (*Prunus mume*), *Ledebouriella divaricata*, and astragalus (*Astragalus membranaceus*).

Acupuncture

In traditional Chinese medicine it is thought that the body has energy pathways known as meridians. Each meridian corresponds to specific internal organs through which it

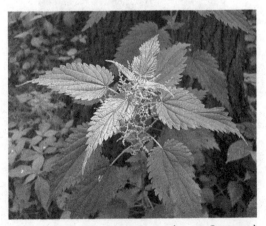

Fig. 5. *Urtica dioica.* (Photo by Uwe H. Friese, Bremerhaven, Germany.)

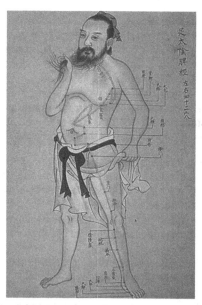

Fig. 6. Acupuncture: ancient drawing of meridian points.

passes (**Fig. 6**). Acupuncture involves the use of hair-fine needles to stimulate specific points on the body along the meridians by removing energy blockages in the meridians and regulating the overall flow of energy so that the body can return to a state of balance and health. Acupressure is a similar method (**Fig. 7**), but instead of needle use, points are pressed or massaged in certain pattern by fingers. Some evidence suggests that acupuncture may be a useful complementary or alternative treatment for people with allergic rhinitis, although not all studies have found any benefit.[62–67] In one study that included 45 people with hay fever, acupuncture worked as well as antihistamines in improving symptoms, and the effects seemed to last longer. One study suggested that combining acupuncture with traditional Chinese herbs did help relieve symptoms. A randomized controlled trial (Acupuncture in Seasonal Allergic Rhinitis [ACUSAR]) that investigates the efficacy of acupuncture in the treatment of seasonal allergic rhinitis (SAR) is currently being conducted in Germany, and results will be available in 2011.[68]

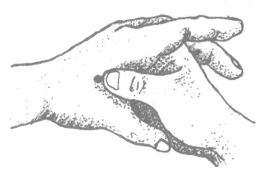

Fig. 7. Acupressure.

Homeopathy

Homeopathy involves the use of herbal preparations in extremely small concentrations that are taken orally in increasing concentrations. The preparation of homeopathic drugs is based on potentiation, with the primary substance specially mixed with a carrier in the ratio 1:10. In a controlled, randomized, strictly double-blind trial with 164 patients, the effectiveness of homeopathically prepared *Galphimia* was investigated in patients with allergic rhinitis. The average duration of treatment was about 5 weeks. Although no statistical significance was achieved, it is remarkable that there was a clear trend for the superiority of *Galphimia* compared with placebo.[69]

Some other known preparations

Nux vomica is used for stuffiness with nasal discharge and dry, ticklish, and scraping nasal sensations with watery nasal discharge and a lot of sneezing; an appropriate person for this remedy is irritable and impatient.

Arsenicum album is used for stuffiness with copious, burning nasal discharge and violent sneezing; an appropriate candidate for arsenicum feels restless, anxious, and exhausted.

Allium cepa is used for frequent sneezing, a lot of irritating nasal discharge, and tearing eyes; people taking this tend to feel thirsty.

Euphrasia is used for bland nasal discharge, with stinging, irritating tears; a suitable person for this remedy has worse nasal symptoms when lying down.

REFERENCES

1. Dykewicz MS, Fineman S, Skoner DP, et al. Diagnosis and management of rhinitis: complete guidelines of the Joint Task Force on Practice Parameters in Allergy, Asthma and Immunology. American Academy of Allergy, Asthma, and Immunology. Ann Allergy Asthma Immunol 1998;81:478.
2. Bachert C. Persistent rhinitis - allergic or nonallergic? Allergy 2004;59(Suppl 76):11.
3. Novak N, Bieber T. Allergic and nonallergic forms of atopic diseases. J Allergy Clin Immunol 2003;112:252.
4. Quan M, Casale TB, Blaiss MS. Should clinicians routinely determine rhinitis subtype on initial diagnosis and evaluation? A debate among experts. Clin Cornerstone 2009;9:54.
5. Meltzer EO, Nathan RA, Derebery J, et al. Physician perceptions of the treatment and management of allergic and nonallergic rhinitis. Allergy Asthma Proc 2009; 30:75.
6. Marple BF, Fornadley JA, Patel AA, et al. Keys to successful management of patients with allergic rhinitis: focus on patient confidence, compliance, and satisfaction. Otolaryngol Head Neck Surg 2007;136:S107.
7. Lockey RF. Rhinitis medicamentosa and the stuffy nose. J Allergy Clin Immunol 2006;118:1017.
8. Simons FE. Chronic rhinitis. Pediatr Clin North Am 1984;31:801.
9. Keyserling HF, Grimme JD, Camacho DL, et al. Nasal septal perforation secondary to rhinitis medicamentosa. Ear Nose Throat J 2006;85:376.
10. Bielory L. Complementary and alternative interventions in asthma, allergy, and immunology. Ann Allergy Asthma Immunol 2004;93:S45.
11. Corey JP, Houser SM, Ng BA. Nasal congestion: a review of its etiology, evaluation, and treatment. Ear Nose Throat J 2000;79:690.
12. Scarupa MD, Kaliner MA. Adjuvant therapies in the treatment of acute and chronic rhinosinusitis. Clin Allergy Immunol 2007;20:251.

13. Johnson DA, Hricik JG. The pharmacology of alpha-adrenergic decongestants. Pharmacotherapy 1993;13:110S.
14. Kushnir NM. Rhinitis medicamentosa. 2009. Available at: http://emedicine. medscape.com/article/995056-overview:medscape. Accessed October 13, 2009.
15. Hatton RC, Winterstein AG, McKelvey RP, et al. Efficacy and safety of oral phenylephrine: systematic review and meta-analysis. Ann Pharmacother 2007;41:381.
16. Kanfer I, Dowse R, Vuma V. Pharmacokinetics of oral decongestants. Pharmacotherapy 1993;13:116S.
17. Burton BT, Rice M, Schmertzler LE. Atrioventricular block following overdose of decongestant cold medication. J Emerg Med 1985;2:415.
18. Escobar JI, Karno M. Chronic hallucinosis from nasal drops. JAMA 1859;247:1982.
19. Hass DJ, Kozuch P, Brandt LJ. Pharmacologically mediated colon ischemia. Am J Gastroenterol 2007;102:1765.
20. Olivier P, Dugue A, Montastruc JL. [Adverse cardiovascular and central neurologic reactions to sympathomimetics used as nasal decongestants: results of the French National Pharmacovigilance Survey]. Therapie 2003;58:361 [in French].
21. Demoly P, Piette V, Daures JP. Treatment of allergic rhinitis during pregnancy. Drugs 1813;63:2003.
22. Using over-the-counter cough and cold products in children. 2008. Available at: http://www.fda.gov/downloads/ForConsumers/ConsumerUpdates/ucm048524. pdf. Accessed October 22, 2008.
23. Dart RC, Paul IM, Bond GR, et al. Pediatric fatalities associated with over the counter (nonprescription) cough and cold medications. Ann Emerg Med 2009;53:411.
24. Vernacchio L, Kelly JP, Kaufman DW, et al. Pseudoephedrine use among US children, 1999–2006: results from the Slone Survey. Pediatrics 2008;122:1299.
25. Reynolds EB. Martindale: the complete drug reference. London: Pharmaceutical Press; 1989.
26. Kobayashi S, Endou M, Sakuraya F, et al. The sympathomimetic actions of L-ephedrine and D-pseudoephedrine: direct receptor activation or norepinephrine release? Anesth Analg 2003;97:1239.
27. Ralston S, Roohi M. A randomized, controlled trial of nasal phenylephrine in infants hospitalized for bronchiolitis. J Pediatr 2008;153:795.
28. Corboz MR, Rivelli MA, Varty L, et al. Pharmacological characterization of postjunctional alpha-adrenoceptors in human nasal mucosa. Am J Rhinol 2005;19:495.
29. Graf P. Long-term use of oxy- and xylometazoline nasal sprays induces rebound swelling, tolerance, and nasal hyperreactivity. Rhinology 1996;34:9.
30. Storms W, Farrar JR. Guaifenesin in rhinitis. Curr Allergy Asthma Rep 2009;9:101.
31. Kuhn JJ, Hendley JO, Adams KF, et al. Antitussive effect of guaifenesin in young adults with natural colds. Objective and subjective assessment. Chest 1982;82:713.
32. Wawrose SF, Tami TA, Amoils CP. The role of guaifenesin in the treatment of sinonasal disease in patients infected with the human immunodeficiency virus (HIV). Laryngoscope 1992;102:1225.
33. Peters-Golden M, Gleason MM, Togias A. Cysteinyl leukotrienes: multi-functional mediators in allergic rhinitis. Clin Exp Allergy 2006;36:689.
34. Ohnishi H, Miyahara N, Gelfand EW. The role of leukotriene B(4) in allergic diseases. Allergol Int 2008;57:291.
35. Piatti G, Ceriotti L, Cavallaro G, et al. Effects of zafirlukast on bronchial asthma and allergic rhinitis. Pharmacol Res 2003;47:541.
36. Lagos JA, Marshall GD. Montelukast in the management of allergic rhinitis. Ther Clin Risk Manag 2007;3:327.

37. Sardana N, Santos C, Lehman E, et al. A comparison of intranasal corticosteroid, leukotriene receptor antagonist, and topical antihistamine in reducing symptoms of perennial allergic rhinitis as assessed through the Rhinitis Severity Score. Allergy Asthma Proc 2010;31:5.

38. Cingi C, Gunhan K, Gage-White L, et al. Efficacy of leukotriene antagonists as concomitant therapy in allergic rhinitis. Laryngoscope 2010;120(9):1718–23.

39. Phan H, Moeller ML, Nahata MC. Treatment of allergic rhinitis in infants and children: efficacy and safety of second-generation antihistamines and the leukotriene receptor antagonist montelukast. Drugs 2009;69:2541.

40. Storms W, Kaliner MA. Cromolyn sodium: fitting an old friend into current asthma treatment. J Asthma 2005;42:79.

41. Henderson WR, Kaliner M. Mast cell granule peroxidase: location, secretion, and SRS-A inactivation. J Immunol 1979;122:1322.

42. Long A, McFadden C, DeVine D, et al. Management of allergic and nonallergic rhinitis. Evid Rep Technol Assess (Summ) 2002;(54):1–6.

43. Meltzer EO. Allergic rhinitis: managing the pediatric spectrum. Allergy Asthma Proc 2006;27:2.

44. Greiner AN, Meltzer EO. Pharmacologic rationale for treating allergic and nonallergic rhinitis. J Allergy Clin Immunol 2006;118:985.

45. Meltzer EO. Efficacy and patient satisfaction with cromolyn sodium nasal solution in the treatment of seasonal allergic rhinitis: a placebo-controlled study. Clin Ther 2002;24:942.

46. Papsin B, McTavish A. Saline nasal irrigation: its role as an adjunct treatment. Can Fam Physician 2003;49:168.

47. Slapak I, Skoupa J, Strnad P, et al. Efficacy of isotonic nasal wash (seawater) in the treatment and prevention of rhinitis in children. Arch Otolaryngol Head Neck Surg 2008;134:67.

48. Govindarajan VS. Capsicum–production, technology, chemistry, and quality. Part III. Chemistry of the color, aroma, and pungency stimuli. Crit Rev Food Sci Nutr 1986;24:245.

49. Bascom R, Kagey-Sobotka A, Proud D. Effect of intranasal capsaicin on symptoms and mediator release. J Pharmacol Exp Ther 1991;259:1323.

50. Marabini S, Ciabatti PG, Polli G, et al. Beneficial effects of intranasal applications of capsaicin in patients with vasomotor rhinitis. Eur Arch Otorhinolaryngol 1991; 248:191.

51. Blom HM, Severijnen LA, Van Rijswijk JB, et al. The long-term effects of capsaicin aqueous spray on the nasal mucosa. Clin Exp Allergy 1998;28:1351.

52. Ciabatti PG, D'Ascanio L. Intranasal capsicum spray in idiopathic rhinitis: a randomized prospective application regimen trial. Acta Otolaryngol 2009; 129:367.

53. Sanico AM, Atsuta S, Proud D, et al. Dose-dependent effects of capsaicin nasal challenge: in vivo evidence of human airway neurogenic inflammation. J Allergy Clin Immunol 1997;100:632.

54. Van Rijswijk JB, Boeke EL, Keizer JM, et al. Intranasal capsaicin reduces nasal hyperreactivity in idiopathic rhinitis: a double-blind randomized application regimen study. Allergy 2003;58:754.

55. Lacroix JS, Buvelot JM, Polla BS, et al. Improvement of symptoms of non-allergic chronic rhinitis by local treatment with capsaicin. Clin Exp Allergy 1991;21:595.

56. Eccles R. Menthol: effects on nasal sensation of airflow and the drive to breathe. Curr Allergy Asthma Rep 2003;3:210.

57. Lee DK, Carstairs IJ, Haggart K, et al. Butterbur, a herbal remedy, attenuates adenosine monophosphate induced nasal responsiveness in seasonal allergic rhinitis. Clin Exp Allergy 2003;33:882.
58. Rehman J, Dillow JM, Carter SM, et al. Increased production of antigen-specific immunoglobulins G and M following in vivo treatment with the medicinal plants *Echinacea angustifolia* and *Hydrastis canadensis*. Immunol Lett 1999;68:391.
59. Weber RW. Stinging nettle. Ann Allergy Asthma Immunol 2003;90:A6.
60. Tanaka A, Ohashi Y, Kakinoki Y, et al. The herbal medticine shoseiryu-to inhibits allergen-induced synthesis of tumour necrosis factor alpha by peripheral blood mononuclear cells in patients with perennial allergic rhinitis. Acta Otolaryngol Suppl 1998;538:118.
61. Das AK, Mizuguchi H, Kodama M, et al. Sho-seiryu-to suppresses histamine signaling at the transcriptional level in TDI-sensitized nasal allergy model rats. Allergol Int 2009;58:81.
62. Brinkhaus B, Witt CM, Jena S, et al. Acupuncture in patients with allergic rhinitis: a pragmatic randomized trial. Ann Allergy Asthma Immunol 2008;101:535.
63. Fleckenstein J, Raab C, Gleditsch J, et al. Impact of acupuncture on vasomotor rhinitis: a randomized placebo-controlled pilot study. J Altern Complement Med 2009;15:391.
64. Jindal V, Ge A, Mansky PJ. Safety and efficacy of acupuncture in children: a review of the evidence. J Pediatr Hematol Oncol 2008;30:431.
65. Kim JI, Lee MS, Jung SY, et al. Acupuncture for persistent allergic rhinitis: a multi-centre, randomised, controlled trial protocol. Trials 2009;10:54.
66. Kong JC, Lee MS, Shin BC. Randomized clinical trials on acupuncture in Korean literature: a systematic review. Evid Based Complement Alternat Med 2009;6:41.
67. Witt CM, Pach D, Brinkhaus B, et al. Safety of acupuncture: results of a prospective observational study with 229,230 patients and introduction of a medical information and consent form. Forsch Komplementmed 2009;16:91.
68. Witt CM, Brinkhaus B. Efficacy, effectiveness and cost-effectiveness of acupuncture for allergic rhinitis - an overview about previous and ongoing studies. Auton Neurosci 2010;157(1–2):42–5.
69. Frei T, Gassner E. Trends in prevalence of allergic rhinitis and correlation with pollen counts in Switzerland. Int J Biometeorol 2008;52:841.

Management of Rhinitis: Guidelines, Evidence Basis, and Systematic Clinical Approach for What We Do

Mark S. Dykewicz, MD

KEYWORDS

- Rhinitis • Medication • Guidelines • Management • Diagnosis
- Treatment

Whereas management of very mild rhinitis may be simply and successfully self-managed by patients using medications available over the counter, most patients with rhinitis who present to medical offices have more severe rhinitis that may need a more comprehensive diagnostic and therapeutic approach. Optimal care may require special diagnostic studies and combination therapies that are arrived at only after trying multiple different medication and therapeutic options. This article presents a systematic approach to office care of rhinitis from the perspective of an allergist-immunologist. To provide an overall framework for more focused discussion of selected topics, a management algorithm is presented (**Fig. 1**), keyed to sections in the article that are organized to follow the algorithm flow. More emphasis is given to discussion of dilemmas that face the specialist or more involved considerations that have been highlighted in recently published guidelines. Although guideline recommendations are discussed (eg, from the US Joint Task Force Rhinitis Parameter update for which this author was co–chief editor),[1] opinions expressed in this review do not necessarily reflect the view of guidelines committees unless specifically stated.

PATIENT WITH RHINITIS SYMPTOMS (ALGORITHM BOX 1)

The first step in the clinical approach to diagnosis of suspected rhinitis is to evaluate symptoms not only to recognize the possible presence of rhinitis and ultimately

Disclosure: Merck provided travel support to present contracted research performed at previous institution.

Allergy and Immunology Unit, Section of Pulmonary, Critical Care Allergy and Immunologic Diseases, Department of Internal Medicine; Center for Human Genomics and Personalized Medicine Research; Wake Forest University School of Medicine Center Boulevard, Winston-Salem, NC 25157, USA

E-mail address: dykewicz@wakehealth.edu

Immunol Allergy Clin N Am 31 (2011) 619–634

doi:10.1016/j.iac.2011.05.002

0889-8561/11/$ – see front matter © 2011 Elsevier Inc. All rights reserved.

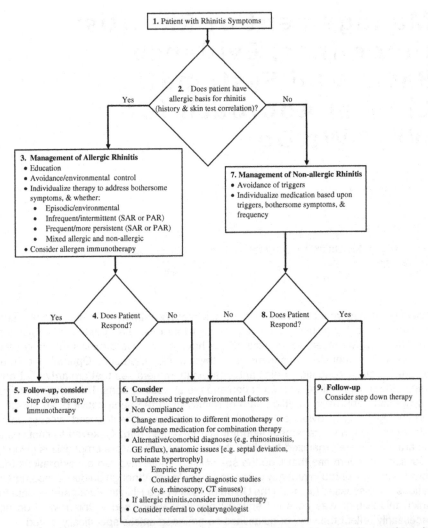

Fig. 1. Management of patients with symptoms of rhinitis. Boxes 1 to 9 are discussed in relevant sections of this article. CT, computed tomography; GE, gastroesophageal; PAR, perennial allergic rhinitis; SAR, seasonal allergic rhinitis.

guide selection of symptom-directed rhinitis therapy but also to assess if there should be consideration of other alternative differential or comorbid conditions such as sinusitis, as is well known, patients with rhinitis can present variably with symptoms of nasal congestion (the most bothersome symptom for many patients), rhinorrhea, sneezing, nasal pruritus, and postnasal drainage. Although it does not assist in the diagnosis of rhinitis per se, rhinitis symptoms should trigger assessment for other comorbid conditions such as asthma (eg, wheezing, cough, and chest tightness).

DOES PATIENT HAVE ALLERGIC BASIS FOR RHINITIS (HISTORY AND SKIN TEST CORRELATION) (BOX 2)

Allergic rather than nonallergic rhinitis is suggested by nasal pruritus; nasal symptoms associated with the presence of seasonal aeroallergens, or with acute exposure to allergens; or the presence of associated ocular symptoms (eg, eye itch).[1] When symptoms are perennial, it becomes more difficult for the clinician to assess from history alone whether rhinitis is allergic or nonallergic, or whether chronic sinusitis may be present. Unilateral nasal symptoms suggest an anatomic issue is present. Physical examination of the nose should be performed to rule out complicating or alternative nasal conditions (eg, nasal polyps, septal deviation), but the appearance of nasal mucosa in allergic and nonallergic rhinitis may be similar. An allergic basis for rhinitis is assessed by correlating history with the presence of specific IgE to aeroallergens, preferably performed by skin testing. Allergy testing is indicated to provide evidence of an allergic basis for the patient's symptoms, to confirm or exclude suspected causes of the patient's symptoms, or to assess the sensitivity to a specific allergen for avoidance measures and/or allergen immunotherapy.[1,2] Data are conflicting about the existence or prevalence of allergic rhinitis due to localized IgE antibody production not associated with positive skin tests.[3]

MANAGEMENT OF ALLERGIC RHINITIS (BOX 3)

The 3 cornerstones of management of allergic rhinitis are (1) allergen avoidance and environmental control to reduce exposure to relevant allergens, (2) pharmacotherapy, and (3) in appropriately selected patients, allergen immunotherapy. Of these 3 modalities, pharmacotherapy has the greatest amount of data that can be applied to clinical decision making, and is therefore the focus of discussion here. However, choosing from medication options for individual patient treatment still requires a clinician's judgment in the application of evidence-based recommendations. Although not discussed further here, education of patients about their rhinitis diagnosis and management obviously is essential to adherence and optimal patient outcome.

Dilemmas in Assessing Evidence for Making Rhinitis Treatment Decisions

Before discussing specific guideline recommendations for selecting medications for rhinitis care, it must be recognized that there are multiple dilemmas and limitations in evaluating the evidence basis for assessing the relative merits of different treatment options—as might apply both to rhinitis patients generally or to an individual patient being treated.

Effectiveness of medications can be assessed by various end points including subjective assessments by patients (eg, ratings of specific symptoms such as nasal congestion or rhinorrhea; aggregate scores of multiple symptoms such as the Total Nasal Symptoms Score [TNSS] that assesses nasal congestion, pruritus, rhinorrhea, sneezing; quality of life assessments based on standardized questionnaire responses [eg, Rhinoconjunctivitis Quality of Life Questionnaire]) and objective physiologic measurements (eg, peak nasal inspiratory flow [PNIF], acoustic rhinometry, and rhinomanometry).[1,2] As has been found in asthma, in rhinitis different subjective and objective end points for assessment do not consistently track together in populations or individuals. This inconsistency can confound making a simple summary assessment of evidence for the relative effectiveness of different medication options, especially when there is heterogeneity of study design and end points.[4] In assessing evidence as might apply to an individual patient predominantly bothered by a particular symptom such as congestion, evidence for greater effectiveness of one medication option versus another for specific relief of congestion may be of far greater importance than the relative impact of these medication options on some other possible end points. In addition, the relative superiority of different treatments may shift over time (eg, after only 1 day vs 2 weeks of continuing treatment). Therefore, in a patient who is bothered by only intermittent rhinitis symptoms and therefore might take a medication occasionally and for short courses, choosing a medication that has quicker onset of action would be more relevant than data from a meta-analysis demonstrating that an alternative medication has greater impact on quality of life after 2 weeks of continuous therapy. Additional dilemmas in applying evidence from clinical trials to an individual include (1) that some rhinitis subpopulations/phenotypes may respond differently to a treatment than other subpopulations (eg, children vs middle aged adults vs senior adults, or patients with mild vs severe disease), and, as may occur in many diseases, (2) that an individual's response may differ from that predicted from group responses. In addition, there often is a very high placebo response rate in rhinitis trials (it is not unusual that >30%–40% of subjects will improve with placebo), so trials with smaller numbers of subjects may have inadequate power to demonstrate a true treatment effect that may be present (Type 2 error).

Differences in How Recent Major Guidelines Assess Evidence

In making management decisions about patients with rhinitis, there are several major national or international treatment guidelines that provide guidance. Probably the two most comprehensive are those of the US Joint Task Force on Practice Parameters (sponsored by American Academy of Allergy, Asthma and Immunology; American College of Allergy, Asthma and Immunology; Joint Council on Allergy, Asthma and Immunology),[1,5] and the Allergic Rhinitis and its Impact on Asthma (ARIA) guidelines (produced by an international, but predominantly European panel).[2,6,7] The most recent updates of these guidelines are firmly based on the systematic review, evaluation, and grading of available scientific evidence about efficacy and safety of rhinitis medications.[1,6,7] However, while recommendations of the major guidelines are generally consistent, some differences do exist, which might be explained by several factors. (1) Different grading schemes are used to evaluate data. ARIA uses a grading scheme (GRADE) that includes additional considerations such as cost and assessed preference of patients for different treatment options.[6,7] By contrast, the US Joint Task Force Parameter[1] generally restricts its recommendations to effectiveness and safety assessments, and avoids making attempts to (a) assess costs (which in the United States can vary greatly over time depending on a patient's insurance coverage, or the change of medication from prescription to over-the-counter status, notwithstanding any other changes in the overall health care system), or (b) patient preference (which can be difficult to objectively assess because of variable influence by multiple factors including marketing, media, cultural environment and physician recommendation to a patient). (2) Some expert opinion is required to make practical recommendations because of existing knowledge gaps that require extrapolation from available evidence, and as just discussed in the previous section, available data can be conflicting and present dilemmas in assessing and weighing the relative importance of discordant findings. The difficulty of assessing published data was recently highlighted by an analysis that cited difficulty obtaining useful information from the published literature because of insufficient reporting of data.[4]

Selection of Medications Using Guideline Recommendations: Need for Individualization

In actual clinical practice, selection of the best phamacotherapeutic options for rhinitis requires individualization with consideration of multiple factors. These factors include age, response to medications tried in the past, patient preference for intranasal versus oral medication, potential effectiveness for the symptoms most bothersome to the patient, symptom severity and seasonality of symptoms, side effects, cost to the patient, the potential for benefiting comorbid conditions such as asthma, and the medication's onset of action affecting its appropriateness for use considering the frequency and duration of symptoms (and corresponding medication use) in a patient.[1]

Considerations in Choosing Medications for Allergic Rhinitis

Table 1 is modified from the table in the US Rhinitis Parameter[1] that lists medication classes with considerations for selecting from different options. Implicit in these statements is the recognition that rhinitis guidelines must provide the clinician some latitude in decision making to accommodate consideration of multiple factors that may be relevant to an individual patient.

Episodic, seasonal and perennial allergic rhinitis; intermittent and persistent rhinitis; frequency and duration of symptoms

Table 2 summarizes the onset of action for principal medication classes, as assessed in the US Rhinitis Parameter, based on review of the published literature and Food and Drug Administration (FDA)-approved product labeling. For a patient who has more infrequent or episodic symptoms, onset of action may be one of the most important considerations in medication selection. This consideration received added focus in the most recent US Rhinitis Parameter[1] with the introduction of the term "episodic" rhinitis, a term that supplements use of the long-standing terms seasonal allergic rhinitis (SAR) and perennial allergic rhinitis (PAR). All 3 terms are derived conceptually from the likely duration and context of aeroallergen exposure. Episodic allergic rhinitis is defined as allergic nasal symptoms "elicited by sporadic exposures to inhalant aeroallergens that are not usually encountered in the patient's indoor or outdoor environment, such as while visiting a farm where there is exposure to horses or while visiting

Table 1
Onset of action of pharmacologic options for allergic rhinitis treatment: US Rhinitis Parameter assessment

Agent/Medication Class	Onset of Action
Anticholinergic, nasal	Rapid, within 15–30 min
Antihistamine, oral	Rapid, within hours
Antihistamine, nasal	15–30 min
Corticosteroids, nasal	Usually within 12 h, may start as early as 3–4 h
Cromolyn, nasal	For ongoing SAR and PAR: onset within 4–7 d Just before episodic allergen exposure, protects for 4–8 h
Leukotriene receptor antagonists (LTRAs)	By second day of daily treatment

Abbreviations: PAR, perennial allergic rhinitis; SAR, seasonal allergic rhinitis.
   Data from Wallace DV, Dykewicz MS, Bernstein DI, et al; The Joint Force on Practice Parameters, representing the AAAAI, ACAAI, JCAAI. The diagnosis and management of rhinitis: an updated practice parameter. J Allergy Clin Immunol 2008;122:S1–S84. PMID: 18662584.

Table 2
Principal medication options for allergic rhinitis for seasonal (SAR) and perennial (PAR) allergic rhinitis (AR): monotherapy

	Therapeutic Considerations
Oral Agents	
Antihistamines, oral (H1 receptor antagonists)	• Continuous use most effective for SAR and PAR, but appropriate for as-needed (PRN) use in episodic or intermittent AR because of relatively rapid onset of action • Less effective for nasal congestion than for other nasal symptoms • Less effective for AR than intranasal corticosteroids (INS), with similar effectiveness to INS for associated ocular symptoms • Because generally ineffective for nonallergic rhinitis, other choices typically better for *mixed* rhinitis • To avoid sedation (often subjectively unperceived), performance impairment, or anticholinergic effects of first-generation antihistamines, second-generation agents generally preferred ○ Of these, desloratacine, fexofenadine, loratadine, without sedation at recommended doses
Corticosteroids, oral	• A short course (5–7 d) may be appropriate for very severe nasal symptoms • Preferred to single or recurrent administration of intramuscular corticosteroids
Decongestants, oral	• Pseudoephedrine reduces nasal congestion • Side effects include insomnia, irritability, palpitations, hypertension
Leukotriene receptor antagonists (LTRAs)	• Montelukast approved for SAR and PAR • Efficacy of LTRA and oral antihistamines similar (with loratadine as usual comparator) • As approved for both rhinitis and asthma; may be considered when both conditions present • Side effects minimal
Intranasal Agents	
Intranasal antihistamines	• Effectiveness for AR equal or superior to oral second-generation antihistamines with clinically significant effect on nasal congestion • Generally less effective than intranasal corticosteroids for nasal symptoms • Clinically significant rapid onset of action (within several hours or less) making them appropriate for PRN use in episodic AR • As azelastine nasal is approved for vasomotor rhinitis, appropriate choice for *mixed* rhinitis • Side effects with intranasal azelastine: bitter taste, somnolence
Intranasal anticholinergic (ipratropium)	• Reduces rhinorrhea but not other symptoms of AR • Appropriate for episodic AR because of rapid onset of action • Side effects minimal, but nasal dryness may occur
Intranasal corticosteroids (INS)	• Most effective monotherapy for AR • Effective for all symptoms of SAR and PAR, including nasal congestion • Usual onset of action is less rapid than oral or intranasal antihistamines, usually occurs within 12 h, and may start as early as 3–4 h in some patients

(continued on next page)

Table 2 *(continued)*	
	Therapeutic Considerations
	• May consider for episodic AR
	• PRN use (eg, >50% days use) effective for SAR
	• More effective than combination of oral antihistamine and LTRA for SAR and PAR
	• Similar effectiveness to oral antihistamines for associated ocular symptoms of AR
	• Appropriate choice for mixed rhinitis, as agents in class also effective for some nonallergic rhinitis
	• Without significant systemic side effects in adults
	• Growth suppression in children with PAR has not been demonstrated when used at recommended doses
	• Local side effects minimal, but nasal bleeding may occur, rare nasal septal perforation
Intranasal cromolyn	• For maintenance treatment of AR, onset of action within 4–7 d, full benefit may take weeks
	• For episodic rhinitis, administration just before allergen exposure protects for 4–8 h against allergic response
	• Less effective than nasal corticosteroids; inadequate data for comparison with leukotriene antagonists and antihistamines
	• Minimal side effects
Intranasal decongestants	• For short-term and possibly for episodic therapy for nasal congestion, but inappropriate for daily use because of risk for rhinitis medicamentosa

Data from Wallace DV, Dykewicz MS, Bernstein DI, et al; The Joint Force on Practice Parameters, representing the AAAAI, ACAAI, JCAAI. The diagnosis and management of rhinitis: an updated practice parameter. J Allergy Clin Immunol 2008;122:S1–S84. PMID: 18662584; and Dykewicz MS, Hamilos DL. Rhinitis and sinusitis. J Allergy Clin Immunol 2010;125(2):S103–15.

a home with pets when a patient has no pet exposure in their own home or work environments."[1]

In view of onset of action, the Parameter recommends consideration of the following medications for treating episodic allergic rhinitis: nasal cromolyn for prophylaxis just before allergen exposure, and for relief of symptoms, nasal anticholinergics (for treatment of rhinorrhea only), oral antihistamines, nasal antihistamines, and nasal corticosteroids. The same medications considered appropriate for relief of symptoms of episodic rhinitis would also be appropriate for use on an as-needed (PRN) basis for treating patients with SAR or PAR who have infrequent symptoms. Because of slower onset of action, leukotriene receptor antagonists (LTRAs) are not recommended specifically for episodic rhinitis or those with infrequent symptoms from SAR or PAR. The ARIA guidelines also recommend that the frequency and duration of symptoms direct selection of therapy for allergic rhinitis, with *intermittent* rhinitis defined as symptoms on fewer than 4 days per week and of less than 4 weeks' duration, and *persistent* rhinitis being applied to patients who have symptoms more frequently or of greater duration. In clinical decision making, this author believes that the ARIA terms intermittent and persistent might be applied to either SAR or PAR, although this is not expressly stated in the US Rhinitis Parameter. It should be noted that the terms SAR and PAR were expressly discouraged by earlier versions of ARIA in favor of the use of intermittent or persistent, noting that an aeroallergen (eg, grass pollen) that occurs seasonally in one region of the world may be detected throughout the year in another region of the world.[6] However, in a partial reversal of previous versions of ARIA, SAR now is used to a limited extent in ARIA's 2010 update.[7] In reconciling recommendations of the different guidelines, the ARIA terms of intermittent and persistent can be viewed to be conceptually analogous to phrasing of *infrequent* and *more frequent* symptoms used in recommendations of the US Practice Parameter. PRN therapy is recommended by guidelines as a treatment option for more infrequent symptoms. However, with regard to the cost implications of continuous therapy versus on-demand therapy, there are recent data that suggest that effective treatment of allergic rhinitis by continuous treatment can reduce overall drug costs (including escape medication) and perhaps more importantly, indirect costs in the form of days absent from work and school.[8]

In an individual patient, recognition that SAR contributes to symptoms is important for pharmacotherapy because this should raise consideration of whether medications should be initiated in anticipation of an allergy season, but then be reduced or discontinued post season.

Although clinicians often assume that the relative effectiveness of medications for SAR can be assumed to translate into relative effectiveness of medications for PAR, this may not necessarily be true. The US FDA requires that in order for medications to receive an indication for the treatment of PAR, studies must be performed in PAR patients and be evaluated for longer treatment periods than for SAR. Although systematic reviews and meta-analyses comparing intranasal corticosteroids and antihistamines have generally shown that nasal corticosteroids provide greater relief of nasal symptoms of allergic rhinitis than other agents,[1,2,9–11] one recent review of published data found that when certain inclusion criteria were used to control for heterogeneity in outcomes used to assess effectiveness, oral antihistamines might be similarly effective to nasal corticosteroids for some patients with PAR.

Mild and more severe rhinitis

As a useful comparative reference point for severity grading schemes that also direct selection of therapy, the US Practice Parameter concurs with the ARIA definition of *mild rhinitis* being rhinitis in the absence of any of the following: sleep disturbance; impairment of daily activities, leisure, and/or sport; impairment of school or work; and symptoms present but not troublesome.[1] The US Parameter (2008) supports the concept that *more severe* rhinitis is defined as more troublesome symptoms or interference with quality of life.

Mixed rhinitis

Among statements in **Table 2**, the Parameter states that nasal antihistamines and nasal corticosteroids are appropriate choices for treating patients with *mixed rhinitis* (those who have both elements of allergic and nonallergic rhinitis), with the explanation that agents in these 2 classes have been demonstrated to benefit both allergic and nonallergic (vasomotor) rhinitis.[1] In explanatory text, the Parameter observes that mixed rhinitis is present in 44% to 87% of patients with allergic rhinitis,[12,13] and is more common than either pure allergic rhinitis or nonallergic rhinitis. However, it should be noted that formal studies have not been conducted to assess whether superior patient outcomes result from prescribing medications selected in consideration that mixed rhinitis is present, compared with selecting medications based on the presence of allergic rhinitis.

Differences in specific recommendations between US Rhinitis Parameter and ARIA
The US Practice Parameter and ARIA make similar recommendations in many respects, for example, concluding that nasal corticosteroids overall are the single most effective agents for treatment of allergic rhinitis. However, there are some significant differences in recommendations.

Compared with ARIA, the US Parameter has a more favorable assessment of intranasal antihistamines and oral LTRAs. The US Parameter cites evidence to recommend nasal antihistamines currently marketed in the United States as treatment options for both SAR and PAR (see **Table 2**).[1] For nasal antihistamines, ARIA gives a "conditional recommendation" for use of nasal antihistamines in both adults and children only for SAR, but for "persistent rhinitis" recommends *against* use of nasal antihistamines, stating that more data about relative efficacy and safety are needed.[6] This issue does bring up the general concept that demonstrating benefit in PAR may be more difficult than in SAR, which this author would argue is another reason to retain the use of the terms SAR and PAR. ARIA states that its recommendation not to use intranasal H1-antihistamines in persistent allergic rhinitis "places a relatively high value on their uncertain efficacy and possible side effects and a relatively low value on a possible small reduction in symptoms."[6]

For LTRAs, the US Parameter notes that montelukast is approved for treatment of SAR and PAR based on controlled studies, although it concludes that effectiveness is similar to oral antihistamines (with loratadine as usual comparator).[1] The Parameter also states that because montelukast is approved for both asthma and allergic rhinitis, it may be considered when both conditions are present. ARIA recommends oral H1-antihistamines over LTRAs for SAR and in preschool children with persistent allergic rhinitis, with this recommendation "placing a relatively high value on avoiding resource expenditure."[7] For reasons noted earlier, the US Practice Parameter avoids applying cost estimates to its recommendations.

DOES THE PATIENT RESPOND? (BOX 4)
When There is Adequate Response to Treatment (Box 5)

When there has been adequate response to treatment, major guidelines recommend that once control of symptoms has been achieved, the clinician should consider stepping down treatment. If SAR is being treated, stepping down when the season ends is a relatively straightforward decision. However, for some pollens there may be persistence of detectable allergen in the air for several weeks beyond the time that significant levels of intact pollen particles are no longer detectable.[14] This factor should be considered in deciding when to advise that a patient reduce or discontinue seasonal medication treatment. Even though a patient may have adequate symptom control on medications used, according to the US Rhinitis Parameter there still may be situations when allergen immunotherapy may be appropriately considered. Specifically according to the Parameter, factors that justify consideration of immunotherapy in addition to responsiveness to medications and avoidance may include severity and duration of symptoms, unacceptable adverse effects of medications, the patient's desire to avoid long-term pharmacotherapy, reduction of the risk of future asthma (particularly in children), and the presence of comorbid conditions such as sinusitis or asthma.[1]

When There is Inadequate Response to Treatment (Box 6)

When initial therapy fails, there should be consideration of whether there are unaddressed triggers or environmental factors. In clinical care, noncompliance/adherence is extremely common, and should probably be one of the first issues assessed when a patient has an inadequate response to prescribed treatment.

Change in rhinitis therapy

The US Rhinitis Parameter recommends that whatever medication is first selected to treat a patient with rhinitis, addition or substitution of another class of medication should be considered if the first medication does not sufficiently control the patient's symptoms.

If the decision is to change from one monotherapy to another, and the first agent tried is known to generally be less effective than a second agent, it certainly seems reasonable to switch to the second agent. However, because there may be heterogeneity in responses to medications and an individual's response may differ from that of mean population responses, it may also be reasonable to switch to an agent that on average may not be demonstrated to be more effective than the first agent tried (eg, change from nasal corticosteroid to nasal antihistamine), but to which an individual patient may have a better response. However, currently there is no robust evidence basis for guiding such decisions.

Another option when a patient does not respond to initial medication monotherapy is to add an additional medication or medications, an approach undoubtedly in common use in the United States.[15,16] However, the use of combination therapy for rhinitis has not always been shown to provide a major therapeutic advantage that outweighs the cost of this approach, and combination therapy may cause decreased compliance.[1,17–19] The most recent update of the US Rhinitis Parameter did attempt to systematically review available data on combination therapy options.[1] **Table 3** lists principal considerations and known evidence basis for selecting different medication combinations for the treatment of allergic rhinitis. There is essentially no evidence from controlled studies to demonstrate that addition of a third or even fourth medication provides additional benefit over that of a 2-medication regimen, although consideration of that add-on strategy is suggested by the US Rhinitis Parameter. The following discussion reviews available data and considerations for the use of 2-medication combination therapy for allergic rhinitis.

Antihistamine, oral with decongestant, oral Both the US Rhinitis Parameter and ARIA cite evidence that demonstrates that this combination provides more effective relief of nasal congestion than antihistamines alone, although the side effects of oral decongestants (insomnia, irritability, palpitations, hypertension) are cited for consideration.[20–25]

Antihistamine, oral with LTRA, oral The US Parameter has assessed that not all studies of the concomitant administration of an LTRA and an antihistamine have shown an additive effect, and in general this approach is less efficacious than administering intranasal corticosteroids as monotherapy.[1,17–19,26] The Parameter states that this medication combination may be considered as an alternative treatment if patients are unresponsive to or not compliant with intranasal corticosteroids. By contrast, ARIA states its review of the evidence finds that the combination of oral H1-antihistamines and LTRAs does not increase the efficacy of any single drug, and that the combination is less effective than intranasal corticosteroids.[2,7,27–29]

Antihistamine, oral with intranasal corticosteroid This combination treatment approach to allergic rhinitis is frequently used in the United States. However, the US Parameter notes that while this combination may be considered, the addition of an oral antihistamine to an intranasal corticosteroid generally has not been demonstrated to provide greater clinical benefit than intranasal corticosteroid monotherapy in

Table 3
Combination medication therapy for allergic rhinitis

	Therapeutic Considerations
Antihistamine, oral with decongestant, oral	• More effective relief of nasal congestion than antihistamines alone
Antihistamine, oral with LTRA, oral	• May be more effective than monotherapy with antihistamine or LTRA, but some evidence finds no additive benefit • Combination less effective than intranasal corticosteroids • An alternative if patients unresponsive to or not compliant with intranasal corticosteroids
Antihistamine, oral with intranasal antihistamine	• Combination may be considered, although controlled studies of additive benefit lacking
Antihistamine, oral with intranasal corticosteroid	• Combination may be considered, although supporting studies limited and many studies unsupportive of additive benefit of adding an antihistamine to an intranasal steroid
Intranasal anticholinergic with intranasal corticosteroid	• Concomitant ipratropium bromide nasal spray with intranasal corticosteroid more effective for rhinorrhea than administration of either drug alone
Intranasal antihistamine with intranasal corticosteroid	• Combination may be considered based on limited data indicating additive benefit • Inadequate data about optimal interval between administration of the 2 sprays • For mixed rhinitis, possible added benefit to combination of intranasal antihistamine with intranasal corticosteroid
LTRA, oral with intranasal corticosteroid	• Subjective additive relief in limited studies, data inadequate

Data from Wallace DV, Dykewicz MS, Bernstein DI, et al; The Joint Force on Practice Parameters, representing the AAAAI, ACAAI, JCAAI. The diagnosis and management of rhinitis: an updated practice parameter. J Allergy Clin Immunol 2008;122:S1–S84. PMID: 18662584; and Dykewicz MS, Hamilos DL. Rhinitis and sinusitis. J Allergy Clin Immunol 2010;125(2):S103–15.

controlled trials or meta-analyses.[1,30,31] The limited amount of data in support of this combination includes one well-controlled study of SAR, in which the addition of cetirizine to intranasal fluticasone propionate led to greater relief of pruritus.[32] In another study, the combination of nasal fluticasone propionate and oral loratadine was superior to fluticasone propionate alone for some patient-rated symptoms.[30] Another study found that at least 50% of patients felt the need to take both intranasal corticosteroids and oral antihistamines to adequately control symptoms of seasonal allergic rhinitis, but this study did not have a placebo control.[33] Based on its review of the literature, ARIA states that insufficient data are available to make a recommendation concerning the combined use of oral H1-antihistamines and intranasal glucocorticosteroids.[2] To fully address the question of whether there is an additive benefit to oral antihistamines over monotherapy with nasal corticosteroids, large numbers of patients (to assure sufficient statistical power) who do not respond adequately to nasal corticosteroids may need to be studied in placebo-controlled trials to assess the effect of the addition of oral antihistamines.

Intranasal anticholinergic with intranasal corticosteroid The US Rhinitis Parameter assesses that concomitant ipratropium bromide nasal spray with intranasal corticosteroid provides more effective relief of rhinorrhea than administration of either drug alone, based on a study using nasal ipratropium with beclomethasone dipropionate.[1,34] In addition to assessing mean rhinorrhea severity, the combination of these agents was found to be superior when assessed by another end point, the mean daily duration of rhinorrhea (number of hours with rhinorrhea from 8 AM to 8 PM).

Intranasal antihistamine with intranasal corticosteroid The US Parameter states that this combination may be considered based on limited data concluding that there is an added benefit to the combination of an intranasal antihistamine with an intranasal corticosteroid.[1,35] A more recently published study also supports use of this combination.[36]

Other considerations
When initial attempts at therapy fail, one should assess whether treatment failure is because of incorrect diagnosis or unrecognized concomitant diagnoses (eg, rhinosinusitis, gastroesophageal reflux). It may be appropriate to begin empiric treatment if the history is suggestive of rhinosinusitis (antibiotics) or gastroesophageal reflux (eg, proton pump inhibitors). Additional diagnostic studies may be required such as fiberoptic nasal endoscopy (rhinoscopy) and/or computed tomography scan of the sinuses. According to the US Parameter, nasal smears for eosinophils are not necessary for routine use in diagnosing allergic rhinitis when the diagnosis is clearly supported by the history, physical examination, and specific IgE diagnostic studies. Nasal smears may be a useful adjunct when nonallergic rhinitis with eosinophilia syndrome or rhinosinusitis is suspected. However, some data suggest that contrary to what may be conventional thinking, nasal corticosteroids are not more likely to benefit patients with perennial nonallergic rhinitis who have nasal smears demonstrating eosinophils, compared with those who do not have eosinophils.[37]

One should also consider referral to an otolaryngologist to assess if surgical intervention may be appropriate for surgical correction of clinically significant nasal septal deviation, turbinate reduction, or concomitant problems such as nasal polyps or chronic sinusitis. In children, indications for adenoidectomy include sleep apnea caused by adenotonsillar hypertrophy, chronic adenoiditis, and chronic sinusitis. If the patient has a clear allergic basis to their rhinitis, allergen immunotherapy should be considered if not done so previously (see discussion on Box 3).

NONALLERGIC RHINITIS
Management of Nonallergic Rhinitis (Box 7)

A full discussion of different forms of nonallergic rhinitis is beyond the scope of this article. However, when an allergic basis for rhinitis has been ruled out, principal considerations would include:

- Nonallergic rhinitis without eosinophilia, sometimes termed idiopathic rhinitis
- Vasomotor rhinitis, a term sometimes used synonymously with nonallergic rhinitis without eosinophilia, but sometimes having the specific connotation that nasal symptoms can be provoked in response to environmental factors, such as changes in temperature or relative humidity, odors (eg, perfumes or cleaning materials), passive tobacco smoke, alcohol, sexual arousal, and emotional factors; for certain irritant triggers are relevant to a patient, avoidance can be recommended
- Gustatory rhinitis with food ingestion; when rhinorrhea is the principal symptom, pre-meal nasal ipratropium would be appropriate treatment
- Nonallergic rhinitis with eosinophilia
- Rhinitis medicamentosa, caused by chronic use of topical nasal decongestant sprays.

Table 4
Monotherapy for nonallergic (idiopathic) rhinitis

Oral Agents	Therapeutic Considerations (for side effects, see Table 2)
Antihistamines, oral (H1 receptor antagonists)	• Generally ineffective for nonallergic rhinitis
Decongestants, oral	• Pseudoephedrine reduces nasal congestion (SS# 70–71)
Intranasal Agents	
Intranasal antihistamines	• Effective for vasomotor rhinitis
Intranasal anticholinergic (ipratropium)	• Effective only for rhinorrhea of nonallergic rhinitis syndromes • Special role for preventing rhinorrhea of gustatory rhinitis
Intranasal corticosteroids	• Effective for some forms of nonallergic rhinitis, including vasomotor rhinitis and nonallergic rhinitis with eosinophilia syndrome

Data from Wallace DV, Dykewicz MS, Bernstein DI, et al; The Joint Force on Practice Parameters, representing the AAAAI, ACAAI, JCAAI. The diagnosis and management of rhinitis: an updated practice parameter. J Allergy Clin Immunol 2008;122:S1–S84. PMID: 18662584; and Dykewicz MS, Hamilos DL. Rhinitis and sinusitis. J Allergy Clin Immunol 2010;125(2):S103–15.

Principal medications that may be useful for nonallergic rhinitis syndromes are listed with therapeutic considerations in **Table 4**. Although many medications effective for allergic rhinitis may be of benefit in some subsets of patients with non allergic rhinitis, LTRAs notably have no demonstrated benefit, and second-generation oral antihistamines are ineffective. First-generation antihistamines may have possible benefit for rhinorrhea because of the anticholinergic effects of these drugs. For patients with rhinitis medicamentosa, discontinuation of nasal decongestant sprays and treatment with either intranasal or systemic corticosteroids may be required.

Does the Patient Respond to Treatment of Nonallergic Rhinitis? (Box 8)

Nonallergic rhinitis that does not respond (Box 6)
Although Box 6 has already been discussed under the algorithm pathway for allergic rhinitis, some of that discussion would also apply to patients with presumptive nonallergic/idiopathic rhinitis. Except for the demonstrated additive benefit of intranasal ipratropium to a nasal corticosteroid for relief of rhinorrhea from nonallergic rhinitis,[34] there are no adequate studies to endorse or guide combination medication treatment for nonallergic rhinitis.

Nonallergic rhinitis that does respond (Box 9)
In follow-up for patients with nonallergic rhinitis who do respond to treatment, step-down therapy should be considered, although the natural course of nonallergic rhinitis may be unpredictable.

SUMMARY

The approach to patients with more severe rhinitis who present to medical offices requires a systematic diagnostic and therapeutic approach that may be guided by the algorithm and discussion provided in this review. Whenever possible, clinical care should be evidence driven, although there are still clinical issues in rhinitis diagnosis and management that are not directly addressed by available data. Although comprehensive clinical guidelines provide a firm foundation for rhinitis care, management ultimately also requires a clinician's judgment to individualize care based on multiple considerations that include age, response to medications tried in the past, patient preference for intranasal versus oral medication, potential effectiveness for the symptoms most bothersome to the patient, symptom severity and seasonality of symptoms, side effects, cost to the patient, and the potential for benefiting comorbid conditions such as asthma.

REFERENCES

1. Wallace DV, Dykewicz MS, Bernstein DI, et al. The Joint Force on Practice Parameters, representing the AAAAI, ACAAI, JCAAI. The diagnosis and management of rhinitis: an updated practice parameter. J Allergy Clin Immunol 2008;122:S1–84. PMID: 18662584.
2. Bousquet J, Khaltaev N, Cruz AA, et al. Allergic rhinitis and its impact on asthma (ARIA) 2008 update (in collaboration with the World Health Organization, GA(2) LEN and AllerGen). Allergy 2008;63(Suppl 86):8–160.
3. Khan DA. Allergic rhinitis with negative skin tests: does it exist? Allergy Asthma Proc 2009;30(5):465–9.
4. Benninger M, Farrar JR, Blaiss M, et al. Evaluating approved medications to treat allergic rhinitis in the United States: an evidence-based review of efficacy for nasal symptoms by class. Ann Allergy Asthma Immunol 2010;104(1):13–29.
5. Dykewicz MS, Fineman S, Skoner DP, et al. Diagnosis and management of rhinitis: complete guidelines of the joint task force on practice parameters in allergy, asthma and immunology. Ann Allergy Asthma Immunol 1998;81:478–518.
6. Bousquet J, Van Cauwenberge P, Khaltaev N. Allergic rhinitis and its impact on asthma. J Allergy Clin Immunol 2001;108:S147–334.
7. Brozek JL, Bousquet J, Baena-Cagnani CE, et al. Allergic rhinitis and its impact on asthma (ARIA) guidelines: 2010 revision. J Allergy Clin Immunol 2010;126: 466–76.
8. Church MK, Watelet JB, Belgian SIGMA Group. Treating allergic rhinitis: continuous versus on-demand regime? Executive summary of the Supportive Initiatives for the Global Management of Allergy (SIGMA): report from the Belgian Working Group. B-ENT 2009;5(Suppl 12):1–25.
9. Stempel DA, Thomas M. Treatment of allergic rhinitis: an evidence based evaluation of nasal corticosteroids versus nonsedating antihistamines. Am J Manag Care 1998;4:89–96.
10. Weiner JM, Abramson MJ, Puy RM. Intranasal corticosteroids versus oral H1 receptor antagonists in allergic rhinitis: systematic review of randomized controlled trials. BMJ 1998;317:1624–9.
11. Yanez A, Rodrigo GJ. Intranasal corticosteroids versus topical H1 receptor antagonists for the treatment of allergic rhinitis: a systematic review with meta-analysis. Ann Allergy Asthma Immunol 2002;89:479–84.
12. Settipane RA. Rhinitis: a dose of epidemiological reality. Allergy Asthma Proc 2003;24:147–54.
13. Settipane RA, Charnock DR. Epidemiology of rhinitis: allergic and nonallergic. Clin Allergy Immunol 2007;19:23–34.
14. Agarwal MK, Swanson MC, Reed CE, et al. Immunochemical quantitation of airborne short ragweed, Alternaria, antigen E, and Alt-I allergens: a two-year prospective study. J Allergy Clin Immunol 1983;72(1):40–5.
15. Blaiss MS. Important aspects in management of allergic rhinitis: compliance, cost, and quality of life. Allergy Asthma Proc 2003;24(4):231–8.

16. Bollinger ME, Diette GB, Chang CL, et al. Patient characteristics and prescription fill patterns for allergic rhinitis medications, with a focus on montelukast, in a commercially insured population. Clin Ther 2010;32(6):1093–102.

17. Pullerits T, Praks L, Ristioja V, et al. Comparison of a nasal glucocorticoid, antileukotriene, and a combination of antileukotriene and antihistamine in the treatment of seasonal allergic rhinitis. J Allergy Clin Immunol 2002;109:949–55.

18. Meltzer EO, Malmstrom K, Lu S, et al. Concomitant montelukast and loratadine as treatment for seasonal allergic rhinitis: a randomized, placebo-controlled clinical trial. J Allergy Clin Immunol 2000;105:917–22.

19. Nayak AS, Philip G, Lu S, et al. Efficacy and tolerability of montelukast alone or in combination with loratadine in seasonal allergic rhinitis: a multicenter, randomized, double-blind, placebo-controlled trial performed in the fall. Ann Allergy Asthma Immunol 2002;88:592–600.

20. Zubizaretta J. Azatadine maleate/pseudoephedrine sulfate repetabs versus placebo in the treatment of severe perennial allergic rhinitis. J Int Med Res 1980;8:395–9.

21. Bronsky E, Boggs P, Findlay S, et al. Comparative efficacy and safety of a once-daily loratadine pseudoephedrine combination versus its components alone and placebo in the management of seasonal allergic rhinitis. J Allergy Clin Immunol 1995;96:139–47.

22. Williams BO, Hull H, McSorley P, et al. Efficacy of acrivastine plus pseudoephedrine for symptomatic relief of seasonal allergic rhinitis due to mountain cedar. Ann Allergy Asthma Immunol 1996;76:432–8.

23. Grossman J, Bronsky EA, Lanier BQ, et al. Loratadinepseudoephedrine combination versus placebo in patients with seasonal allergic rhinitis. Ann Allergy 1989;63:317–21.

24. Wellington K, Jarvis B. Cetirizine/pseudoephedrine. Drugs 2001;61:2231–40 [discussion: 2241–2].

25. Berkowitz RB, McCafferty F, Lutz C, et al. Fexofenadine HCl 60 mg/pseudoephedrine HCl 120 mg has a 60-minute onset of action in the treatment of seasonal allergic rhinitis symptoms, as assessed in an allergen exposure unit. Allergy Asthma Proc 2004;25:335–43.

26. Rodrigo GJ, Yanez A. The role of antileukotriene therapy in seasonal allergic rhinitis: a systematic review of randomized trials. Ann Allergy Asthma Immunol 2006;96:779–86.

27. Wilson AM, O'Byrne PM, Parameswaran K. Leukotriene receptor antagonists for allergic rhinitis: a systematic review and meta-analysis. Am J Med 2004;116:338–44.

28. Wilson AM, Orr LC, Sims EJ, et al. Effects of monotherapy with intranasal corticosteroid or combined oral histamine and leukotriene receptor antagonists in seasonal allergic rhinitis. Clin Exp Allergy 2001;31:61–8.

29. Saengpanich S, deTineo M, Naclerio RM, et al. Fluticasone nasal spray and the combination of loratadine and montelukast in seasonal allergic rhinitis. Arch Otolaryngol Head Neck Surg 2003;129:557–62.

30. Ratner PH, van Bavel JH, Martin BG, et al. A comparison of the efficacy of fluticasone propionate aqueous nasal spray and loratadine, alone and in combination, for the treatment of seasonal allergic rhinitis. J Fam Pract 1998;47:118–25.

31. Barnes ML, Ward JH, Fardon TC, et al. Effects of levocetirizine as add-on therapy to fluticasone in seasonal allergic rhinitis. Clin Exp Allergy 2006;36:676–84.

32. Di Lorenzo G, Pacor ML, Pellitteri ME, et al. Randomized placebo-controlled trial comparing fluticasone aqueous nasal spray in mono-therapy, fluticasone plus

cetirizine, fluticasone plus montelukast and cetirizine plus montelukast for seasonal allergic rhinitis. Clin Exp Allergy 2004;34:259–67.

33. Juniper EF, Guyatt GH, Ferrie PJ, et al. First-line treatment of seasonal (ragweed) rhinoconjunctivitis: a randomized management trial comparing a nasal steroid spray and a nonsedating antihistamine. CMAJ 1997;156:1123–31.

34. Dockhorn R, Aaronson D, Bronsky E, et al. Ipratropium bromide nasal spray 0.03% and beclomethasone nasal spray alone and in combination for the treatment of rhinorrhea in perennial rhinitis. Ann Allergy Asthma Immunol 1999;82: 349–59.

35. Ratner PH, Hampel F, Van Bavel J, et al. Combination therapy with azelastine hydrochloride nasal spray and fluticasone propionate nasal spray in the treatment of patients with seasonal allergic rhinitis. Ann Allergy Asthma Immunol 2008;100(1):74–81.

36. Hampel FC, Ratner PH, Van Bavel J, et al. Double-blind, placebo-controlled study of azelastine and fluticasone in a single nasal spray delivery device. Ann Allergy Asthma Immunol 2010;105(2):168–73.

37. Webb DR, Meltzer EO, Finn AF Jr, et al. Intranasal fluticasone propionate is effective for perennial nonallergic rhinitis with or without eosinophilia. Ann Allergy Asthma Immunol 2002;88:385–90.

Index

Note: Page numbers of article titles are in **boldface** type.

A

Acrivastine, 514, 517, 529
Acupressure, 613
Acupuncture, 612–613
Adenoid hypertrophy, 446
Air filters, for allergen removal, 500
Allergen avoidance, **493–507**
    allergen characterization and, 494–497
    allergen sensitization diagnosis and, 497
    measures for, 498–503
Allergen immunotherapy. *See* Specific allergen immunotherapy.
Allergic rhinitis
    allergen avoidance in, **493–507**
    antihistamines for, **509–543**
    asthma and, 481–483
    corticosteroids for, 552–553
    eczema and, 485–486
    food allergy and, 486–487
    immunotherapy for, **561–599**
    pathophysiology of, **433–439**
    sinusitis and, 483–485
    treatment algorithm for, **619–634**
Allergic Rhinitis and its Impact on Asthma (ARIA), 482, 622, 627
Allium cepa, 614
Alternaria allergens, 496
Alternative treatments, 610–614
Anaphylaxis, in immunotherapy, 578
Anticholinergics, 450–451, 629–630
Antigen-presenting cells, in rhinitis, 434
Antihistamines, for rhinitis, **509–543,** 624, 628, 630
    development of, 509–510, 512–513
    in children, 528–531
    in elderly persons, 463
    in lactation, 533
    in pregnancy, 529, 532
    intranasal, 521, 525–528
    mechanism of action of, 510–511
    nonallergic, 449–450
    oral, 511, 514–524
        corticosteroids with, 521
        dosing of, 518–519

Immunol Allergy Clin N Am 31 (2011) 635–644
doi:10.1016/S0889-8561(11)00075-0
0889-8561/11/$ – see front matter © 2011 Elsevier Inc. All rights reserved.
immunology.theclinics.com

Printed in the United States
By Bookmasters